Clinics in Developmental Medicine No. 134

CNS MAGNETIC RESONANCE IMAGING
IN INFANTS AND CHILDREN

© 1995 Mac Keith Press
526/529 High Holborn House, 52–54 High Holborn, London WC1V 6RL

Set in Times and Avant Garde on QuarkXPress

First published in this edition 1995

British Library Cataloguing-in-Publication data:
A catalogue record for this book is available from the British Library

ISSN: 0069 4835
ISBN: 0 898683 01 8

Printed by The Lavenham Press Ltd, Water Street, Lavenham, Suffolk
Mac Keith Press is supported by **Scope** (formerly The Spastics Society)

Clinics in Developmental Medicine No. 134

CNS Magnetic Resonance Imaging in Infants & Children

Edited by

ERIC N. FAERBER

Department of Radiology

St Christopher's Hospital for Children

Philadelphia

1995

Mac Keith Press

Distributed by **CAMBRIDGE**
UNIVERSITY PRESS

AUTHORS' APPOINTMENTS

DANIELLE K. BOAL, MD

Associate Professor of Radiology and Pediatrics, Pennsylvania State University; *and* Chief, Pediatric Radiology, University Hospital, Milton S. Hershey Medical Center, Hershey, PA, USA

SHARON E. BYRD, MD

Associate Professor of Radiology; *and* Head, Division of Neuroradiology, Northwestern University Medical School, The Children's Memorial Hospital, Chicago, IL, USA

PATRICIA C. DAVIS, MD

Associate Professor of Radiology, Emory University School of Medicine; *and* Director, Magnetic Resonance Imaging, Egleston Children's Hospital, Atlanta, GA, USA

KATHLEEN D. EGGLI, MD

Associate Professor of Radiology and Pediatrics, Pennsylvania State University; *and* Attending Pediatric Radiologist, University Hospital, Milton S. Hershey Medical Center, Hershey, Pennsylvania, PA, USA

THOMAS ERNST, PhD

Senior Research Scientist in Physics, Magnetic Resonance Department, Radiologische Universitaatsklinik, Freiburg, Germany

ERIC N. FAERBER, MB, BCh, DMRD

Director of Radiology, St Christopher's Hospital for Children; *and* Professor of Diagnostic Imaging, Temple University; *and* Clinical Professor of Radiologic Sciences, School of Medicine of the Medical College of Pennsylvania and Hahnemann University, Philadelphia, PA, USA

KENNETH D. HOPPER, MD — Associate Professor of Radiology, Pennsylvania State University; *and* Chief of Body Imaging/Radiology Research, Milton S. Hershey Medical Center, Hershey, PA, USA

MICHELE H. JOHNSON, MD — Assistant Professor of Radiology, Diagnostic and Therapeutic Neuroradiology, Medical College of Virginia, Virginia Commonwealth University, Richmond, VA

ROLAND KREIS, PhD — Scientific Assistant, Department for Magnetic Resonance Spectroscopy and Methodology, University of Bern, Switzerland

BENJAMIN C.P. LEE, MD, FRCR(UK), MRCP(Eng) — Associate Professor of Radiology, Mallinckrodt Institute of Radiology, Washington University School of Medicine; *and* Director of Pediatric Neuroradiology, St Louis Children's Hospital, St Louis, MO, USA

ROBIN E. OSBORN, DO — Director of Neuroradiology and Magnetic Resonance, Department of Radiology, Mercy Medical Center, Springfield, OH, USA

BRIAN D. ROSS, MD — Professor of Clinical Medicine, University of Southern California; *and* Director of Magnetic Resonance, Huntingdon Medical Research Institutes, Pasadena; *and* Visiting Associate, California Institute of Technology, Los Angeles, CA, USA

JOHN L. SHERMAN, MD — Clinical Associate Professor of Radiology, University of Colorado, Denver, CO; *and* Clinical Professor of Radiology, Uniformed Services University of the Health Sciences, Bethesda, MD; *and* Medical Director, MRI of Colorado, Colorado Springs, CO, USA

JOEL D. SWARTZ, MD

Professor of Radiologic Sciences, Medical College of Pennsylvania; *and* Chairman, Department of Radiology, Germantown Hospital, Philadelphia, PA, USA

A. ARIA TZIKA, PhD

Research MR Scientist, Children's Hospital, Boston, MA; *and* Assistant Professor of Radiology, Harvard Medical School, Boston, MA, USA

THEODORE VILLAFANA, PhD

Professor, Director of Radiation Physics and Safety division, Medical College of Pennsylvania, Philadelphia, PA, USA

PHILIP S. YUSSEN, MD

Director of MRI and Neuroradiology, Graduate Hospital, City Avenue Hospital Division, Philadelphia, PA; *and* Adjunct Assistant Professor of Radiology, Medical College of Pennsylvania, Philadelphia, PA; *and* Medical Director, Open MRI Center, Bala Cynwyd, PA; *and* Medical Director, Haverford MRI, Haverford, PA, USA

CONTENTS

FOREWORD

Τα παντα ρει και ουδεν παγιωζ εχει.
Everything flows and nothing remains unchanged.

Herakleitos

The explosion of information in the field of diagnostic imaging has opened an unimaginable wealth of the most dramatic demonstration of human anatomy and pathology. Physicians find themselves in an unprecedented race to absorb rapidly expanding knowledge, judge its clinical impact, and compare it with existing technology, in an environment of ever increasing pressure to conserve precious resources. The applications, strengths and limitations of each new modality, often unforeseen, need to be subjected to careful scrutiny.

MRI has emerged as the most powerful instrument of understanding non-invasively the structure and function of the central nervous system. Physicians can now see clearly what could only be suspected indirectly just a few years ago.

This volume, produced by Dr Eric Faerber and a constellation of experts in the field, is the most comprehensive work on the application of MRI in the understanding of central nervous system disorders in infants and children. It covers succinctly the absolutely essential technical features of MRI, preparation of the young patient for the procedure, and all aspects of the vast spectrum of neurologic disease in the young, including the orbit and spine. The evolving role of MRI spectroscopy is also covered, by authors in the forefront of advances in this area.

No physician could accomplish putting together this material better than Dr Faerber, a student of medicine in many continents with an impressive list of credentials in Pediatric Radiology and Neuroradiology. Anyone with interest in the neurosciences will find this volume to be packed with precious information, and an invaluable companion in keeping abreast.

On a personal note, I had the privilege of working very closely with Dr Faerber when he was a fellow at the New England Medical Center in Boston. In return, I learned quite a lot from reading this superb book edited by a former student.

JOHN C. LEONIDAS, MD,
Chief of Pediatric Radiology,
Schneider Children's Hospital,
Long Island Jewish Medical Center;
Professor of Radiology and Pediatrics,
Albert Einstein College of Medicine,
New York, NY

PREFACE

> Will the future ever arrive? . . . Should we continue to look upwards?
>
> Victor Hugo (1802–1885)

The centennial of the discovery of X-rays by Wilhelm Roentgen on November 8, 1895 is fast approaching. Ever since this momentous event in medical history the field of radiology has pursued a relentless path forward. The applications within the sphere of neuroimaging have continued to be exciting. Plain radiography was soon followed by pneumoencephalography, ventriculography, myelography and angiography. The addition of radionuclide imaging and ultrasound were further valuable additions to the neuroimaging armamentarium. The subsequent introduction of computed tomography (CT) was hailed universally as the most important event since the discovery of X-rays, making a major impact on diagnostic imaging.

The future of neuroimaging suddenly appeared to have arrived, only to be replaced by the development of magnetic resonance imaging (MRI). Although MRI is a relatively new imaging modality for diagnostic purposes, the basic physical principles have been long understood, dating back to the description of magnetic properties of the nucleus in 1924. The experimental magnetic work in 1945 on solids by Edward Purcell at Harvard University and on liquids by Felix Block at Stanford University culminated in the sharing of the Nobel Prize in 1952 for their research.

The aim of this monograph is to describe the basic physical principles of MRI and the essential MRI features of the major disease processes involving the central nervous system and orbits in infants and children.

I am deeply grateful to the many people who have willingly assisted me in the preparation of the text. All of the contributors have demonstrated enthusiasm and diligence in the preparation of their chapters. The late Dr Henry Baird was the guiding force behind the monographs in CT and MRI, and will always be a source of inspiration to me. Dr Martin Bax, Dr Pamela Davies, Pat Chappelle and Michael Pountney of Mac Keith Press have been model editors displaying much encouragement and patience.

I wish to thank my associates and friends who have all been extremely helpful in the fields of radiology and the neurosciences: Barbara Wolfson, Eleanor Smergel, Bruce Greenberg, Evan Geller, Kristin Crisci, Warren Grover, Daniel Miles, Catherine Foley, Augustin Legido, Paul Kanev, Karen Bierbrauer, Lois Martyn, Joseph Kubacki, Glenn Isaacson, Ellen Deutsch, Jean-Pierre de Chadarevian and Nellie Karmazin. I wish to acknowledge the assistance of my friends and colleagues Te-Hua (Ros) Liu, Joel Swartz, Philip Yussen, and Michele Johnson. Calvin Bland, Kevin Hammeran and Carolyn Ballard of Administration, St Christopher's Hospital for Children, have always been attentive to our needs.

Superb technology assistance has been provided by Daniel Benson, Diane Siderio, Christine Melanson, Debra Brown, Angela Prioleau, Lisa McGrogan and Sharon O'Brien.

Our MRI nursing staff, Carole Aspinall and Ruth Adams have, as always, been invaluable for their skilled expertise in patient care and sedation.

Shirlene Davis and Veronica Horn have been pillars of strength in the preparation of this manuscript. The assistance of Michael Faerber is also much appreciated.

My special thanks to my wife Esme and children Jennifer and Michael for their continued love, support and encouragement.

ERIC FAERBER
Philadelphia, 1995

1
PRINCIPLES OF MAGNETIC RESONANCE IMAGING

Theodore Villafana

Magnetic resonance imaging (MRI) represents a very powerful tool not only for imaging anatomic detail, but also for the evaluation of tissue states, tissue function and motion dynamics. This sets MRI quite apart from computerized tomography (CT) where the principal result is an anatomical view. The only similarity between MRI and CT is that both produce cross-sectional images. The physical principles underlying the two imaging modalities are entirely different. CT scanning depends on the X-ray attenuation properties of tissues which in turn are dependent on tissue atomic number and physical density. MRI, on the other hand, depends on the magnetic spin properties of hydrogen nuclei in tissues and how these nuclei recover after excitation with radio frequency (RF) electromagnetic waves. The great advantage that MRI offers over CT scanning is the greater sensitivity to subtle differences in tissue types as well as tissue chemical states.

Figure 1.1 illustrates the overall MRI process. We see a patient within a strong external magnetic field (designed B_0). This magnetic field usually ranges from 0.3 to 2.0 Tesla. [The tesla is a unit of magnetic field strength and is abbreviated with the letter T. Alternatively, field strength can be expressed in units of Gauss (10,000 Gauss = 1 Tesla). For comparison purposes the earth's magnetic field is about 0.5 Gauss.] The B_0 field serves to align the hydrogen nuclei within the body into two specific equilibrium states. RF waves are then directed into the body which excites this equilibrium state. In time the individual nuclei revert back to equilibrium and the excitation energy is released from the body in the form of RF energy. This energy is detected with special antenna receiver coils and a signal related to that excitation energy state is generated. We therefore can follow the time course from excitation to relaxation. The time it takes for hydrogen nuclei to relax back to the equilibrium state is expressed by the two time parameters T_1 and T_2. These relaxation times depend on the specific tissues and pathological tissue states within which the hydrogen nuclei find themselves. That is, hydrogen nuclei have different T_1 and T_2 values in edema, in water, in tumor, in white matter disease, etc. Images can be produced with proper spatial localization of these signals, and diagnostic decisions made.

The MR process can be broken down into four distinct steps as follows: (i) preparatory alignment; (ii) RF excitation; (iii) signal measurement; (iv) spatial localization. Each of these will be studied in turn.

Preparatory alignment
The basic physical principle upon which MRI depends is the fact that around every

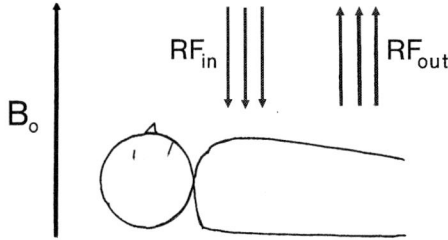

Fig. 1.1. The basic MR process involves beaming radio frequency (RF) energy into the patient, who lies within a strong external magnetic field B_0. The RF energy excites the hydrogen nuclei. As the nuclei relax, RF energy is released. Decay time of the detected RF energy is characteristic of the various tissues within the patient and constitutes the basis for imaging and for distinguishing between tissues.

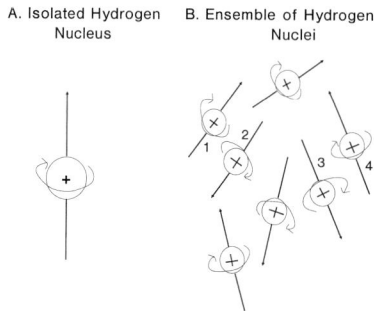

A. Isolated Hydrogen Nucleus   B. Ensemble of Hydrogen Nuclei

Fig. 1.2. *(A)* Spinning hydrogen nucleus comprising a single positively charged proton. Circular spin of the electrical charge results in a dipole magnetic field or magnetic moment oriented perpendicular to the plane of rotation. *(B)* Individual nuclear spins are oriented at random in space. As a consequence, any one nuclear magnetic field is cancelled by some other oppositely directed field, as *e.g.* 1 and 2, or 3 and 4.

moving charge there exists a magnetic field. For instance, when a negatively charged electron moves along a wire conductor a circular magnetic field exists around that wire. This is the basis for many electrical instruments. In MRI we are interested in hydrogen nuclei. These are composed of simple, positively charged protons, which rotate (so-called 'nuclear spin'). The circular motion of a rotating proton results in a linear magnetic field, as seen in Figure 1.2A. As such the nucleus behaves as a miniature dipole magnet exhibiting a north and a south pole. We also refer to these as magnetic vectors. Nuclei other than hydrogen can also display such dipole fields, though these are usually much weaker. Generally, nuclei having both an odd number of protons and an odd number of neutrons have a stronger net nuclear magnetic field due to their nuclear spin characteristics. In bulk tissues these miniature magnets are aligned randomly, and no net magnetism exists around the tissue in that the magnetic field around any one nucleus is counterbalanced and cancelled by some other nearby nucleus which is aligned exactly opposite (Fig. 1.2B).

Things change dramatically when the anatomical tissue is placed in a strong external magnetic field (B_0). Specifically two things occur: (i) each nucleus aligns either parallel

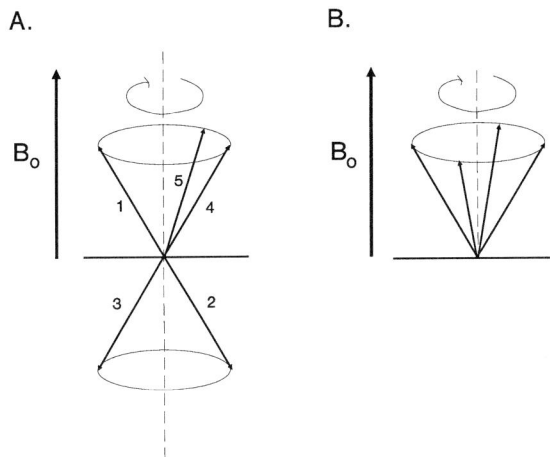

Fig. 1.3 *(A)* At any given image point, the randomly oriented nuclear spins when subjected to a strong external magnetic field B_0 align either parallel to B_0 or anti-parallel (or opposite) to B_0. In either case they precess around B_0. Parallel vectors cancel with anti-parallel vectors, as *e.g.* 1 with 2, and 3 with 4. Vector 5 represents a parallel aligned residual vector which has not cancelled with an anti-parallel vector. *(B)* The parallel state being a lower energy state is slightly greater populated and there are some residual vectors remaining. These precess randomly (out of phase) around B_0 and represent vectors which effectively enter into the MR process.

(along the external magnetic field) or antiparallel (opposite the external magnetic field); (ii) the magnetic vector aligns at some angle to the external field and precesses around that field. The interaction of forces between the external B_0 field and the nuclear magnetic field allows for two energy states, one with an alignment of the magnetic vector along (or parallel to) the external B_0 field and the other aligned in the opposite direction to the B_0 field (antiparallel). These two oppositely directed magnetic states are illustrated in Figure 1.3A. If equally populated, these would completely cancel themselves out and no net magnetism would result. For instance, vector 1 cancels with vector 2, vector 3 cancels with vector 4, etc. Fortunately, the parallel state is a lower energy state and there is a slight excess population of nuclei in that direction. Typically there are one to two residual vectors per million depending on the magnitude of the external field as compared to the antiparallel state (vector 5 in Fig. 1.3A). Though only a small percentage of the original they are still considerable in number, and are sufficient to yield a useable MR signal after suitable excitation and detection. This population of nuclei aligned parallel to the external field represents the equilibrium, ground (or unexcited) nuclear state.

In addition to pointing either parallel or antiparallel, the magnetic vector of each nucleus aligns at some angle to the B_0 field and commences to precess around B_0 as also seen in Figure 1.3A. This precessional motion is similar to the wobble of a spinning top. The precessional frequency (F) is called the Larmor frequency and is directly proportional to the external magnetic field (B_0) as $F = KB_0$ (the Larmor equation), where K is a constant (the gyromagnetic ratio) specific for each nucleus. Hydrogen, for example,

3

TABLE 1.1
Larmor frequencies and magnetic
field strength

B_0 (Tesla)	Frequency (MHz)
0.3	12.77
0.5	21.28
1.0	42.56
1.5	63.84
2.0	85.12

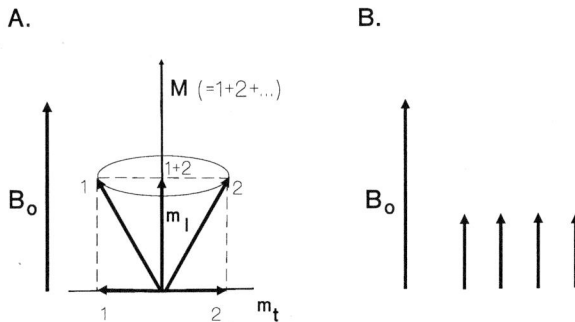

Fig. 1.4. *(A)* Spinning vectors can be broken down into longitudinal components (m_l), which produce the bulk magnetization vector M (*e.g.* vectors 1 and 2 add up along the longitudinal axis), and transverse components m_t which are randomly directed and hence (as with vectors 1 and 2) tend to cancel out. *(B)* At equilibrium every image point can be characterized by magnetization aligned parallel to the direction of the external magnetic field B_0, that is, m_l = max, and m_t = 0.

has a value of 42.56 MHz/T. Table 1.1 shows precessional frequencies associated with various Tesla strength systems. As shown in Figure 1.3B the individual vectors at an image point precess randomly around B_0, acting independently with respect to each other. We say they are out of phase.

We can break down the randomly precessing vectors to either the longitudinal axis or the transverse axis. The projection onto the longitudinal axis, *i.e.* the direction of the external magnetic field, we call the longitudinal magnetization, m_l. These add up as seen in Figure 1.4*a* and constitute the bulk magnetization (M) vector. Projected onto the transverse axis (transverse magnetization, m_t), all vectors cancel out since they are out of phase and precess randomly (all directions are equally probable) (vectors 1 and 2 in Fig. 1.4A). Thus, at equilibrium: m_l = maximum; m_t = 0.

Since longitudinal magnetizations add up and transverse magnetizations cancel out, every image point of the patient can be characterized with a series of single magnetic vectors parallel to the external field B_0 as seen in Figure 1.4B.

In clinical practice, the external magnetic field is supplied by a permanent, a resistive

A. 90° Tip

B. 180° Tip

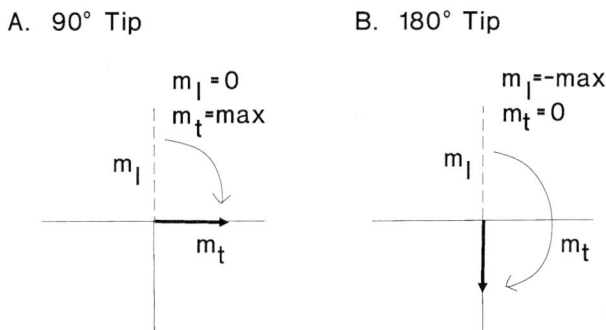

Fig. 1.5. *(A)* The result of a 90° tip is to drive m_l to zero and m_t to a maximum. This is the opposite of the equilibrium state where m_l = max and m_t = zero. Maximum m_t is produced because RF excitation drives all the vectors into phase and they all add up on the transverse axis *(bold arrows)*. M_t maximum will produce a strong signal. *(B)* The result of a 180° tip is to drive m_l to a negative maximum; however, m_t is zero since no transverse projection exists. No initial signal will result, therefore, from the 180° tip angle.

or a superconducting magnet. Field strengths vary from 0.3 to 2.0 T and greater. In the past, there has been active discussion as to which magnetic field strength is optimal for imaging. It is now generally felt that clinical MR body imaging is probably optimal between 0.5 and 1.0 T and head imaging is optimal up to at least 1.5 T. It is also clear that for spectroscopic applications higher field strengths of 1.5–2.0 T or greater are preferable.

Radio frequency excitation
We have seen that when the patient is placed within the MRI gantry and subjected to B_0 magnetic field the hydrogen nuclei rapidly align into an equilibrium configuration. The next step is to excite and disturb this equilibrium and to study the timing characteristics of how the nuclei relax back to equilibrium. These relaxation rates are characteristic of the tissue and tissue states (presence of edema, tumor, etc.).

In order to excite the nuclei, an electromagnetic RF wave is passed into the tissues. Electromagnetic waves have rapidly varying electric and magnetic fields associated with them. It is the magnetic field component that is of importance in MRI. These waves have a wide spectrum of frequencies. However, the wave frequency must match the Larmor frequency of the precessing nuclei. It is only under this matching condition that resonance absorption occurs between the magnetic component of the RF wave and the precessing magnetic vector of the aligned nuclei. The excitation that results manifests as a tipping of the bulk magnetization vector in space (Fig. 1.5). The duration and intensity of the pulse determines the angle through which the vector is tipped. 90° and 180° tipping angles are commonly utilized clinically.

Excitation results in shifting the magnetization away from the longitudinal axis and onto the transverse axis. For instance, in the case of a 90° tip, the transverse magnetization maximizes while the longitudinal component decreases to zero (Fig. 1.5A). Figure 1.5B shows what happens when the tip angle is 180°: in this case, m_l goes to a negative

5

maximum, while $m_t = 0$, since there is no transverse component of magnetization. In general, one can tip the magnetization vector to any angle desired. More recent high speed MRI applications utilize smaller tip angles in the range of 10° to 50°.

Regardless of the amount of magnetic vector tipping (or degree of excitation), when the RF energy ceases, the magnetic fields are all in phase, that is, they are all spinning in step with each other. Under these conditions the individual vectors no longer precess randomly but rather are brought into phase, acting as one large vector.

After excitation the nuclei at each point in the medium proceed to recover back to their original thermal equilibrium or unexcited state (original longitudinal alignment of the bulk magnetization vector with the external static magnetic field). This recovery occurs via two specific interaction mechanisms with specific timing rate characteristics for particular tissues. These rates are referred to as the T_1 and T_2 relaxation rates.

Signal measurement

To determine the T_1 and T_2 characteristics of the various tissues, a signal which varies according to T_1 and T_2 must be measured. As already emphasized, the signal obtained is directly related to the transverse magnetization produced by the RF excitation. This leaves the questions, What form does the signal take? How do we measure it? and How is it related to T_1 and T_2?

Measurement is accomplished by means of a wire coil that serves as an antenna to detect the MR signal. This is the same coil used to generate the RF waves which were originally beamed into the patient to cause nuclear excitation. In general, an electrical signal is induced in any wire coil by a changing magnetic field as a function of the rate of that change and the direction of that change relative to the coil orientation as well as the magnitude of the magnetic field. The greater the component of change perpendicular to the coil (lying in the transverse plane in our case), the greater the signal induced. This can be summarized by saying that the MR signal can be detected by a suitable coil, and that the signal strength consists, as stated before, of that component of the magnetization which lies in the transverse plane. In our specific case the spinning vectors constitute a changing magnetic field. In the equilibrium condition there is no net transverse magnetization and therefore no net signal. Upon excitation, m_l is tipped away from the longitudinal plane and into the transverse plane: then all the precessing vectors are in phase and suddenly a strong signal is developed. We can now compare the equilibrium state with the excited state as follows:

Equilibrium state	Excited state
m_l = max	m_l = 0
m_t = 0	m_t = max
Result = no net signal	Result = net signal

The T_1 and T_2 relaxation times are measures of how the excited state relaxes to the equilibrium state, *i.e.* how quickly m_l recovers back to its maximum value (T_1) and how quickly m_t decays back to zero (T_2). In all cases we can tell the degree of excitation or relaxation by a measurement of m_t. This latter point must be re-emphasized. That is, the

A.

B.

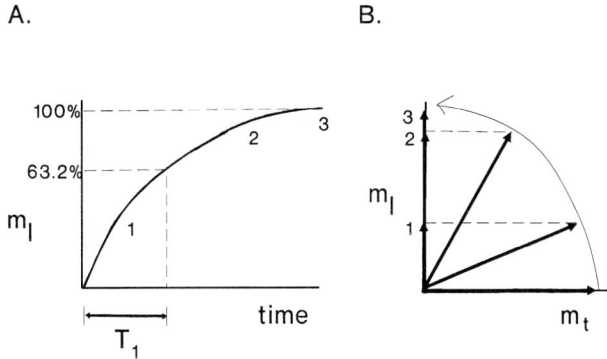

Fig. 1.6. *(A)* With time, the longitudinal magnetization m_l recovers exponentially back to its original value. T_1 represents the time it takes to recover back to 63.2 per cent of the original m_l. Points 1 and 2 are other intermediate recovery points. Point 3 represents full recovery of the original m_l. *(B)* The recovery of m_l shown as the excited state *(bold arrow)* returns and vectors move from the 90° position through various intermediate angles given by points 1 and 2. Position 3 represents full recovery of m_l.

measurable signal in MRI is entirely dependent on the magnitude of m_t. It is this signal which yields information on the time course of relaxation.

T_1 recovery

After the cessation of the RF excitation pulse the magnetization vector which had been tipped, *e.g.* through 90°, begins to recover back to the equilibrium ground state. The time it takes to recover to this state is characteristic of the chemical milieu the hydrogen nuclei find themselves in. This recovery process is exponential in nature and is depicted in Figure 1.6A. Points 1 and 2 are intermediate relaxation levels. Point 3 represents full recovery where m_l is maximal. T_1 is defined as the time necessary to recover to 63.2 per cent of the original 100 per cent longitudinal magnetization. Figure 1.6B shows how the originally tipped vector gradually recovers back to 100 per cent m_l through the same intermediate points and finally to full recovery at point 3.

T_1 typically is measured in hundreds of milliseconds for biological tissues and varies greatly with magnetic field strength and temperature. The mechanism by which m_2 recovers depends on the individual spinning nuclei interacting with the overall molecular thermal environment or lattice around it. We refer to this as spin–lattice interactions. Here, the protons carried along within one molecule randomly interact with others, gradually losing their excitation energy and reverting back to the original equilibrium longitudinal alignment. We see that T_1 is related to the time it takes for zero m_l to revert back to the original m_l = max.

T_2 decay

After excitation there is another relaxation mechanism at play. In addition to spin–lattice interactions which determine T_1 there are what are called spin–spin interactions which

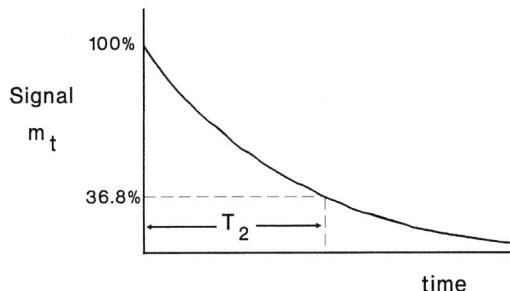

Fig. 1.7. The maximum signal occurs immediately after RF excitation when all the vectors are in phase along m_t. With time, vectors separate out and dephase. This results in the signal decaying exponentially back to the dephased state where $m_t = 0$. The time it takes to decay down to 36.8 per cent of the original value is called the T_2 time.

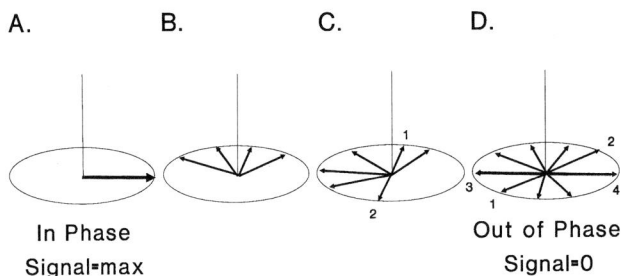

Fig. 1.8. Events leading to dephasing in the m_t plane. *(A)* Initial 90° tip yield m_t = max, where all the vectors are in phase. *(B–D)* As time goes on, vectors dephase, that is, they no longer act as one vector but rather separate out. In this process, the signal goes from a maximum at *(A)* to zero at *(D)*. As a result, they begin to cancel each other out, as vectors 1 and 2 in *(C)*. Eventually, complete dephasing and hence complete cancellation occurs. That is, m_t reverts to zero *(D)* as any one vector will cancel some other oppositely directed vector, *e.g.* vectors 1 and 2, or 3 and 4.

determine T_2. Here each nucleus interacts with the other nuclei in its immediate neighborhood within the same molecule. This results in a transfer of energy between the interacting nuclei and a consequent dephasing of the individual spins. That is, some slow down, some speed up, and the vectors no longer act together but precess randomly and start cancelling each other out. Thus all the nuclei—which were originally in phase (having the same precessional frequency) after RF excitation, with maximum m_t and therefore a maximum signal—start to separate out and become dephased. As described earlier, signal strength at any instant is determined exclusively by the projection of the magnetic vector onto the horizontal plane (transverse magnetization). As this transverse magnetization is lost (*i.e.* as relaxation occurs and nuclei revert to random orientation in a transverse plane), the signal decays. By measuring the signal decay we can determine T_2.

T_2 is defined as the time necessary for dephasing to cause a 63.2 per cent loss of signal (Fig. 1.7). In general, T_2 is measured in the tens of milliseconds and is therefore significantly shorter than T_1. Because it is so short, the T_2 dephasing action rapidly takes the detectable signal to zero even though longitudinal relaxation may not yet have been completed. Since this dephasing depends on intra- rather than intermolecular interactions, the magnitude of T_2 is generally very insensitive to magnetic field strength and temperature, whereas the opposite is true for T_1.

Transverse magnetization decay due to spin–spin interactions is further illustrated in Figure 1.8. There we see the original in-phase vector producing M_t = maximum. As time goes on the precessing vectors separate out and start dephasing, cancelling each other out (as vectors 1 and 2 in Figure 1.8C) with consequent signal reduction. What is occurring is that nuclei in different molecular milieux interact differently and therefore experience different intramolecular magnetic fields; hence, spins rapidly dephase with a concomitant loss in signal. Eventually the vectors are completely dephased and all cancel out (vector 1 with oppositely directed vector 2, 3 with 4, etc. in Fig. 1.8D) and the equilibrium condition of $M_t = 0$ is re-established.

Magnetic field inhomogeneities—$T_2\star$
The magnets in our gantries do not produce perfectly uniform magnetic fields over the full patient volume. Therefore, each image point in the field experiences a slightly different magnetic field strength and the nuclei at each point precess at a slightly different Larmor frequency. These local inhomogeneities in the external magnetic field provide a second spin–spin interaction mechanism that causes dephasing of the transverse magnetization. This means that although all the spins are in phase immediately after the excitation pulse, the local inhomogeneities tend to cause further dephasing beyond that due to true T_2, and an even more rapid transverse magnetization decay results. This dephasing relaxation is referred to as $T_2\star$ (T_2 star) and usually overshadows the true T_1 and T_2 relaxation behavior. It should be emphasized that $T_2\star$ is contributed to by a number of phenomena, and it incorporates not only the true T_2 and any dephasing due to the local magnetic inhomogeneities but also other dephasing mechanisms as well. These are discussed below.

Figure 1.9 shows both true T_2 decay and the much shorter $T_2\star$ decay. Hypothetical signal effects due to T_1 recovery are indicated by a broken line because in practice the signal variation due to T_1 is completely masked by $T_2\star$ and T_2 decay and thus its signal (net projection on m_t axis) is not obtainable directly. T_2 in turn is masked by the presence of $T_2\star$. The $T_2\star$ decay curve is referred to as the free induction decay (FID) curve. It is obtained by simply exciting the nuclear state and observing the resultant signal decay. The FID is always governed by all sources of dephasing present in the system.

In summary then we can state that the excitation of nuclear spin states drives M_l to zero and M_t to a maximum and returns a strong signal. After excitation the nuclear spins relax back to their equilibrium state and the signal decays away. T_1 is a measure of M_l recovery via spin–lattice interactions and T_2 a measure of M_t decay via spin–spin interactions. $T_2\star$ decay is a complicating dephasing mechanism due to many other things including local magnetic inhomogeneities. The MR signal detected after suitable RF

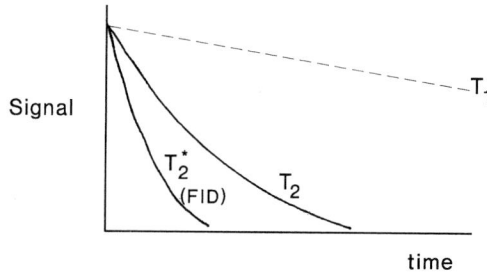

Fig. 1.9. Decay time of m₁ signal. T_2 is shorter than T_1 by about a factor of 10 (tens of milliseconds *vs.* hundreds of milliseconds). $T_{2\star}$ is shorter still by another factor of approximately 10. Signal due to T_1 *(dashed line)* is hypothetical in that it is masked by the presence of T_2 and $T_{2\star}$. The $T_{2\star}$ decay is also referred to as the free induction decay (FID) curve.

TABLE 1.2
Pulse sequences

Approach	Pulse sequence	Weighting
Partial saturation	Repeated 90° pulses	Proton density at long TR; T_1 at short TR
Inversion recovery	180° pulse followed by 90° pulse	Mainly T_1
Spin echo	90° pulse followed by 180° pulse	T_1, T_2 or proton density

excitation depends on T_1, T_2 and $T_{2\star}$, in addition to the overall number of hydrogen nuclei (proton density) present at each image point.

The fundamental problem in the MR process is to provide for an excitation sequence that minimizes $T_{2\star}$ and yields image data specific for (or at least weighted for) either T_1, T_2 or proton density parameters. It is desirable to minimize $T_{2\star}$ because this is influenced mainly by the quality of the magnet rather than the more important tissue characteristics.

To unravel T_2 from T_1 or $T_{2\star}$, one must design various RF pulse sequences. Designing a pulse sequence usually involves specifying a particular excitation flip angle followed by some delay time followed by a series of other pulses all designed to emphasize or weight either T_1, $T_{2\star}$ or proton density. The sequence is repeated line by line to build up an image. For instance, a 256×256 matrix image will normally require repeating the sequence 256 times. The time interval between repetitions (called the repetition time) is also a key parameter which determines the degree of weighting.

The three common sequences typically employed in clinical imaging are shown in Table 1.2. The critical parameter in these sequences is the delay times between the pulses and the repetition time (TR) between pulse sequences. We will see that since different tissues have different relaxation times, the repetition rate as well as the delay times between pulses can be used to enhance these differences. Of the three pulse sequences, the spin–echo sequence is by far the most clinically important. The relationship between delay times and TR will become clear as we address the spin–echo process.

Spin echo

The spin echo sequence can yield images which emphasize T_1, $T_{2\star}$ or proton density tissue characteristics. However, to achieve this we must eliminate or minimize the $T_{2\star}$ dephasing effects. This is done with a 90° pulse followed by some delay time. During this delay time the signal goes to zero due to $T_{2\star}$. We then follow with a 180° pulse which undoes the inhomogeneity dephasing, and a recovery of the signal results. We call this signal an echo. The time interval between the 90° pulse and the peak echo signal time is called the echo time (TE). The 180° pulse was given at exactly half this time (TE/2) and represents the delay time after the initial 90° pulse. The sequence can thus be described as being a 90°, TE/2, 180° sequence (Fig. 1.10).

To understand how the echo signal devoid of $T_{2\star}$ influence is accomplished, we must understand the basic effects of magnetic inhomogeneities. In Figure 1.11A, we see two adjacent protons. Both experience exactly the same B_0 field (no inhomogeneities). Vectors here are seen to be in phase after cessation of RF pulse. They will dephase only under the influence of magnetic fields provided by neighboring spins, that is, true T_2. In Figure 1.11B, the two spins are affected by inhomogeneities fixed in the magnet. That is, one spin may experience the true field B_0, while an adjoining spin may experience a slightly different magnetic field $B_{0\pm}$. The Larmor equation determines the precessional frequency for each spin. If each point has a slightly different B_0 field, then it will have a slightly different precessional frequency. In Figure 1.11B, this results in vectors dephasing not only due to true T_2 but also due to the magnetic inhomogeneities.

A key point here is that magnetic inhomogeneity dephasing is fixed in nature, while true T_2 dephasing is due to the random interactions between spins. Therefore, one way to undo the effect of $T_{2\star}$ is to reverse the action of the inhomogeneities. This is illustrated in Figure 1.12. Here we see that after the 90° pulse, dephasing begins and M_t starts to go to zero via $T_{2\star}$. The local magnetic inhomogeneity relaxation component of $T_{2\star}$, however, is not random, while true T_2 relaxation is entirely random. This forms the basis for distinguishing between T_2 and $T_{2\star}$. Since the magnetic inhomogeneities are fixed in space they add a fixed perturbation to the spin states. We first pulse the system 90°, then allow the spins to relax for a certain time (TE/2), then give a 180° pulse such that all the spins are flipped to the opposite side of the plane as shown in Figure 1.12B. The random components after such a flip (not shown in the figure) continue to dephase randomly. The fixed non-random components, however, add perturbations exactly opposite to those exerted in the first half of the pulse sequence. As a result, the magnetic inhomogeneities undo their influence and the vectors begin to rephase and zero themselves out as seen in Figure 1.12B,C. However much the vectors were dephased via $T_{2\star}$ before the 180° pulse they are now rephased back to the starting position. The result is a signal that the true T_2 would have had in time TE if no $T_{2\star}$ interference had been present. That is, the signal builds up to the value corresponding to true T_2 as if there had been no $T_{2\star}$. Since it is a

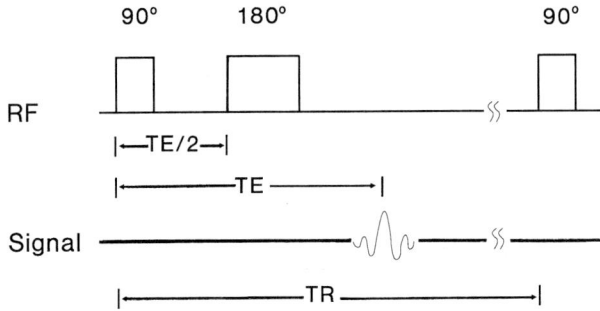

Fig. 1.10. Timing of events in a spin echo sequence. The 180° rephasing pulse is given at TE/2, the maximum signal occurring at TE. The repetition time TR is the time interval between 90° pulses.

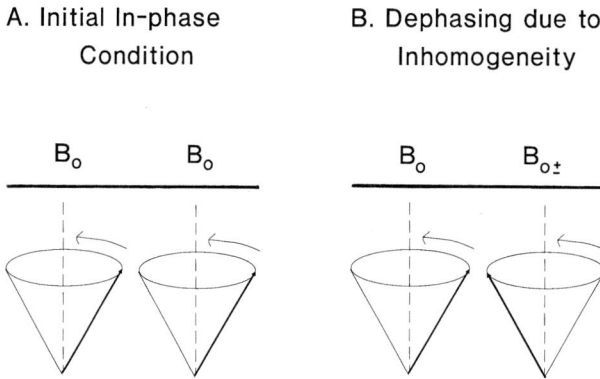

Fig. 1.11. *(A)* Two neighboring spins in phase after cessation of RF pulse. If both experience the same B_0 they will eventually dephase due to interactions with neighboring spins only. *(B)* Two neighboring spins, one under the influence of B_0 and the other under the influence of a slightly different magnetic field $B_{0\pm}$. Each will begin to precess at a different frequency given by the Larmor equation; dephasing will be due to $T_{2\star}$, which is made up of true T_2 and the corrupting magnetic inhomogeneities.

recovered signal which echoes back it is referred to as the spin echo.

After time TE, dephasing reinitiates and the signal once again declines. This is further illustrated in Figure 1.12D where we see that echo magnitude decays after TE but can be rephased to give another peak echo at time 2TE. It is very common to obtain two images one at an early TE and one at a later TE. Since images have different TE times each will show some different characteristic of the tissues (parameter weighting).

The signal strength depends on the choice of TE as well as on the repetition time. Standard spin echo sequences utilize TEs between 20 and 100 ms long. The echo received corresponds to one line in the image. This sequence must be repeated for whatever times there are lines in an image (256 times for a 256×256 matrix image). TR times can vary from relatively short (500 ms) to relatively long (2500 ms). The choice of TE and TR determines the parameter weighting.

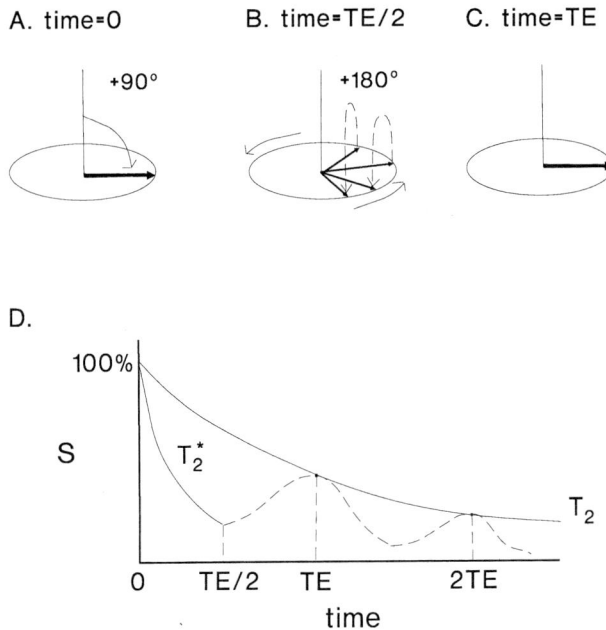

A. time=0   **B. time=TE/2**   **C. time=TE**

+90°   +180°

D.

100%

S

T_2^*

T_2

0   TE/2   TE   2TE

time

Fig. 1.12. Sequence of events in spin echo procedure. *(A)* Initial 90° pulse yields maximum m_t and maximum signal. *(B)* After some time (TE/2) the fast and slow non-random components which are due to local magnet inhomogeneities separate themselves out. A 180° pulse is then given which shifts vectors as shown. Non-random components proceed to rephase, with fast and slow components catching up with each other and cancelling out. *(C)* The non-random components which were driving signal to zero have rephased themselves. When this occurs, signal obtained is exclusively due to true T_2. *(D)* Time course of signal. At t = 0 signal is a maximum. At TE/2 the 180° rephasing pulse is given. Signal starts echoing back. At time TE the maximum echo signal occurs corresponding to signal strength of T_2 if no $T_{2\star}$ had been present. The process can be repeated and another echo can be received at time 2TE. Note that signal strength for later echoes is lower.

To understand how the signal strength depends on TR, refer to Figure 1.13. As usual a 90° flip will yield a large signal (bold arrow, Fig. 1.13A), since m_t is a maximum. If TR is short (STR), the spins recover only slightly before the next 90° pulse. The broken vector, representing partial recovery at this point, indicates that spins have dephased (due to $T_{2\star}$) and no net projection on m_t is possible. When the next 90° pulse is given to repeat the sequence, the vectors rephase and a net projection on m_t occurs. In this partial recovery case a relatively small signal S_{STR} is produced (Fig. 1.13B). If TR is long (LTR) the spins will have more closely recovered back to equilibrium. A subsequent 90° flip then results in a greater signal S_{LTR} (Fig. 1.13C). If a very long TR (VLTR) is used such that spins have fully recovered to the longitudinal axis then a subsequent 90° flip will yield a full signal (S_{VLTR}) as seen in Figure 1.13D. Corresponding graphical representations for STR, LTR and VLTR are shown in Figure 1.13E,F,G.

13

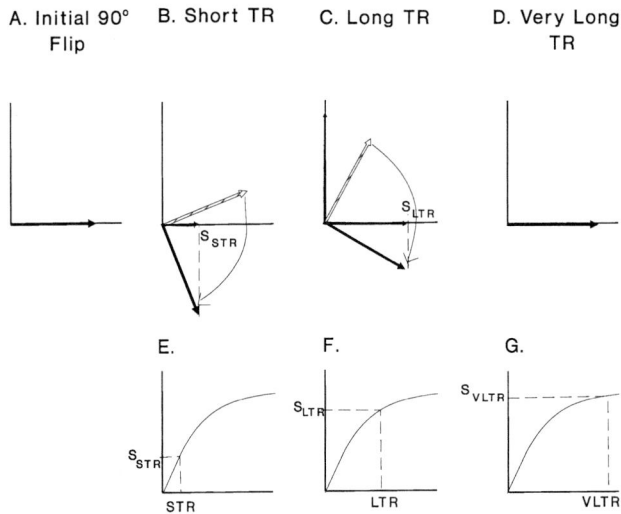

Fig. 1.13. Signal strength is dependent on TR. *(A)* Maximum signal occurs after 90° flip. Subsequent 90° flips will catch the vectors at some point in their return to the fully relaxed position along the longitudinal axis. *(B)* For short TR (STR), recovery has been minimal and subsequent 90° flip rephases vectors and yields relatively small signal S_{STR}. The dashed vector implies a dephasing yielding no signal, while the bold vector implies vectors are fully in phase yielding a possible signal. *(C)* For long TR (LTR), recovery may be nearly complete, in which case a subsequent 90° flip yields relatively large m_t and larger signal S_{LTR}. *(D)* For very long TR (VLTR), recovery is complete and 90° RF yields maximum signal. *(E, F, G)* Formation of signal along recovery curve as a function of TR, yielding same conclusions as *(B)*, *(C)* and *(D)* respectively.

Parameter weighting

In practice, different tissue states are better visualized by emphasizing T_1, T_2 or proton density characteristics. The timing of TE and TR can be chosen such that one of these parameters is weighted as compared to the others. In fact the image actually produced is going to depend critically on the choice of TE and TR and the subsequent parameter weighting which results.

T_1 WEIGHTING

Figure 1.14 illustrates how T_1 weighting is obtained. Here we see two tissues, one with a short T_1 (ST_1) and one with a long T_1 (LT_1). Depending on the choice of TR, one sees that the difference in signal between the tissues is greatly affected. For instance, at VLTR there is virtually no difference in signal and one could not distinguish between the two tissues (no image contrast). Some difference is seen at an intermediate TR (ITR), but at a short TR (STR) the relative difference between the two tissues gets even greater. At STR, for instance, we see that the short T_1 tissue yields a signal about twice as large as the long T_1 tissue. Note that even though signal difference is greater, the overall signal strength is lower for shorter TR. Low strength affects the signal-to-noise ratio (SNR) parameter. The SNR is the basic imaging performance parameter in MRI.

14

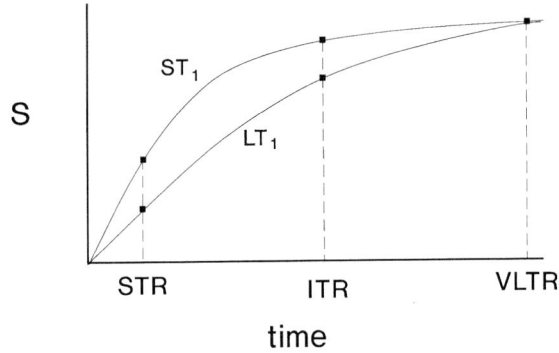

Fig. 1.14. T_1 parameter weighting, showing signals from two tissues, one with short T_1 (ST_1) and one with long T_1 (LT_1). Signal difference between the two tissues (image contrast) after 90° RF excitations depends on TR. At very long TR (VLTR) there is little if any difference between tissues and little contrast results, though signals are high. At short TR (STR) the difference is seen to be twice that at intermediate TR (ITR).

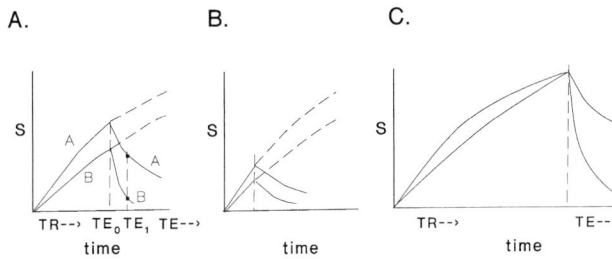

Fig. 1.15. Effect of TE on weighting. *(A)* For a given TR, different tissues (*e.g.* curves A, B) will yield signals of varying strength depending on their T_2 values and the TE chosen. At TE_0 the observed difference depends entirely on T_1 differences; at TE_1 the difference, depicted as large, depends on T_2 of the respective tissues. *(B)* At shorter TR, the initial signal differences at TE_0 are relatively large when first given the 180° rephasing pulse and dependent wholly on T_1. As TE increases, that dependency decreases, but initial T_1 influence is still felt for longer TE. *(C)* At very long TR there is essentially no initial T_1 difference, and differences observed as TE progresses are due strictly to T_2.

T_2 WEIGHTING

TE affects both T_1 and T_2 weighting in that after any given TR the possible signal from any tissue decays with time. The longer the TE the less emphasis there is on the T_1 difference between the tissues and the greater the emphasis on the T_2 differences. At TE_0 in Figure 1.15A we see a given difference. Images at this point have no T_2 dependency since no TE time has elapsed to separate out T_2 characteristics. Only the T_1 influence is present. At some time later, *e.g.* TE_1, the T_1 influence is not as dominant. Rather, the image differences are more dependent on the T_2 characteristics of tissue. This is because initial differences at TE_0 decay away as TE increases. In Figure 1.15A, we see a relatively large signal difference between tissues A and B at TE_1, as compared to TE_0: this is due to

15

TABLE 1.3
Brightest tissue as a function of parameter weighting and choice of TR and TE

	T_1 weighting	T_2 weighting	Proton weighting
TR	Short	Long	Long
TE	Short	Long	Short
Brightest tissue	Short T_1	Long T_2	High proton density

the large difference in T_2 decay between the two tissues. In general, as TE increases, the T_1 characteristics become less important and the T_2 differences dominate more. Again, notice that the magnitude of signal is less as TE is increased and SNR is therefore also reduced.

Finally, in Figure 1.15B, at short TR, we see that the initial signal difference at TE_0 is greatly influenced by T_1. As TE increases such as at TE_1, differences are more T_2 dependent but still have some T_1 dependency because of the initial conditions. At very long TR where T_1 weighting is negligible, the signal with subsequent TE will depend solely on TE, and T_2 differences become even greater as TE is increased further (Fig. 1.15C).

PROTON WEIGHTING

Any two tissues would be expected to have different amounts of hydrogen nuclei because of their differing chemical make-up. The tissue with more hydrogen nuclei (greater spin density) would yield a greater signal since more nuclei would be participating in the MR process. This is shown in Figure 1.16, where tissue A with greater spin population projects a greater m_t and greater signal upon a 90° flip as compared to tissue B. Tissue A would then appear brighter on a proton weighted image. To emphasize such a difference longer TRs are used because, as this minimizes T_1 weighting and the starting off position for the flip is closest to the longitudinal axis, we then obtain both strong signals (high SNR) and maximum spin density differences.

Table 1.3 summarizes what has to be done to TR and TE to obtain parameter weighting. We see that T_1 weighting is obtained by minimizing T_2 at short TE and maximizing T_1 and proton density with short TR. T_2 weighting is obtained by minimizing proton density (long TR) and maximizing T_2 (long TE). Proton weighting is obtained by minimizing T_1 at long TR and minimizing T_2 at short TE. This table also indicates which tissue is brightest under the various weighting schemes.

One further complicating factor is introduced by the fact that different tissues have different spin densities as well as different T_1 and T_2 characteristics. This accounts for much of the gray scale inversions seen in MRI, as depicted in Figure 1.17. If tissue B has a short T_1 but low spin density, then at short TR (STR) it would be brighter than tissue A. If a longer TR (LTR) is used (spin density weighting) then the gray scale will be inverted and tissue A will be brighter than tissue B. Likewise, as seen in Figure 1.17B, if one has a

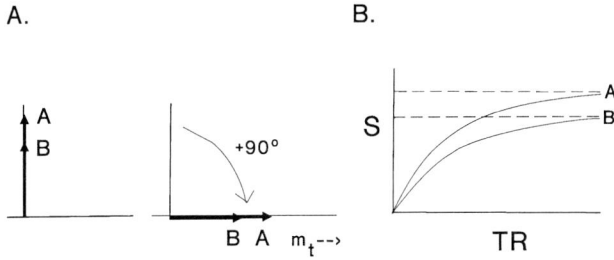

Fig. 1.16. *(A)* Spin density weighting is obtained at long TR where spins have fully recovered; after subsequent 90° excitations, the only difference in signals between tissues (*e.g.* A, B) will be dependent on the number of protons present. The greater the proton number, the greater the m_l and the greater the possible signal. *(B)* Graph showing same conclusion as *A* in that after very long TR both tissues A and B are fully recovered and differences in signal are due to spin density.

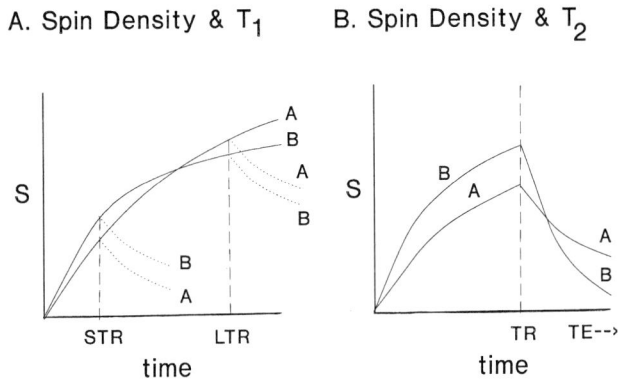

Fig. 1.17. Gray scale inversions from differences in spin densities. *(A)* Tissue 2 has higher spin density than tissue 1. At short TR (STR) tissue B is brighter than A. At long TR (LTR) tissue A is brighter than B. *(B)* Gray scale inversions from differences in T_2. At a given TR, tissue B is brighter than A for short TE. At long TE, tissue A is brighter than tissue B.

given initial difference between tissues A and B with B being the brightest at a given TR time, then the shorter T_2 tissue (B) will eventually yield less signal and will appear darker than the longer T_2 tissue (A).

Spatial localization

We have seen how the MR signal is produced and how it decays with time. To be of value in forming an image, the signal must be localized to a specific three dimensional point in space. Only in this way will each point in the image be identified. The problem is that the signal produced comes from the total volume excited. To spatially localize the signal to an image point, a series of magnetic field gradients are superimposed on the static magnetic field such that each point in the medium experiences a different but con-

17

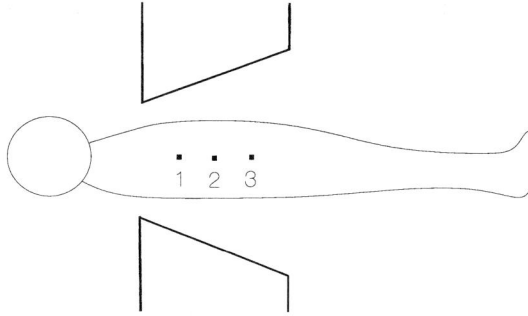

Fig. 1.18. Hypothetical magnet configured to give a linearly varying gradient of magnetic field over patient. At point 1, since the pole faces are closer the magnetic field is stronger and hence the Larmor precessional frequency is higher than at points 2 and 3. The slice selection gradient would selectively excite only this slice. In practice, gradients are obtained with special gradient coils rather than by pole face shaping.

A. After Slice Selection   B. After Phase Encoding

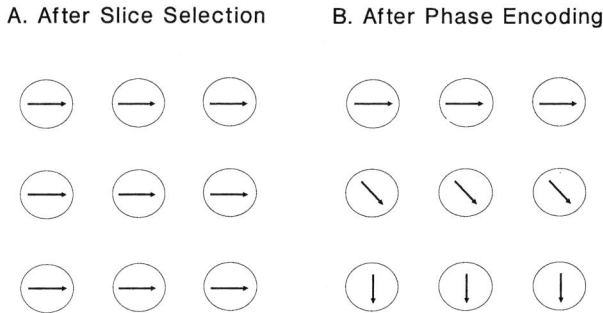

Fig. 1.19. Phase encoding gradient. *(A)* Slice selection gradient lines up all magnetizations in the transverse plane. *(B)* Application of phase encoding gradient will alter the precessional frequency along each row so that each row will end up with a different phase and can be distinguished from any other row. The final read out gradient, which is in frequency, completes the coding process in the third dimension.

trolled and known field strength. Gradient refers to the situation wherein the magnetic field B_0 varies linearly from one end of the field to the other. Since each point has a different magnetic field it has a different resonance frequency and a specific phase. It can be selectively excited and selectively detected. In essence, we have coded each position in space with a specific frequency or phase, by which we can identify them. For localization in three dimensions, three gradients are necessary: (i) slice selection gradient; (ii) phase encoding gradient; (iii) read out gradient.

Normally the slice selection and read out gradients encode frequency, while the phase encoding gradient obviously encodes phase. To help understand this process, refer to Figure 1.18. Here we see a hypothetical magnet system which because of its configuration produces a linearly varying magnetic field. Points 1, 2 and 3 have progressively lower magnetic fields because of their progressively larger distance from the magnet pole face, and hence each will have a different resonance frequency as determined by the Larmor equation. If information from the slice plane incorporating point 1 is desired, then one beams the specific frequency associated with that plane, so that only protons within that slice will be excited. Subsequent signals must therefore originate from this slice, and localization has been accomplished in this one dimension. The variation of magnetic field strength for this case (z direction) is referred to as the slice selection gradient. In a similar manner, two additional gradients are progressively applied to accomplish the x and y localization within the slice. Rather than having a magnet with pole faces configured like that shown in Figure 1.18, the three gradients referred to above are produced by incorporating special electrical coils in the gantry. These gradient coils can produce the linear magnetic field variation pattern that needs to be superimposed on the main magnetic field.

To accomplish the final localization in space, frequency and phase data (often referred to as 'K space') are converted to spatial position information by means of a mathematical technique known as Fourier transformation. After applying the slice selection gradient, the phase encoding gradient is applied followed by the read out gradient. The Fourier transform operation is applied to the data acquired over these latter two directions, producing what is called two dimensional Fourier transform (2DFT) acquisition.

Figure 1.19 shows what happens when a phase encoding gradient is applied. In Figure 1.19A all points in a 3×3 matrix in the image plane have been tipped 90° and are aligned initially as indicated. Figure 1.19B shows the result of applying the phase encoding gradient. Since each point sees a different magnetic field along Y, each will rotate at a slightly different frequency during the time the gradient is on. The gradient acting on the vectors along any column Y will cause them to advance a certain amount depending on the gradient strength at that particular point. As a result, vectors at each level along Y will be at slightly different positions or phases with respect to each other. We therefore have coded one more dimension, but this time in phase. Lastly, a third gradient is applied which codes along the final axis. This is referred to as the read out gradient and encodes frequency. The combination of phase encoding and read out gradients is repeated for each line of the image. After the application of the three gradients and the collection of all signals one may then go on to excite other slices. In each case one must apply the specific Larmor frequency associated with these slice levels.

Slice thickness and acquisition strategies
How do we produce different slice thicknesses? This is a relatively simple matter. Figure 1.20 shows two possible approaches. First, since distance is coded by frequency one can simply apply a range of frequencies corresponding to the thickness desired. As seen in Figure 1.20A a frequency range A′–D′ will produce thickness A–D. Correspondingly, a smaller frequency range B′–C′ will yield a thinner thickness B–C. The second approach consists of keeping the frequency range constant (Δf) but varying the gradient. A shallow gradient, for instance, will produce slice thickness A–D (Fig. 1.20B), while a steeper gradient will result in a thinner slice thickness B–C.

Rather than acquire information one slice at a time, the above process can be extended to a three-dimensional acquisition approach. In either case, the planar or volume

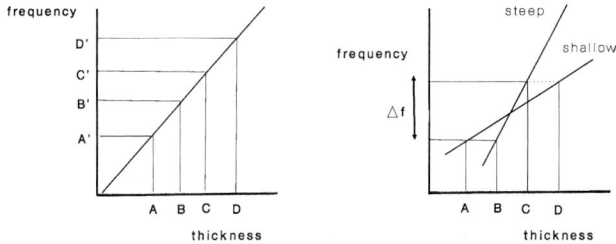

A. Changing Frequency   B. Changing Gradients

Fig. 1.20. Two methods of varying slice thickness. In all cases the slice thickness excited is due to the range of frequencies beamed into the patient and the gradient. *(A)* Varying the frequency. For a given gradient, a frequency range A′–D′ will give a slice thickness of A–D, while a lower frequency range B′–C′ will give a thinner slice B–C. *(B)* Varying the gradient. For a given frequency range, a shallow gradient yields a slice thickness A–D, while a steep gradient gives a thinner slice B–C.

acquired data must always be analysed via Fourier transforms (2 DFT for planar and 3 DFT for volume acquisition) to convert frequency and phase information to a signal value calculated for each pixel point in space.

To get maximum information in the least amount of time, one can utilize the relatively long repetition times inherent in each sequence during which no information is being gathered to pulse other anatomic levels and obtain other image planes and therefore accomplish multiplanar acquisition. Likewise, different TEs can be employed in the spin echo sequences to yield multi-echo reconstructions at specific anatomical levels as well. Clinically we utilize both multi-echo and multiplanar image acquisition spin echo approaches.

Finally, in all cases having a signal value at each image position an appropriate gray scale can be assigned to produce a visible image. Imaging display and windowing functions for MR is very similar to that done in computerized tomography with CT signal numbers. However, one major difference as compared to computerized tomography is that MR signal intensity values are not absolute and therefore do not correspond to any particular tissue. They may be used only for relative comparisons within a given image.

Fast echo imaging

From the beginning there has been an emphasis on accomplishing the MR scan process in shorter and shorter time. Just where, in the scan process, can we cut down on scan and examination time? The time (T) it takes to accomplish a given scan is given by: $T = N_y \cdot TR \cdot NEX$, where N_y is the number of phase encoding steps (*i.e.* the matrix size), TR is the repetition time for each line, and NEX is the number of excitations (number of images) which have been acquired and averaged together. Remember that in 2D Fourier transform MRI the image is acquired line by line, one line corresponding to one phase encoding step (*e.g.* 256 lines for a 256 × 256 matrix). If the number of phase encoding

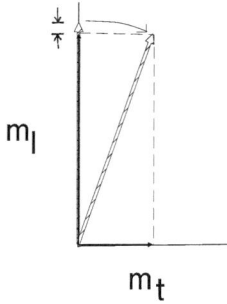

Fig. 1.21. A partial flip angle produces a relatively small change in m_l but a relatively large m_t and resulting signal.

steps is reduced, then a spatial resolution loss would result due to fewer image lines. TR in general is long (about 1000–2000 ms) and would seem to be a good candidate for reduction. However, the reason it is long is to allow the longitudinal magnetization to recover fully to assure a large signal. Also, to make TR short is to introduce T_1 weighting into the image which may not be desirable. As for the NEX component, it is necessary to repeat the whole acquisition process a number of times and average the data to reduce the noise in the final image. As the signal to noise performance of MRI units has improved, the need for multiple acquisitions has been reduced. However, if NEX is reduced further a signal noise penalty ensues. From the above it seems that every attempt to reduce scan times leads to some undesirable effect. There are, however, other possibilities. One of these is to reduce the flip angle. The logic is simple: if the flip angle is small, the required recovery time is also short and the TR times can be reduced. Figure 1.21 shows what happens if instead of a 90° initial flip, only a partial flip is excited. The important idea here is that even though the longitudinal magnetization is hardly affected the transverse magnetization is still appreciable and hence an appreciable signal can be generated. In this way TR times can be shortened substantially. The partial flip approach is always combined with gradient echoes to accomplish relatively short scan times. Not only is the 180° RF pulse time consuming, it turns out it cannot effectively be used with initial excitation flip angles of less than 90°. The gradient echo (GRE) approach replaces the spin echo process.

To understand the GRE approach, one must remember that spin echo requires a 180° rephasing RF pulse. Rephasing is necessary to remove the dephasing produced by the local magnetic inhomogeneities in the magnet. However, it also serves to remove the dephasing due to any other inhomogeneity including that produced by the gradients themselves. In the GRE approach, rather than apply a 180° pulse, the gradients are reversed. This will accomplish the required rephasing due to the gradients. Local magnetic inhomogeneities, however, are not removed. As a result, final images with GRE are weighted by $T_{2\star}$. Remember, though, that $T_{2\star}$ does carry T_2 information. Modern magnet homogeneity is so good that T_2 forms an appreciable part of $T_{2\star}$, and the GRE approach is now possible.

A number of other fast scan approaches have been introduced recently. One of these is the partial Fourier (or partial NEX) method. In this approach, scan times can be reduced by up to 50 per cent. This is accomplished by means of mathematical techniques

TABLE 1.4
Magnet types: advantages and disadvantages

Type	Advantages	Disadvantages
Permanent	Reduced electrical costs; reduced fringe fields	Heavy weight; limited field strength
Air core resistive	Relatively low cost	Limited field strength; non-uniform, unstable magnetic field
Iron core resistive	Reduced fringe fields	Limited field strength; electrical costs
Superconducting	High magnetic field strength; reduced electrical costs	Cost of cryogens; fringe fields

that necessitate only approximately half the number of lines along the phase encoding gradient. The full image data set can be computed from these lines due to mathematical symmetries inherent in the data. The fastest of all approaches, however, is the echo planar process. The details of this process are beyond the scope of this chapter; suffice it to say that in this approach all of the MRI data are collected using just one excitation rather than a multiple number of phase encoding steps. The approach has the potential of reducing scan times down to the millisecond level.

Instrumentation

The heart of MRI instrumentation comprises the gantry supplying the external B_0 field, the series of coils which are used to generate and detect RF energy, and the gradient coils used to position signals in three dimensional space. Some of the more important aspects of this instrumentation are discussed below.

Magnet types

There are a variety of ways by which strong magnetic fields can be generated. These are listed in Table 1.4 along with their advantages and disadvantages. Two general classifications can be identified: permanent, and electromagnetic (Fig. 1.22). Permanent magnets are just that; their magnetism cannot be turned off. Likewise, they use no electrical power to sustain their magnetic field. Such magnets tend to weigh a great deal (*ca.* 100 tons) and they are limited in how strong a magnetic field can be generated. They are usually configured in an 'H' shape as seen in Figure 1.22A. The B_0 magnetic field is directly across the pole faces in such configurations.

Electromagnets are produced whenever a current flows through a coil of wire. Early MR units consisted of a series of simple coils ('Helmholtz coils') in air and were termed air core resistive magnets (Fig. 1.22B). The B_0 magnetic field is directed along the center of the coil system. These early units were also very restricted in terms of magnetic field strength. Typically they ran to a maximum of 0.15 T. Additionally, the fields they generated were non-uniform and unstable. These resistive air core magnets are no longer used clinically.

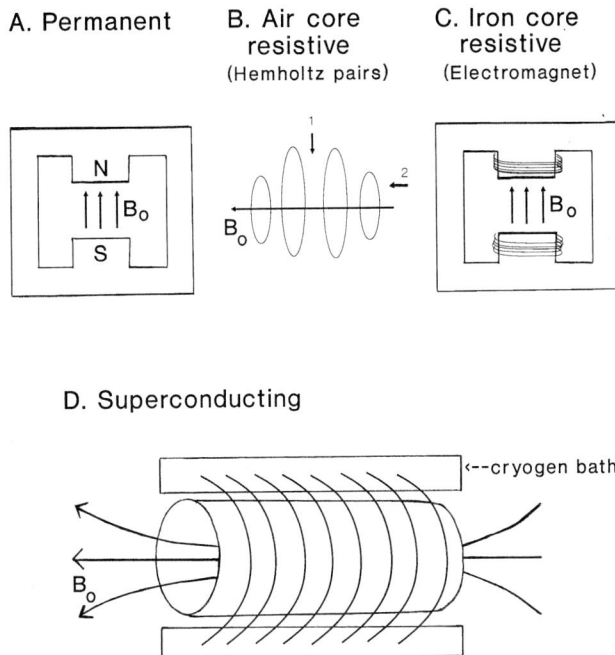

A. Permanent   B. Air core   C. Iron core
                  resistive   resistive
               (Hemholtz pairs)   (Electromagnet)

N
↑↑↑ B_0
S

B_0

↑↑ B_0

D. Superconducting

<--cryogen bath

B_0

Fig. 1.22. Different magnetic configurations. *(A)* Permanent magnet. B_0 field lined up between pole faces. Minimal fringe fields produced. *(B)* Air core magnet, made up of Helmholtz coil pairs. B_0 field down center of coils. Patient can be inserted either along 1 or along 2. Fringe fields extend beyond coils. *(C)* Iron core resistive magnet. B_0 field created between pole faces when current flows around iron core. Relatively weak fringe fields result. *(D)* Superconducting magnet. Coil around gantry is bathed in cryogen. B_0 field goes out through gantry opening to environs. Considerable fringe fields may exist outside the gantry depending on the magnetic shielding provided.

Iron core resistive magnets are usually configured in an 'H' shape similar to permanent magnets. They consist of coils of wire wound around a magnetic material (Fig. 1.22c). When current flows in the wire coils, the magnetic field is established between the two pole faces. The iron core serves to intensify this magnetic field. As a result, higher strength magnets are available with this technology (up to 0.4 T) as compared to air core systems. Likewise the magnetic fields generated are more stable and uniform than air core systems.

Finally, superconducting systems (Fig. 1.22d) employ coils immersed in a cryogen. In this state, current flows without resistance and very strong magnetic fields—from 0.5 T to 2.0 T and beyond—can be generated. Note that the B_0 magnetic field is directed along the center of the gantry.

One important aspect of magnet configuration is the fact that permanent and iron core resistive magnets produce magnetic fields which are highly concentrated within the gantry but weak beyond the gantry. Air core and superconducting systems, on the other hand, generate their magnetic fields well beyond the gantry area. This is important in siting the MR unit since these extraneous magnetic fields, referred to as fringe fields, can affect

TABLE 1.5
Types of coils used in MRI

Coil	Types	Application
Main field coils	Helmholtz pairs	For air core resistive magnets (<0.2 T)
	Around magnetic material	For mid-field systems (0.1–0.3 T)
	Helical superconducting	For high field systems (0.5–2.0 T)
Gradient coils	Generic coils	To produce 3-dimensional spatial localization of MR signals
Radio frequency excitation/detection	Body, head and local coils (saddle shape, bird cage types)	To produce RF energy and detect emitted RF signal from patient. Many local coils detect only
Shim coils	Simple coils	To help produce uniform magnetic field within gantry

nearby electronic instrumentation (including cardiac pacemakers). They also interact with ferrous material in the environment such that the magnetic field may be warped back at the patient position within the gantry, thereby affecting image quality. Fringe fields in general must be no greater than 5 Gauss in accessible areas. Permanent and iron core systems accomplish this quite close to the gantry. For superconducting systems there are various approaches to reduce fringe fields. One is to build a large iron shield around the magnet or possibly within the walls of the scan room. Another is the so-called self-shielding approach. Here, thick iron slabs are placed immediately around the magnet to absorb the magnetic field. Depending on the size of the room, additional shielding in the walls of the room may or may not be necessary. Another possible approach is to generate oppositely directed magnetic fields to neutralize the fringe fields.

Coils
MRI utilizes a number of coils to accomplish the scan process. Table 1.5 summarizes these.

The main field coils, as described previously, are associated with producing the strong external magnetic field, B_0. These coils are wrapped either over the gantry length (superconducting systems) or around the magnetic core (electromagnet systems).

RF coils are those necessary to generate the RF energy to be broadcast into the patient. They are also used to detect the RF energy emitted by the patient during the spin relaxation period. These coils are sometimes referred to as body or head coils.

Surface coils (or local coils) are smaller RF coils placed directly over the region of interest on the patient. Local coils greatly enhance both the SNR and spatial resolution characteristics of the image. SNR is improved because coils are very close to the region emitting the RF energy and so more signal is collected. Spatial resolution is improved because a full matrix is being applied to a smaller volume and each pixel is smaller. Local coils are typically configured to detect RF and not necessarily to broadcast it, though the latter is possible.

Gradient coils are configured within the gantry. Their function, of course, is to provide for the sequential application of field gradients in order to provide for three-dimensional spatial localization of data. The fields they produce are such that a linear variation in magnetic field is superimposed on the original B_0 field.

Shim coils are placed at various locations within the gantry. Their function is to provide a means of making more uniform the magnetic field within the gantry. Computer programs are available which, if given data as to the initial homogeneity of the B_0 field, will determine how much current should flow through the various shim coils to smooth the B_0 field further. These small shim magnetic fields can be applied at various points within the gantry to compensate for inhomogeneities not only in the magnet itself but also due to the presence of ferrous objects outside the gantry.

Imaging performance
How much information does the image convey and what are the factors affecting it? We have seen that the actual appearance of the images depends critically on the choice of TE and TR and therefore on which tissue characteristics one is weighting for. The image quality parameter involved here is that of image contrast, which is a measure of how distinguishable the various tissues are. As well as SNR, referred to earlier, two further factors must be mentioned which affect image quality. These are spatial resolution and the possible presence of artifacts in the image. These will be discussed in turn.

Image contrast
Image contrast refers to the differences seen between the various tissues or tissue states and more specifically the differences seen as determined by whether the image is T_1, T_2 or spin density weighted. In Figure 1.14 we saw that T_1 differences varied with TR. There is essentially no T_1 contrast at very long TR after full spin recovery, while shorter TR yields increasing T_1 contrast. Note, however, that greater T_1 contrast has lower signal magnitude and thus greater noise. If one were interested in spin density contrast one would employ a long TR (see Fig. 1.16) and in fact also enjoy high signals and low noise. For T_2 contrast we have seen that relatively long TEs are necessary. In the standard multi-echo acquisition one obtains an early image (short TE) which is more spin density contrast weighted and a later image (longer TE) which is more T_2 weighted. It is clear, however, that later echoes have lower signal amplitudes (Fig. 1.12D) and therefore more noise.

Signal to noise ratio
One may theoretically expect a certain contrast for a particular set of TEs and TRs. However, the final image may have superimposed upon it random signal fluctuations that hinder the ability of the system to distinguish and display the expected contrast. The SNR is formed by obtaining the ratio of the average signal magnitude and the noise magnitude as seen in Figure 1.23A. In Figure 1.23B, the difference between high and low SNR is shown. In the presence of noise, low image contrast structures are easily lost.

The signal fluctuations, which constitute the noise, come from various sources. The main source is random and is dependent on the magnitude of signal detected. Electronic

A.

Signal | average signal magnitude

noise magnitude

distance

B.

Signal

High SNR

Low SNR

distance

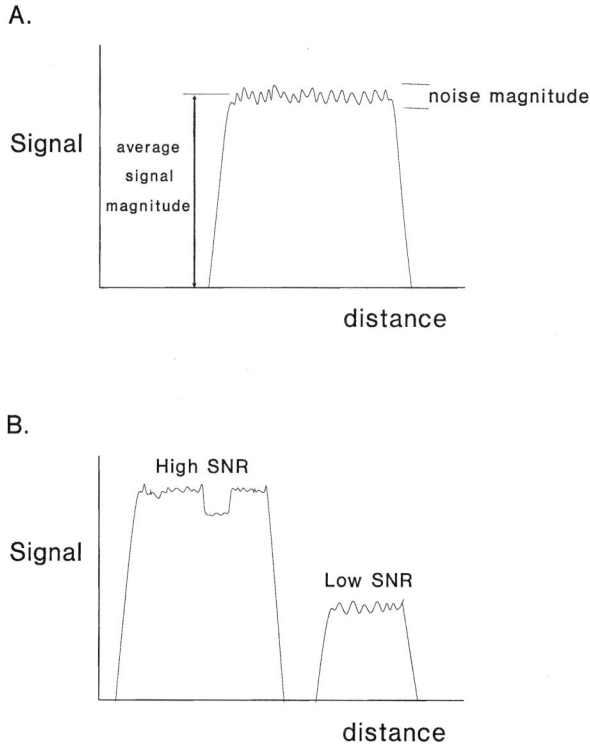

Fig. 1.23. Signal to noise ratio (SNR). *(A)* The SNR is defined as the ratio of the average signal magnitude to the noise magnitude across the image. *(B)* High *vs.* low SNR. At high SNR the noise is relatively small as compared to low SNR. A small signal variation is easily seen at high SNR but is lost at low SNR.

noise constitutes another source. One also has noise introduced by the patients themselves due to the small fluctuating magnetic fields caused by the naturally occurring electrical currents in their own bodies. In well engineered systems the random signal-dependent noise is by far the most important.

Sometimes we also refer to a contrast to noise ratio (CNR). This measure is even more specific as a descriptive image quality in that it refers to the effects of noise on the observable contrast, that is, the distinguishability of tissues.

It is important to note that SNR increases not only with increasing TR and decreasing TE but also with increasing NEX as the B_0 field is increased. In addition, SNR is increased as thicker slices are chosen, as pixel sizes are increased and as matrix sizes are decreased. These latter points will be discussed in the following section. Figure 1.24 shows the effects of high and low SNR for distributions of TR and TE. There is progressively less noise for long TR and short TE (Fig. 1.24A). If the system is inherently noisier (Fig. 1.24B), this hinders the ability to separate signals from different tissues. SNR becomes progressively worse, as expected, at short TR and long TE.

A. Relatively High SNR

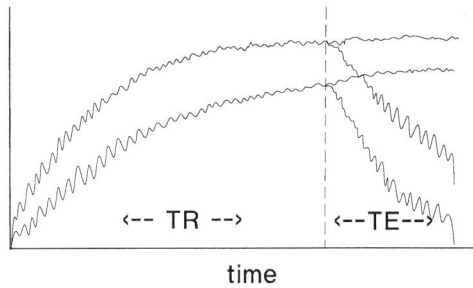

time

B. Relatively Low SNR

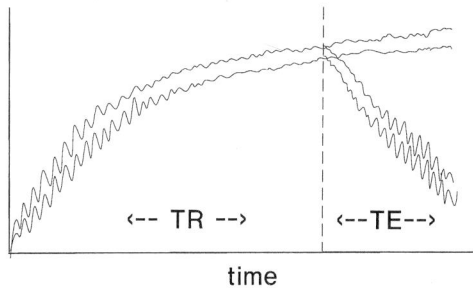

time

Fig. 1.24. Illustration on variations of SNR at the various TR and TE levels for two different tissues. Specifically, noise increases as TR decreases and TE increases. *(A)* At high SNR the two tissues are distinguishable. *(B)* At low SNR the two tissues start to become indistinguishable for low TR and high TE.

Spatial resolution

Spatial resolution refers to the image performance of a system under optimal conditions, *i.e.* how small a detail is observable under conditions of very high contrast and negligible noise. The primary factor affecting spatial resolution is the size of the image pixel. In MRI, as with all digital imaging, the image is processed in terms of little discrete image elements called pixels. An image expressed as having a 256×256 matrix, for instance, would comprise an array of 256 pixels in both the vertical and horizontal directions. For a given field of view (FOV), the pixel size would equal the FOV divided by the matrix size, *e.g.* a 256×256 matrix and a 250 mm FOV implies a pixel size $(250/256) = 0.98$ mm. To increase spatial resolution one would have to increase the matrix size or decrease the FOV. A penalty ensues, however, when pixel size is decreased. Specifically, smaller pixel sizes imply fewer hydrogen protons available to provide signal, and noise increases. Likewise, as FOV decreases, pixels also decrease in size and we see the same phenomenon. Finally, spatial resolution is also affected by the slice thickness. Thinner slices imply that a particular tissue is better visualized since there are fewer other tissues contributing to the

TABLE 1.6
Common artifacts and their causes

Artifact	Appearance	Methods used to minimize
Motion	Series of repetitive ghost-like images projected along the phase encoding gradient direction; usually results in noisier images	• Restrict motion • Shorter scan time • Change phase encoding gradient direction • Presaturation pulses • Motion compensation
Truncation	Series of repetitive images parallel to surface having abrupt signal change	Smaller pixels (larger matrix size)
Wrap around (aliasing)	Presence of anatomic structure superimposed on image (due to exciting an anatomic region but then not sampling it)	Ensure that entire sample in field of view is both excited and signal sampled
Chemical shift	Water and lipid structures separate due to slightly different frequencies. Black and white bands result	• Use large pixel sizes, *i.e.* chemical shift falls within pixel dimensions • Use smaller fields of view. • Use lower field strengths

signal coming from the whole volume of the pixel (called a voxel). The thinner the slice, the smaller the voxel and the greater the relative signal from a given small structure; hence, the more able one is to visualize it. Again, however, the problem of noise arises in that thinner slices also imply fewer hydrogen protons available to contribute to the signal.

As in any other imaging modality, there are a number of ways to express spatial resolution. Examples are line pairs per millimeter and 'modulation transfer functions', but the easiest and most straightforward way is by specifying pixel size as above.

It should be realized that although a larger matrix size may improve spatial resolution it also increases the scan time and the time required for computer processing and image reconstruction, as well as the necessary storage space (*e.g.* a 512×512 matrix needs four times more storage capacity than a 256×256 matrix and twice the scan time), implying a need for more powerful computers.

Artifacts
There are many sources of possible artifacts in MRI. Only the more clinically important ones are discussed here. These are summarized in Table 1.6.

MOTION ARTIFACTS
Just as in CT scanning and indeed classical radiological imaging, motion degrades the MR image. There is, however, a distinct pattern to motion artifacts in MRI. The Fourier transform data processing is such that a moving structure is imaged as a series of repetitive, ghostlike images. What is happening is that the signal from the moving object is being spread out in space along the phase encoding gradient (PEG). This gradient is primarily affected because it is this direction over which the scan time is spread, that is, there is a long TR time between successive PEGs. Not only do the ghost images obscure

28

(a)   (b)

(c)   (d)

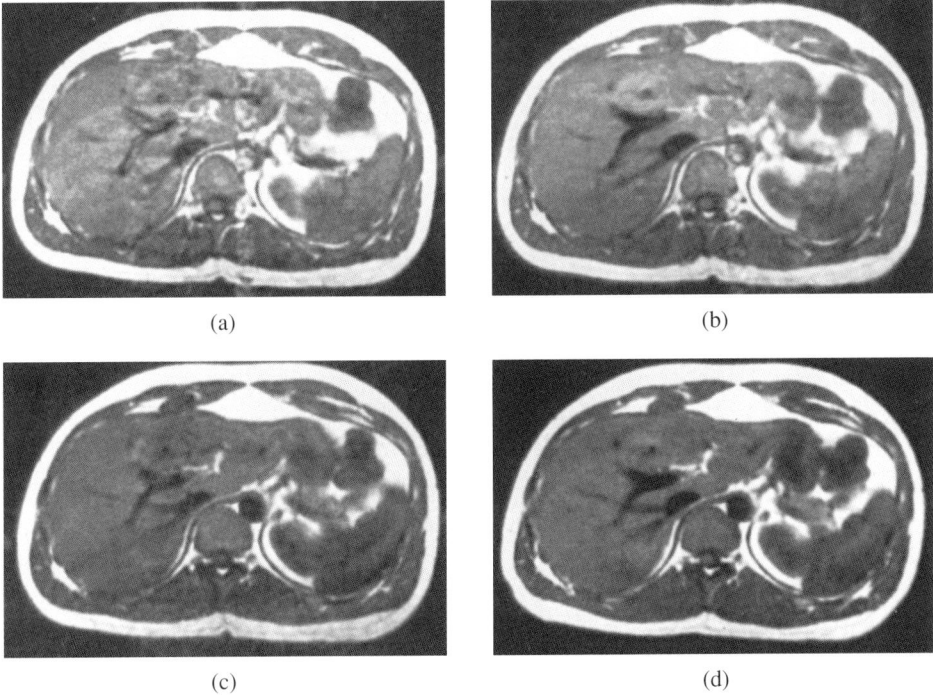

Fig. 1.25. Blood flow motion artifacts. *(a)* Ghosting appears for all abdominal blood vessel signals in phase encoding direction. *(b)* Saturation superior to slice produces flow voids and eliminates ghosting from aorta and hepatic arteries. *(c)* Saturation inferior to slice eliminates ghosting from venous flow (inferior vena cava and hepatic veins). *(d)* Bilateral saturation producing flow voids and eliminating all flow artifacts. (Scans courtesy of General Electric Corp.)

structures of interest, but the moving structure itself, because of its diminished signal, has diminished visualization. Finally, as in classical imaging, blurring is increased with motion.

There are a number of ways to reduce motion artifacts. One way, of course, is to provide for physical restraints or somehow reduce scan time. Some of the fast scan techniques which reduce scan time to at least the point where the patient can hold their breath would be of obvious value here. Shorter scan times, though, may also mean a reduction in overall signal and hence in SNR. Another approach is to align the PEG with respect to the moving structures so that ghosts generated either go out of the image plane, or fall in a direction which does not obscure critical structures from being visualized. Another way which has become very popular is the technique of presaturation. In this approach the volume containing the moving structure is saturated with RF energy in such a way that it cannot return a signal and thus cannot create ghost images. This approach is limited to moving structures within volumes that are not required to be visualized, for example, a structure entirely out of the plane or a structure within the desired plane but which can be blocked off.

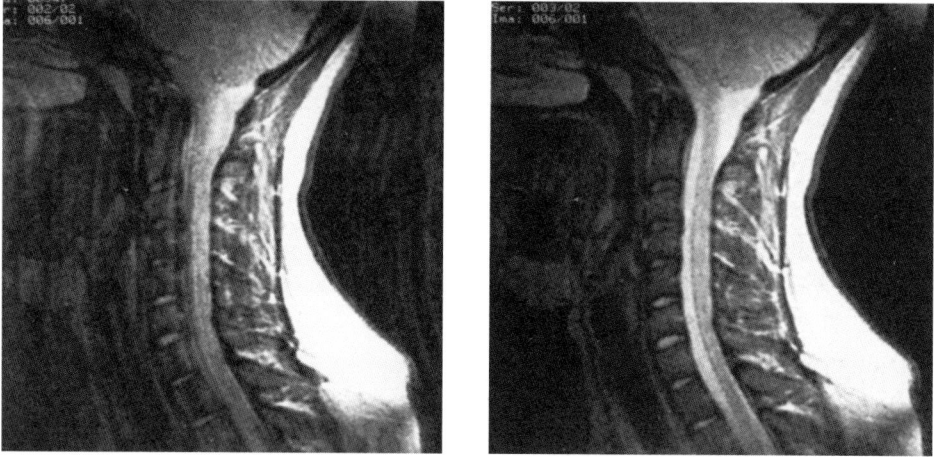

Fig. 1.26. Effect of CSF pulsation in a T$_2$-weighted cervical spine image. *(Left)* No flow compensation; *(right)* with flow compensation. (Images courtesy General Electric Corporation.)

One further approach is known as 'motion gating acquisition', where imaging is timed to coincide with the point of least motion by monitoring, for instance, the patient's breathing cycle (respiratory gating) or heartbeat (cardiac gating). The technique is to allocate image data from a particular part of cycle where motion artifact is minimal, *e.g.* when the blood is flowing the lowest. Notice that gating approaches usually increase scan times as well as set-up times.

Finally, various software and data allocation schemes are available which can reduce the effects of motion. For instance, if the position of a given point at a given moment is known, then data are allocated to that point. Since image points, as they move, sit in different parts of the gradient, then knowledge of point position (via motion detector) will allow correct ordering of the gradients. This latter approach and similar ones have been called various acronyms by MR vendors, *e.g.* 'rope', 'cope' and 'exorcist'.

Figure 1.25*b* shows the effects of presaturation on motion artifacts. Here, the region superior to the slice of interest is presaturated. As a result, ghosting from the aorta and hepatic arteries is eliminated producing arterial flow voids. Figure 1.25*c* shows the effect of presaturation inferior to the slice. Here the ghosting from venous flow (inferior vena cava and hepatic veins) is eliminated. Figure 1.25*d* shows the result of presaturating both inferiorly and superiorly to the slice. All ghosting is then eliminated. Figure 1.26 shows motion artifacts due to pulsating CSF with and without flow compensation.

Truncation artifacts

Truncation artifacts are seen as a series of repetitive ripples outlining the contours of sharp borders or sharp discontinuities in signal intensity such as at the cranium or at sub-cutaneous fat (Fig. 1.27). Such ripples mask important image information. An example of

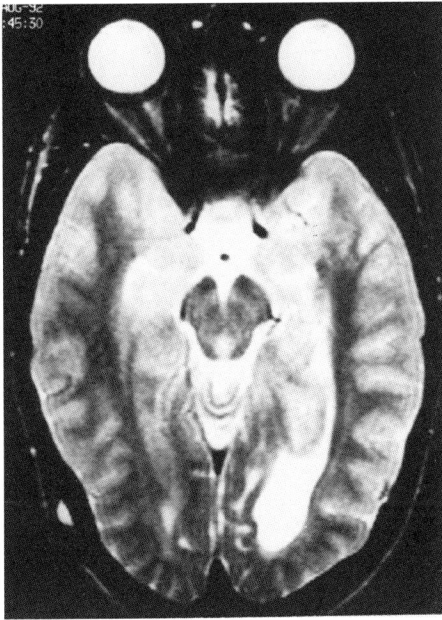

Fig. 1.27. Illustration of Gibbs truncation artifact. These artifacts occur at sharp high signal tissue boundaries. Here the artifact is seen as repetitive lines or ripples following the contours of the skull and subcutaneous fat. These artifactual lines disappear as matrix size increases (pixel sizes decrease).

a possible problem arising from truncation artifacts is the appearance of a ripple along the cord mimicking a syringomyelia.

Truncation artifacts can occur in either the phasing encoding or frequency gradient direction. The source of these artifacts is related to the way the echo signal data are sampled. Specifically, it is due to the fact that the echo signal train may not be sampled out to its fullest extent but rather is truncated and signal values of zero arbitrarily substituted. This discontinuity of data can also be averaged away but that would introduce an unwanted and unacceptable general loss of spatial resolution. The most straightforward way of minimizing the truncation artifact is to extend echo sampling time. This can be done by increasing the number of phase encoding steps (increase matrix size/decrease pixel size).

CHEMICAL SHIFT ARTIFACT

As already stated, hydrogen protons have a fixed Larmor frequency as a function of B_0. Depending on the particular molecular structure, the precession frequency can be shifted away from the expected Larmor frequency. For instance, hydrogen protons in lipids (CH_2 groups) are shifted to a higher frequency with respect to those in water by about 3.5 parts per million (220 Hz at 1.5 T). Shift is along the frequency gradient direction. The result is the formation of a black band at one end of the structure due to a gap in signal formed by the shift of fat signal relative to water and a bright area at the other end of the structure where images overlap (Fig. 1.28). Clinically the appearance of this artifact can be used to advantage if it is necessary to determine whether lipid content is present. One method of

31

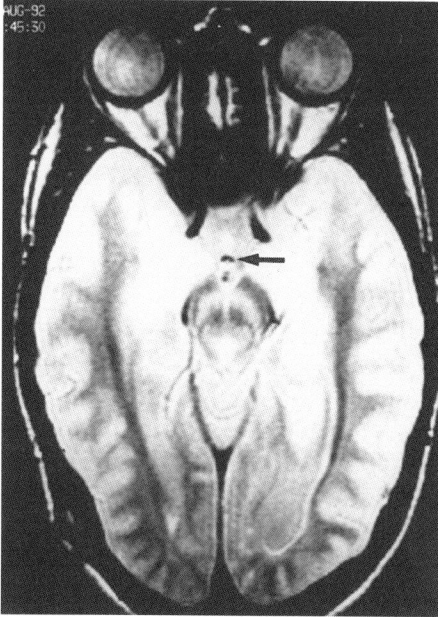

Fig. 1.28. Illustration of chemical shift on a hypothalamic lipoma as evidenced by artifactual signal void *(arrow)*. This void disappeared when a fat suppression technique was employed.

minimizing this artifact is via fat suppression techniques. One can identify bright or dark bands as being artifactual and due to chemical shift by reversing the polarity of the gradient and observing whether bands interchange from one end to the other. The chemical shift artifact becomes more significant at higher B_0 field strengths.

WRAP-AROUND (ALIASING) ARTIFACTS

Wrap-around or aliasing artifacts occur if part of the anatomy receives the initial 90° RF pulse but then is not within the gradient field of view for the rephasing pulse. In this case signal from these tissues 'wrap around' to the other side of the patient. As a result, the anatomy is misplaced on the image. This is illustrated in Figure 1.29 where the mandibular region is cut off from the top of the image and reappears superimposed at the bottom. These artifacts are avoided by ensuring a large enough field of view to make sure that tissues receive both initial excitation and rephasing pulses and are subsequently sampled correctly.

SUSCEPTIBILITY ARTIFACTS

Any ferrous or otherwise magnetic material in the body is going to warp the magnetic field in its vicinity. This inhomogeneity will cause rapid dephasing and loss of signal, resulting in the formation of signal voids in the image as well as image distortion. Examples of sources of susceptibility artifacts include cobalt in mascara, dental prostheses, iron specks or metallic implants, clips, etc. Susceptibility artifacts are particularly bothersome in gradient echo imaging since 180° rephasing as is found for spin echo imaging is

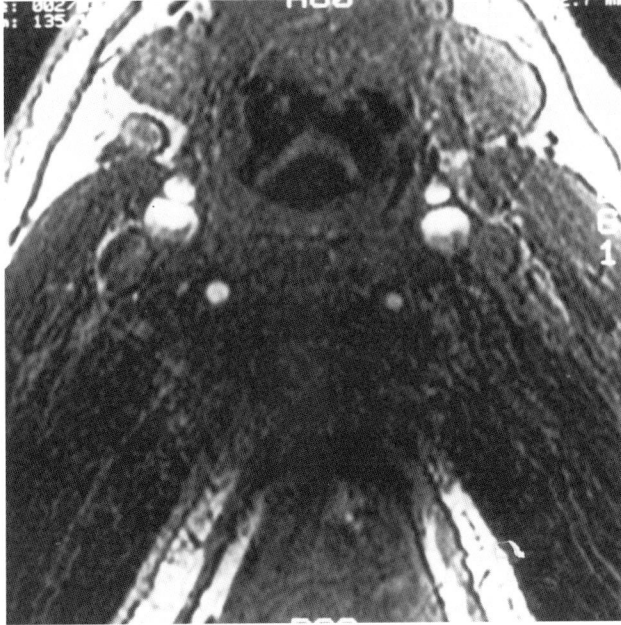

Fig. 1.29. Wrap-around artifact. Axial 3D time of flight view through carotid artery bifurcation. Scan had been done with small field of view to maximize resolution. The mandibular region is seen to wrap around from the top of the image back down to the bottom.

missing. In GRE imaging only the gradient inhomogeneity is rephased. All other sources of inhomogeneities including susceptibility effects stay in the images as artifacts.

Other MRI applications

There are a number of other exciting applications of MRI which have either established their practicality (*e.g.* MR angiography) or have significant potential for the future (MR spectroscopy, perfusion/diffusion imaging).

Magnetic resonance angiography

In addition to T_1, T_2 and spin density, a fourth parameter critical in MRI is motion. Considerations on motion were at first based on how to eliminate it and the bothersome ghost artifacts which were formed. It was soon realized that there was important information related to the motion of structures in an MR image, in particular, the motion and flow characteristics of blood and CSF. In fact, images just of flow can be obtained yielding angiographic information. Both 'time of flight' and 'phase contrast' information is capitalized on to obtain angiographic information.

The time of flight approach relies on the fact that the signal detected is dependent upon how fast and how far the blood flowed within the signal gathering time. The phase contrast approach is based on the observation that motion serves to produce a dephasing

33

effect among the spinning nuclei and consequently a loss of signal. Signal flow differences therefore produce phase differences which result in image signal differences.

MR spectroscopy
Molecular spectroscopy is based on the fact that hydrogen protons sitting in different molecules have slightly different precessional frequencies. This represents a molecule-dependent chemical shift which can be detected and quantitated. Spectral distributions can then be made showing relative abundance of the various biologically important molecules such as ATP.

Perfusion/diffusion imaging and other applications
Function imaging is now becoming increasingly used. Here the perfusion and diffusion characteristics of tissues yield important information. Techniques to fuse and register together images from different imaging modalities have also been developed. Examples include fusing positron emission tomography images or radionuclide scan images onto MR images.

A full description of motion effects, magnetic resonance angiography, spectroscopy and perfusion/diffusion studies is beyond the scope of this book but the interested reader is referred to the literature (see below).

ACKNOWLEDGEMENT

I would like to acknowledge Dr Scott Faro for providing some of the clinical artifact images.

BIBLIOGRAPHY

Bradley, W.G. (1992) 'Flow phenomena.' *In:* Stark, D.D., Bradley, W.G. (Eds.) *Magnetic Resonance Imaging. 2nd Edn.* Chicago: Mosby Year Book.

Edelman, R.R., Mattle, H.P., Atkinson, D.J., Hoogewoud, H.M. (1990) 'MR angiography.' *American Journal of Roentgenology,* **154**, 937–946. *(Review article.)*

Matson, G.B., Weiner, M.W. (1992) 'Spectroscopy.' *In:* Stark, D.D., Bradley, W.G. (Eds.) *Magnetic Resonance Imaging. 2nd Edn.* Chicago: Mosby Year Book.

2
SEDATION, PATIENT MONITORING AND CONTRAST MEDIA

Eric N. Faerber

The increasing use of the newer imaging modalities, computed tomography (CT) and magnetic resonance imaging (MRI), has led to a corresponding need for sedation in many infants and children, since optimal imaging depends on lack of patient motion during study. Advances in technology have brought about a dramatic reduction in CT scan time, but for MRI the scan time is still much longer. The necessity for multiplanar scans with multiple pulse sequences followed by further imaging after injection of contrast medium may result in a lengthy examination.

Selection of patients for sedation
Infants beyond the neonatal period and children up to the age of 7–8 years generally require sedation. Neonates at our hospital are usually sedated and given nothing by mouth for two hours prior to the study. Children over 8 years of age usually do not require sedation; however, emotional lability, hyperactivity and mental retardation will influence the need for it.

Preparation of patients
When the MRI scan is scheduled on an outpatient basis at our hospital, the parents (or legal guardians) are questioned about previous allergies and drug reactions, history of apnea which would preclude oral sedation, and any recent previous intracranial or spinal surgery with placement of ferromagnetic clips. They are advised to keep their child without food or drink for four hours prior to the study.

When the child and parents arrive at the MRI suite they are met by the radiology nurse. The patient's weight is recorded, a medical history is obtained with reference to allergies, food and drug reactions, asthma, liver and renal disease, and sickle cell disease and related conditions, and vital signs including pulse and respiratory rate are obtained. Children with an upper respiratory tract infection or fever are rescheduled.

The parents are then shown an album containing an array of color photographs that sequentially depict all the phases of a child undergoing an MRI scan; a hand-out explaining the study is also available. The concept of a pictorial display was devised at our hospital, and these albums are available for both CT and MRI scans. Parents report them to be both informative and reassuring. Older children are also encouraged to view the photographs in order to alleviate any anxieties.

The child is administered sedation orally by the radiology nurse 30–45 minutes prior to the procedure. Inpatients are similarly sedated by hospital nursing staff at a time predetermined with the MRI nurses and technologists.

Choice of sedation

The sedative of choice should ideally have the following properties: ease of administration, consistency of action, safety, rapid action with complete immobilization, and controllable duration of action (Thompson *et al.* 1982). There is no single ideal sedative to fulfil all these criteria. The choice of sedation varies from hospital to hospital and is dependent on numerous variables such as ease and comfort with use of the chosen sedative, availability of nursing and medical staff, and imaging equipment.

At our hospital, chloral hydrate is used almost exclusively for sedation of patients undergoing MRI. This regimen is described in detail below, followed by details of alternative choices.

Chloral hydrate

This is the most widely used sedation agent in North American pediatric centers (Keeter *et al.* 1990). Chloral hydrate is a halogenated hydrocarbon metabolized primarily in the liver. Excretion is mostly through the hepatobiliary system but also partly through the kidneys.

It is available in oral (liquid or capsule) and rectal suppository forms. The liquid form administered orally or by nasogastric tube is the preferred method at our hospital because of ease of administration and safety of action. Use of rectal suppositories has been limited because of frequent evacuation and less reliable absorption. Chloral hydrate is considered the safest, most effective agent for sedation in most infants and young children (Boyer 1992), although its use has recently been challenged because of a potential carcinogenic effect (American Academy of Pediatrics 1993). Contraindications to the use of chloral hydrate are allergy, CNS and respiratory depression, and hepatic or renal failure.

The dosage of oral chloral hydrate used in our department is 50 mg/kg for neonates and 80–100 mg/kg in infants and older children, the same as for CT (Faerber 1986), with a maximum of 2.5 g (Greenberg *et al.* 1993*a*). Analysis of sedation data in 300 infants and children between 1 month and 11 years of age receiving oral choral hydrate for MRI scans revealed successful sedation in 91 per cent of the patients (Greenberg *et al.* 1993*a*). There was a 96 per cent success rate in children aged 4 years or younger and an 81 per cent success rate in children older than 4 years.

Thioridazine

Thioridazine is a phenothiazine with sedative properties. It has been successfully used at our hospital as an adjunct to chloral hydrate in infants and children who had a hyperactivity reaction with chloral hydrate. These patients fall into two categories: (i) those with previously failed sedation using chloral hydrate alone, and (ii) mentally retarded children.

Thioridazine is administered in a dose of 2–4 mg/kg, with a maximum of 100 mg, two hours prior to the MRI examination. Chloral hydrate is then administered 30 minutes prior to the study, in a dose of 50–100mg/kg with an upper limit of 2.5g.

Analysis of sedation data of 104 infants and children ranging in age from 4 months to 17 years who received the combination of thioridazine and chloral hydrate at our hospital revealed successful MRI studies in 89 per cent of patients overall and in 92 per cent of those who were mentally retarded (Greenberg *et al.* 1993*b*).

Pentobarbital (pentobarbitone)
Pentobarbital is a short-acting barbiturate frequently used for sedation during CT and MRI (Merrick *et al.* 1991, Hubbard *et al.* 1992). It may be administered intravenously or intramuscularly in doses of up to 6mg/kg (Strain *et al.* 1986). With intravenous administration, onset of sedation is rapid (under 60 seconds), and the recovery time is shorter than with chloral hydrate (Strain *et al.* 1986). Hubbard *et al.* (1992) found no significant difference between intravenous pentobarbital and oral chloral hydrate in the ability to sedate pediatric patients for CT and MRI. In this series the incidence of minor complications was the same for both regimens.

'Cardiac cocktail' (CM3)
This mixture, which consists of meperidine (pethidine) (25mg/mL), chlorpromazine (6.25mg/mL) and promethazine (6.25mg/mL), has been used for neuroimaging procedures in a dose of 0.1mL/kg up to a maximum of 2mL. In some cases it may not be suitable due to a potential for respiratory depression (Thompson *et al.* 1982), and because it also decreases the seizure threshold it is not recommended for patients with a history of seizures.

Diazepam
Intravenous diazepam, which is rapid acting and decreases the respiratory rate, is useful for calming anxious adults for MRI. However, it is often ineffective for sedation of children (Kuharik 1990) and it is unsafe in the higher doses required to achieve satisfactory immobilization (Thompson *et al.* 1982).

General anesthesia
General anesthesia is not routinely used for MRI. It is reserved for those patients in whom sedation has previously failed or is considered unsafe. In the early days of MRI, ventilators could not be used in the imaging room because of their ferromagnetic materials. Many of the technical problems have now been solved. Induction for anesthesia is usually performed outside the scanning suite, with the patient then being transferred back to the imaging area. The MRI unit (depending on the manufacturer) may have a detachable table on which the patient may undergo induction. Successful MRI procedures under general anesthesia are the result of collaborative team work between members of the radiology, anesthesiology and nursing teams.

Monitoring
After administration of the sedative of choice, the child is kept in the sedation room with

the overhead lights dimmed. The child may lie either in a parent's lap in a rocking chair or on a stretcher until asleep. If an intravenous line is needed for contrast medium administration it will be inserted at this time; ideally this will be around 15–20 minutes after administration of chloral hydrate where that is the sedative of choice.

The child is then transferred to the MRI scanning room. Monitoring is essential for all infants and children requiring sedation, and this has been greatly facilitated by the availability of CO_2 monitors that measure expired carbon dioxide content and pulse oximeters, numerous types of which are now commercially available. Skin burns have been reported from coiled monitoring wires touching a sedated patient lying in the changing magnetic flux (Kanal *et al.* 1990). Shielding devices are available to prevent skin burns, as well as interference with pulse oximetry and degradation of MR images.

Preterm infants require particular attention to maintenance of body temperature. An air bag that is warmed to body temperature may be used (McArdle *et al.* 1987), or a plastic wrap and prewarmed towels (Barkovich 1988). A stockinette cap prevents heat loss from the head.

When the MR study is completed, the images are routinely checked by radiology personnel (resident, fellow or attending) to ensure that they are satisfactory. Additional scans may be obtained provided the patient is still sedated if there has been patient movement during the study. Additional pulse sequences or imaging planes may be needed due to the detection of pathologic features, or if contrast medium administration is required.

The discharge criterion for outpatients is that they must be arousable with intact protective reflexes.

Contrast agents
MRI affords an exquisite display of anatomy and pathology; however, non-contrast MRI demonstrates very high sensitivity with lack of specificity (Hesselink and Press 1988).

The intravascular contrast agents used for MRI are paramagnetic compounds. When placed in a magnet such substances tend to align in parallel with the external magnetic field, but when it is removed they lose this alignment, returning to a random orientation. The phenomenon of proton relaxation enhancement occurs by shortening the T_1 and T_2 relaxation times. The T_1 shortening process predominates resulting in enhancement.

The paramagnetic contrast agents are composed of a metal ion (gadolinium) and a chelating agent. Gadolinium is an element in the lanthanide (rare earth) group, discovered by the Finnish scientist, Gadolin, in 1794. It must be chelated because of its toxicity (Weinmann *et al.* 1984*a*). The chelating agent most widely used is diethylenetriamine-penta-acetic acid (DTPA). The generic name of this ionic agent is Gd-DTPA, also known as gadopentetate dimeglumine. In the USA, this was first approved for use by the Food and Drug Administration (FDA) in 1988. Two non-ionic gadolinium MRI contrast agents have subsequently been approved by the FDA for use in adults, and approval is pending for their use in children. These are gadoteridol and gadodiamide, both administered intravenously.

Gd-DTPA is now the most widely used contrast agent for MRI on the North American continent. It is produced as a water soluble dimeglumine salt. In the chelated form it behaves similarly to iodinated contrast media (Powers *et al.* 1988). After intravenous administration of contrast medium there is rapid distribution in the intravascular and extracellular fluid spaces of the body except where the intact blood–brain barrier (BBB) prevents it from entering the extravascular space (Hesselink and Press 1988). Localization of contrast medium occurs in structures without a BBB, such as the choroid plexus, pituitary gland and stalk, and cavernous sinus. Vascular enhancement is more variable on MRI than on CT because of flow, and is most obvious in venous structures where small veins are noted to enhance more than larger ones (Saini *et al.* 1991). Large arteries do not usually show significant enhancement unless blood flow is pathologic (Saini *et al.* 1991). The tentorium and falx enhance in 50 per cent of cases, with lesser enhancement seen than on CT (Kilgore *et al.* 1986).

The normal spinal cord, nerve roots and intravertebral discs do not enhance. There is, however, variable enhancement in the region of the ventral and dorsal nerve root ganglia, especially in the lumbar region and epidural venous plexus (Saini *et al.* 1991).

If the BBB is disrupted, the molecules of contrast agent diffuse into the interstitial compartment producing T_1 shortening and enhancement on T_1-weighted images (Runge *et al.* 1985). Gd-DTPA is useful in delineating tumor nidus from edema, residual tumor, metastatic disease, subacute nature of infarcts, activity in multiple sclerosis, vasculitis and inflammatory disease (Elster *et al.* 1989).

Spinal applications for the use of contrast medium in T_1-weighted sequences are the evaluations of intramedullary and intradural extramedullary lesions and evaluation of the postoperative spine (Saini *et al.* 1991).

Gd-DTPA is rapidly excreted by the kidneys with more than 80 per cent of the contrast agent in the urine within three hours after intravenous injection (Weinmann *et al.* 1984*b*). The usual recommended dose is 0.1 mmol/kg.

The varied application and safety of use of Gd-DTPA in children have been well documented (Bird *et al.* 1988, Powers *et al.* 1988, Cohen *et al.* 1989, Elster and Rieser 1989, Elster 1990). Although minor side-effects are common, major adverse reactions are rare. The paramagnetic contrast agents can be cautiously administered to patients with renal compromise, although their safety for use in pregnant or nursing mothers has yet to be established.

REFERENCES

American Academy of Pediatrics Committee of Drugs and Committee on Environmental Health (1993) 'Use of chloral hydrate for sedation in children.' *Pediatrics*, **92**, 471–473.

Barkovich, A.J. (1988) 'Techniques and methods in pediatric magnetic resonance imaging.' *Seminars in Ultrasound, CT and MR*, **9**, 186–191.

Bird, C.R., Drayer, B.P., Medina, M., Rekate, H.L., Flom, R.A., Hodak, J.A. (1988) 'Gd-DTPA-enhanced MR imaging in pediatric patients after brain tumor resection.' *Radiology*, **169**, 123–126.

Boyer, R.S. (1992) 'Sedation in pediatric neuroimaging: the science and the art.' *American Journal of Neuroradiology*, **13**, 777–783.

Cohen, B.H., Bury, E., Packer, R.J., Sutton, L.N., Bilaniuk, L.T., Zimmerman, R.A. (1989) 'Gadolinium-DTPA-enhanced magnetic resonance imaging in childhood brain tumors.' *Neurology*, **39**, 1178–1183.

Elster, A.D. (1990) 'Cranial MR imaging with Gd-DTPA in neonates and young infants: preliminary experience.' *Radiology*, **176**, 225–230.

—— Rieser, G.D. (1989) 'DTPA-enhanced cranial MR imaging in children: initial clinical experience and recommendations for its use.' *American Journal of Neuroradiology*, **10**, 1027–1030.

—— Moody, D.M., Ball, M.R., Laster, D.W. (1989) 'Is Gd-DTPA required for routine cranial MR imaging?' *Radiology*, **173**, 231–238.

Faerber, E.N. (1986) *Cranial Computed Tomography in Infants and Children. Clinics in Developmental Medicine No. 93.* London: Spastics International Medical Publications.

Greenberg, S.B., Faerber, E.N., Aspinall, C.L., Adams, R.C. (1993*a*) 'High-dose chloral hydrate sedation for children undergoing MR imaging: safety and efficacy in relation to age.' *American Journal of Roentgenology*, **161**, 639–641.

—— —— Radke, J.L., Aspinall, C.L., Adams, R.C., Mercer-Wilson, D.D. (1993*b*) 'Use and limitation of thioridazine as an adjunct to chloral hydrate sedation in the difficult-to-sedate child undergoing MR imaging.' *Radiology*, **189**, (Suppl.), 182–183. (Abstract.)

Hesselink, J.R., Press, G.A. (1988) 'MR contrast enhancement of intracranial lesions with Gd-DTPA.' *Radiologic Clinics of North America*, **26**, 873–887.

Hubbard, A.M., Markowitz, R.I., Kimmel, B., Kroger, M., Bartko, M.B. (1992) 'Sedation for pediatric patients undergoing CT and MRI.' *Journal of Computer Assisted Tomography*, **16**, 3–6.

Kanal, E., Shellock, F.G., Talagala, L. (1990) 'Safety considerations in MR imaging.' *Radiology*, **176**, 593–606.

Keeter, S., Benator, R.M., Weinberg, S.M., Hartenberg, M.A. (1990) 'Sedation in pediatric CT: national survey of current practice.' *Radiology*, **175**, 745–752.

Kilgore, D.P., Breger, R.K., Daniels, D.L., Pojunas, K.W., Williams, A.L., Haughton, V.M. (1986) 'Cranial tissues: normal MR appearance after intravenous injection of Gd-DTPA.' *Radiology*, **160**, 757–761.

Kuharik, M.A. (1990) 'Sedation, anesthesia, and patient monitoring.' *In:* Cohen, M.D., Edwards, M.K. (Eds.) *Magnetic Resonance Imaging in Children.* Philadelphia: B.C. Decker, pp. 75–81.

McArdle, C.B., Richardson, C.J., Nicholas, D.A., Mirfakhraee, M., Hayden, C.K., Amparo, E.G. (1987) 'Developmental features of the neonatal brain: MR imaging. Part I. Gray–white matter differentiation and myelination.' *Radiology*, **162**, 223–229.

Merrick, P.A., Case, B.J., Jagjivan, B., Stackman, T.J. (1991) 'Care of pediatric patients sedated with pentobarbital sodium in MRI.' *Pediatric Nursing*, **17**, 34–38.

Powers, T.A., Partain, C.L., Kesslar, R.M., Freeman, M.W., Robertson, R.H., Wyatt, S.H., Whelan, H.T. (1988) 'Central nervous system lesions in pediatric patients: Gd-DTPA-enhanced MR imaging.' *Radiology*, **169**, 723–726.

Runge, V.M., Clanton, J.A., Price, A.C., Wehr, C.J., Herzer, W.A., Partain, C.L., James, A.E. (1985) 'The use of Gd-DTPA as a perfusion agent and marker of blood–brain barrier disruption.' *Magnetic Resonance Imaging*, **3**, 43–55.

Saini, S., Modic, M.T., Hamm, B., Hahn, P.F. (1991) 'Advances in contrast-enhanced MR imaging.' *American Journal of Roentgenology*, **156**, 235–252.

Strain, J.D., Harvey, L.A., Foley, L.C., Campbell, J.B. (1986) 'Intravenously administered pentobarbital sodium for sedation in pediatric CT.' *Radiology*, **161**, 105–108.

Thompson, J.R., Schneider, S., Ashwal, S., Holden, B.S., Hinshaw, D.B., Hasso, A.N. (1982) 'The choice of sedation for computed tomography in children: a prospective evaluation.' *Radiology*, **143**, 475–479.

Weinmann, H-J., Brasch, R.C., Press, W-R., Wesbey, G.E. (1984*a*) 'Characteristics of gadolinium-DTPA complex: a potential NMR contrast agent.' *American Journal of Roentgenology*, **142**, 619–624.

—— Laniado, M., Mützel, W. (1984*b*) 'Pharmacokinetics of Gd-DTPA/dimeglumine after intravenous injections into healthy volunteers.' *Physiological Chemistry and Physics and Medical NMR*, **16**, 167–172.

3
BRAIN ANATOMY

Philip S. Yussen and Joel D. Swartz

A typical MRI study of the brain starts with a sagittal pilot image (Fig. 3.1) which is used to prescribe a series of images from the cranial base to the vertex in the axial plane. These are then supplemented by imaging in additional planes, usually sagittal or coronal, depending on the clinical question. In this chapter, sample images are presented to demonstrate basic MRI anatomy of the brain from base to vertex (Figs. 3.2–3.15), supplemented by both coronal (Figs. 3.16–3.18) and sagittal (Figs. 3.19–3.20) imaging.

Embryologically, by the fourth gestational week three vesicles have formed at the rostral segment of the neural tube. The highest vesicle corresponds to the forebrain or prosencephalon, the middle one to the midbrain or mesencephalon, and the third to the hindbrain or rhombencephalon. The forebrain will further divide into the telencephalon (cerebral hemispheres) and a more centrally placed diencephalon. The hindbrain also further divides into the more superiorly placed metencephalon (future pons and cerebellum) and the myelencephalon (future medulla). Early in gestation, the brain has a smooth surface, then, as the fetus develops, cortical sulcation can be recognized. The presence of cortical sulci and gyri leads to a vast increase in the surface area of the brain.

The major lobes of the hemispheres are the frontal, parietal, temporal and occipital lobes. The frontal and parietal lobes are separated by the central sulcus which defines the more anteriorly placed precentral gyrus (motor strip) and the postcentral gyrus (sensory strip). The centrally placed parieto-occipital fissure separates the parietal and occipital lobes. The boundary between the temporal and occipital lobes is not as clearly defined.

The subcortical ganglionic structures include the lentiform nuclei, comprising the globus pallidus medially and putamen laterally, the caudate nucleus which follows the course of the lateral ventricles, the amygdala which is located at the anterior margin of the temporal horn, and the thalamus. The internal capsule, a white matter structure, separates the medially placed caudate and thalamic nuclei from the more laterally positioned globus pallidus and putamen. Additionally, extrinsic to the putamen lies the thin claustrum, also a gray matter structure. The external and extreme white matter capsules respectively separate the putamen from the claustrum and the claustrum from the insular cortex of the temporal lobe.

The ventricular system comprises the paired lateral ventricles plus the midline third and fourth ventricles. The lateral ventricles can be divided into the frontal horns anteriorly, the paramedian lateral ventricular bodies, and the occipital and temporal horns. The lateral ventricular atria denote the junction of the lateral ventricular bodies with the occipital and temporal horns. The third ventricle is situated between the two thalami, inferior to the corpus callosum and underlying cisterna vellum interpositum. At the floor of the third ventricle lie the hypothalamus and more posteriorly placed subthalamus. The thalamus, hypothalamus, subthalamus and epithalamus comprise the diencephalon.

The important structures of the suprasellar cistern include the infundibular stalk and the immediately adjacent optic chiasm anteriorly. The circle of Willis lies within the suprasellar cistern. The parasellar cavernous sinuses contain the cavernous carotid arteries, as well as cranial nerves III, IV, V1, V2 and VI. Cranial nerve I (olfactory) lies along the inferior surface of the frontal lobe in a paramedian location.

The brainstem consists of the diencephalon, midbrain, pons and medulla. Cranial nerve III exits from the ventral surface of the midbrain, whereas cranial nerve IV crosses and exits the brainstem immediately inferior to the inferior colliculi. Cranial nerve V exits the pons laterally and extends anteriorly toward Meckel's cave. Cranial nerve VI exits ventrally near the junction of the pons and medulla. Cranial nerves VII and VIII exit laterally at the junction of the pons and medulla and enter the internal auditory canals. Cranial nerves IX–XII exit from the medulla.

The cerebellum is situated posterior to the pons and medulla and consists of the paired cerebellar hemispheres and midline vermis. The cerebellar tonsils are noted inferomedially, extending toward the foramen magnum. Between the cerebellar tonsils lies the vallecula which communicates with the fourth ventricle via the foramen of Magendie. The lateral recesses of the fourth ventricle also communicate with the subarachnoid space bilaterally via the foramina of Luschka.

The major white matter tracts communicating with the cerebellum are the paired superior, middle and inferior cerebellar peduncles, the largest of which are the middle peduncles. The cerebral peduncles represent the inferior extension of hemispheric white matter tracts through the internal capsule to the brainstem. This tract crosses at the level of the medulla. The cerebral peduncles are well demonstrated anteriorly at the level of the midbrain. The complex limbic system consists of cortical tissue in the cingulate and parahippocampal gyri with contributions from the thalamus, hypothalamus, amygdala and fornix. It is thought that this system performs a variety of complex functions including emotion.

FURTHER READING

Degroot, J. (1987) 'Functional neuroanatomy by magnetic resonance imaging.' *In:* Brant-Zawadski, M., Norman, D. (Eds.) *Magnetic Resonance Imaging of the Central Nervous System.* New York: Raven Press, pp. 115–121.

Faerber, E.N. (1986) 'Normal anatomy.' *In: Cranial Computed Tomography in Infants and Children. Clinics in Developmental Medicine No. 93.* London: Spastics International Medical Publications, pp. 18–28.

Rumeau, C., Gouaze, A., Salamon, G., Laffont, J., Gelbert, F., Einseidel, H., Jiddane, M., Farnarier, P., Habib, M., Perot, S. (1988) 'Identification of cortical sulci and gyri using magnetic resonance imaging: a preliminary study.' *In:* Gouaze, A., Salamon, G. (Eds.) *Brain Anatomy and Magnetic Resonance Imaging.* Berlin: Springer-Verlag, pp. 11–30.

Scott, W.R., Hanaway, J. (1987) 'Correlative anatomy of the brain.' *In:* Taveras, J.M., Ferrucci, J.T. (Eds.) *Radiology: Diagnosis–Imaging– Intervention, Vol. 3.* Philadelphia: J.B. Lippincott, pp. 1–25.

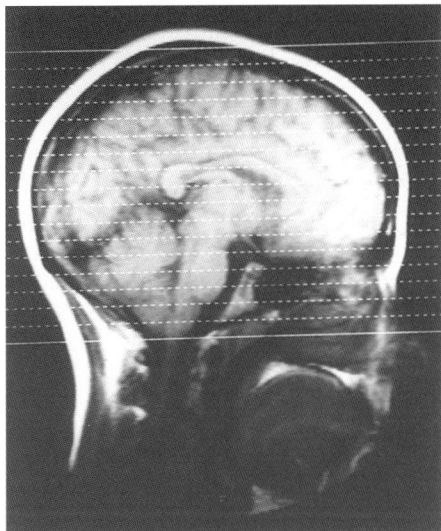

Fig. 3.1. Midline T_1 sagittal pilot image demonstrating slice positions 1–17 (Figs. 3.2–3.15).

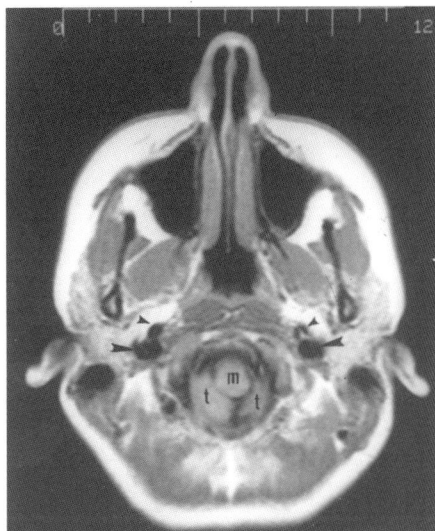

Fig. 3.2. Slice 1. (T_1 axial.) Note lower medulla (m); cerebellar tonsils (t); internal carotid arteries *(small arrowheads)*; internal jugular veins *(large arrowheads)*.

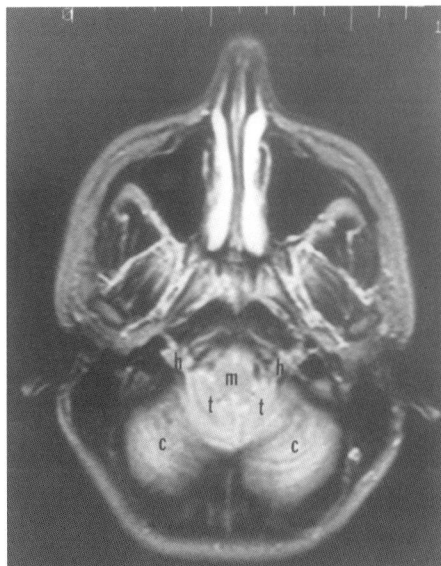

Fig. 3.3. Slice 2. (T_2 axial.) Note medulla (m); cerebellar tonsils (t); cerebellar hemispheres (c); hypo-glossal canals (h).

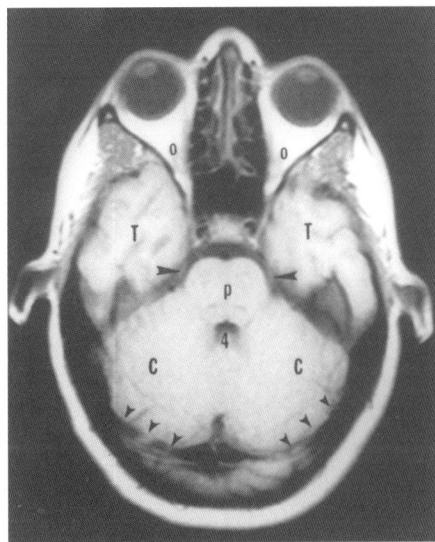

Fig. 3.4. Slice 5. (T_1 axial.) Note cerebellar hemispheres (C); temporal lobes (T); fourth ventricle (4); pons (p); transverse venous sinuses *(small arrowheads)*; pre-ganglionic Vth cranial nerves *(large arrowheads)*; optic nerves (o).

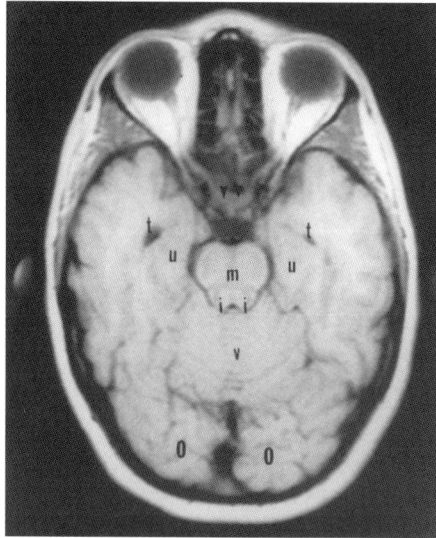

Fig. 3.5. Slice 6. (T$_1$ axial.) Note occipital lobes (O); cerebellar vermis (v); inferior colliculi (i); midbrain (m); uncus (u); temporal horns (t); sella turcica *(arrowheads)*.

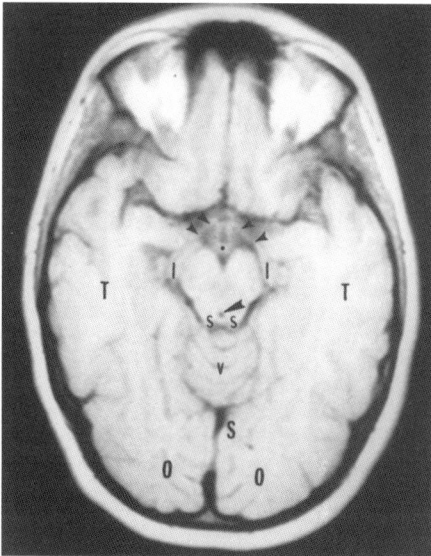

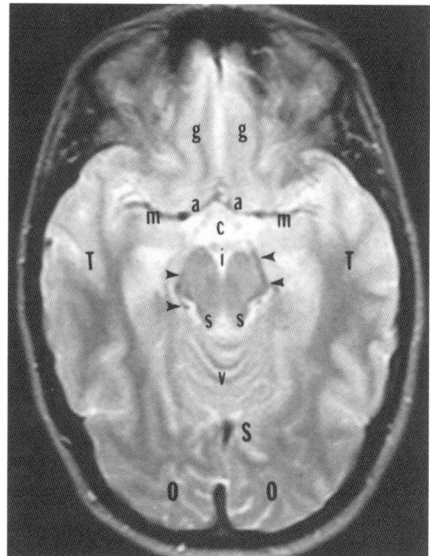

Fig. 3.6. Slice 7. *(Left)* T$_1$ axial. Note occipital (O) and temporal (T) lobes; straight sinus (S); vermis (v); superior colliculi (s); lateral geniculate bodies (l); cerebral aqueduct *(large arrowhead)*; optic tracts *(small arrowheads)*; mammillary bodies *(dot)*. *(Right)* T$_2$ axial. Note occipital (O) and temporal (T) lobes; straight sinus (S); vermis (v); superior colliculi (s); posterior cerebral arteries *(arrowheads)*; interpeduncular cistern (i); suprasellar cistern (c); anterior cerebral arteries (a); middle cerebral arteries (m); gyrus rectus (g).

44

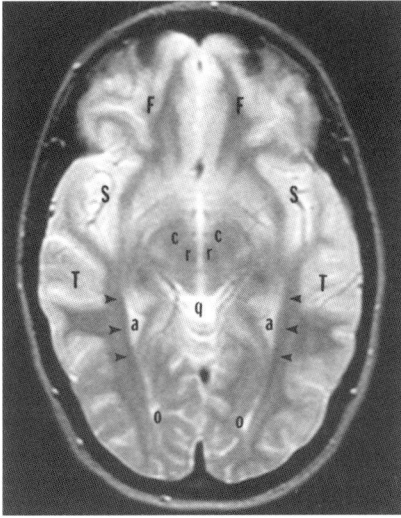

Fig. 3.7. Slice 8. (T$_2$ axial.) Note frontal (F) and temporal (T) lobes; sylvian fissures (S); occipital horns (o); lateral ventricular atria (a); cerebral peduncles (c); red nuclei (r); quadrigeminal plate cistern (q); position of optic radiations *(arrowheads)*.

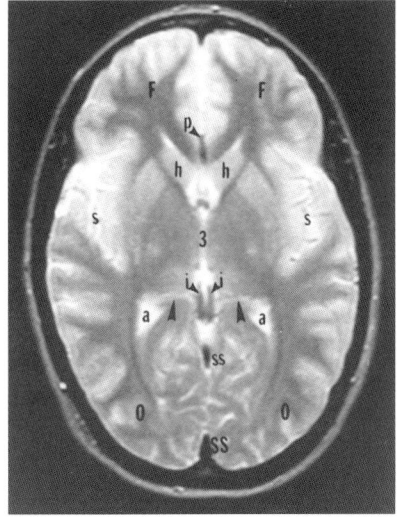

Fig. 3.8. Slice 9. (T$_2$ axial.) Note frontal (F) and occipital (O) lobes; superior sagittal sinus (SS); straight sinus (ss); third ventricle (3); lateral ventricular atria (a); sylvian fissures (s); internal cerebral veins (i); choroidal fissures *(large arrowheads)*; pericallosal arteries (p); caudate heads (h).

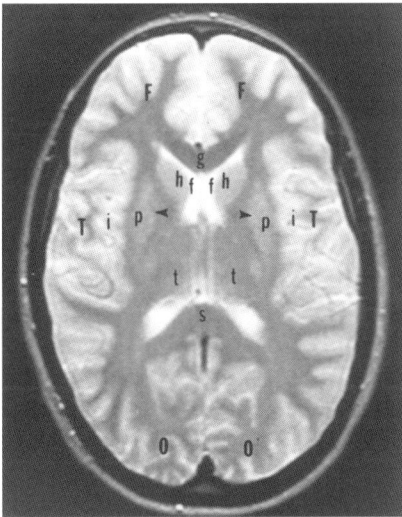

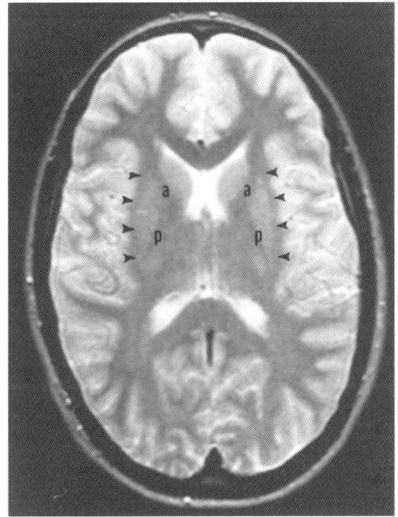

Fig. 3.9. Slice 10. *(Left)* T$_2$ axial. Note frontal (F), temporal (T) and occipital (O) lobes; thalami (t); genu (g) and splenium (s) of the corpus callosum; insular cortex (i); putamen (p); globus pallidus *(arrowheads)*. *(Right)* T$_2$ axial. Note anterior (a) and posterior (p) limbs of the internal capsule; lateral ganglionic structures including external capsule, claustrum and extreme capsule *(arrowheads)*.

45

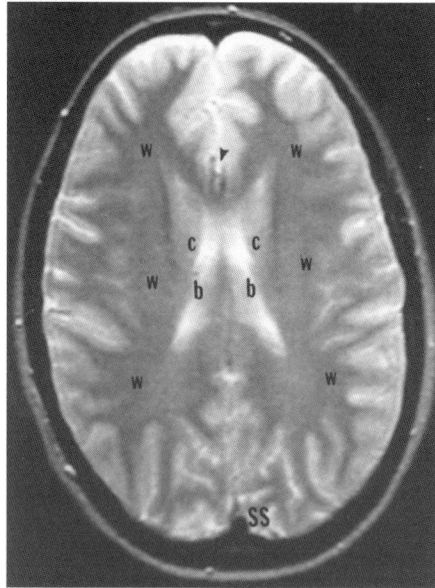

Fig. 3.10. Slice 11. (T$_2$ axial.) Note hemispheric white matter (w); bodies of the lateral ventricles (b); caudate nuclei (c); superior sagittal sinus (SS); pericallosal arteries *(small arrowhead)*.

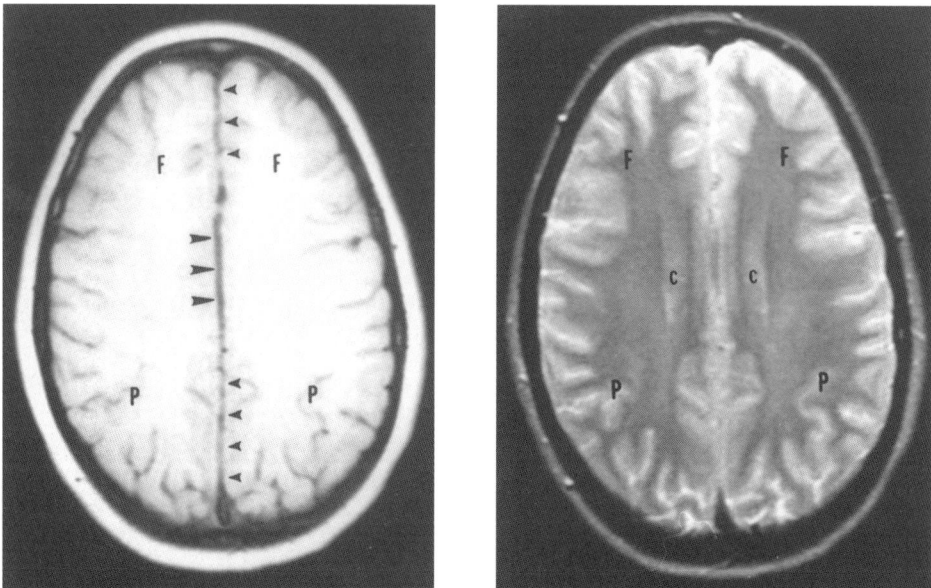

Fig. 3.11. Slice 12. (*Left*—T$_1$ axial; *right*—T$_2$ axial.) Note frontal (F) and parietal (P) lobes; bodies of the caudate nuclei (c); position of the falx *(small arrowheads)*; position of pericallosal arteries *(large arrowheads)*.

46

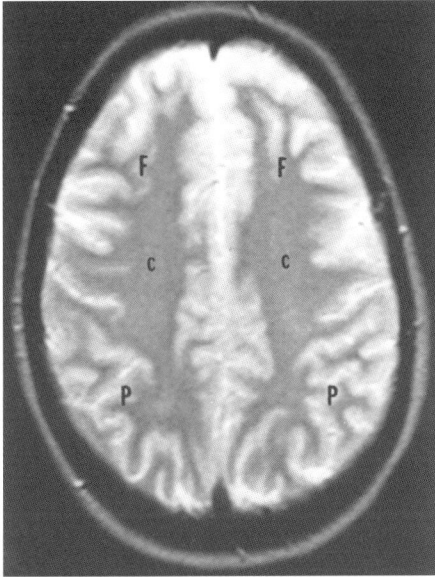

Fig. 3.12. Slice 13. (T$_2$ axial.) Note frontal (F) and parietal (P) lobes; white matter of corona radiata (c).

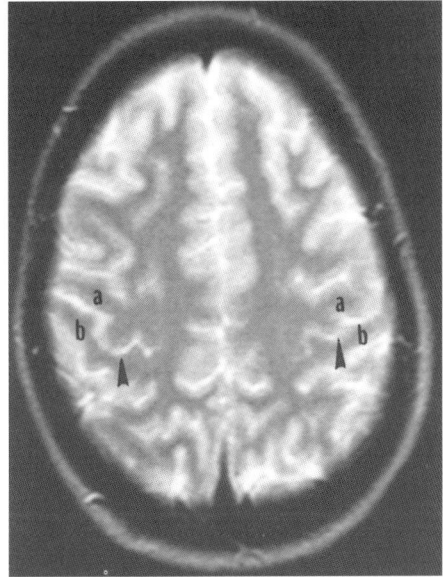

Fig. 3.13. Slice 14. (T$_2$ axial.) Note precentral (a) and postcentral (b) gyri; central sulcus *(arrowheads)*.

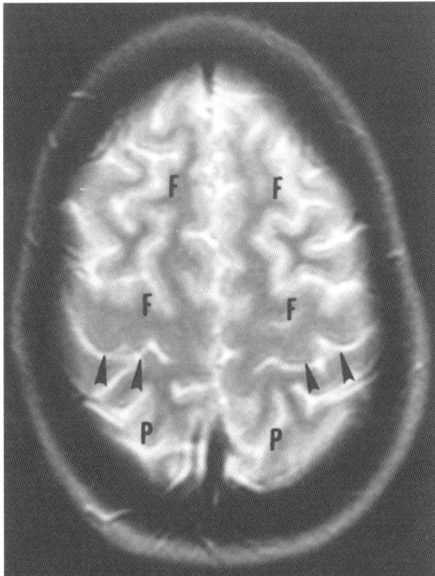

Fig. 3.14. Slice 15. (T$_2$ axial.) Note frontal (F) and parietal (P) lobes; central sulcus *(arrowheads)*.

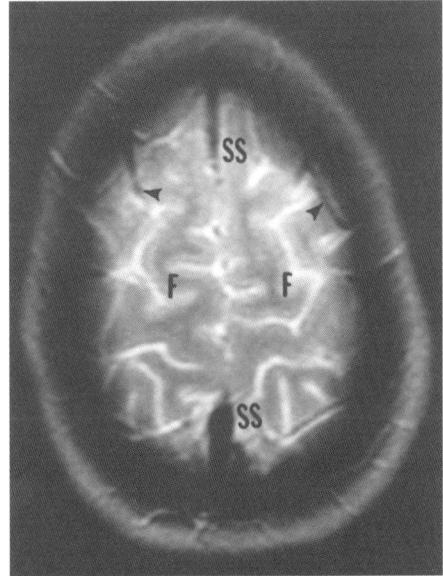

Fig. 3.15. Slice 16. (T$_2$ axial.) Note frontal lobes (F); superior sagittal sinus (SS); cortical veins *(arrowheads)*.

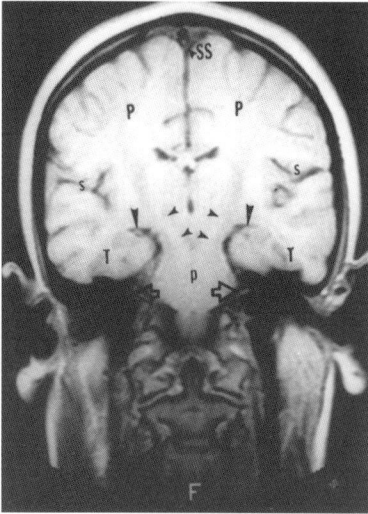

Fig. 3.16. T$_1$ coronal image at the level of the pons. Note temporal (T) and parietal (P) lobes; superior sagittal sinus (SS); pons (p); sylvian fissures (s); choroidal fissures *(large arrowheads)*; position of corticospinal tract *(small arrowheads)*; internal auditory canals *(open arrows)*.

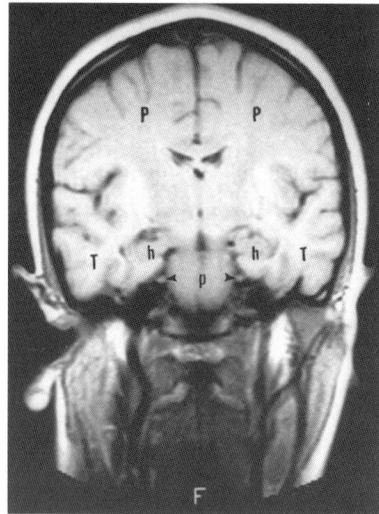

Fig. 3.17. T$_1$ coronal image at the level of the anterior pons. Note temporal (T) and parietal (P) lobes; hippocampus (h); pons (p); pre-ganglionic Vth nerves *(arrowheads)*.

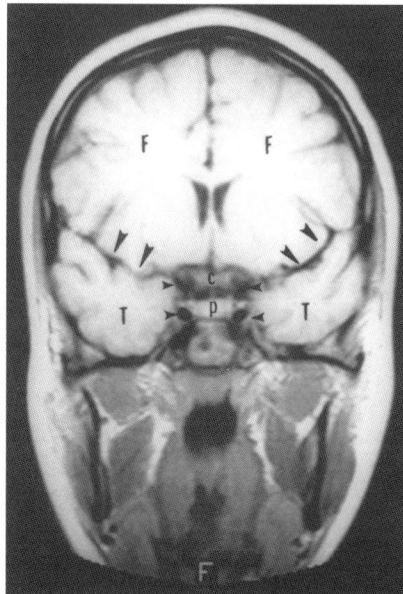

Fig. 3.18. T$_1$ coronal image at the level of the sella. Note frontal (F) and temporal (T) lobes; sylvian fissures *(large arrowheads)*; cavernous carotid arteries *(small arrowheads)*; optic chiasm (c); pituitary (p).

48

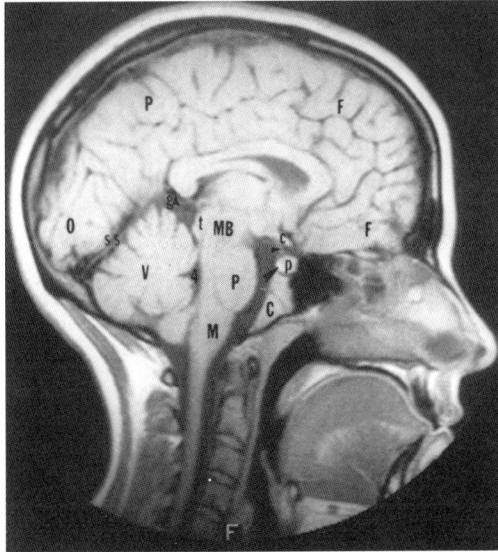

Fig. 3.19. Midline T$_1$ sagittal image. Note frontal (F), parietal (P) and occipital (O) lobes; midbrain (MB); tectum (t); pons (P); medulla (M); cerebellar vermis (V); fourth ventricle (4); vein of Galen (g); straight sinus (ss); optic chiasm (c); infundibular stalk *(small arrowhead)*; pituitary (p); posterior pituitary *(large arrowhead)*; clivus (C).

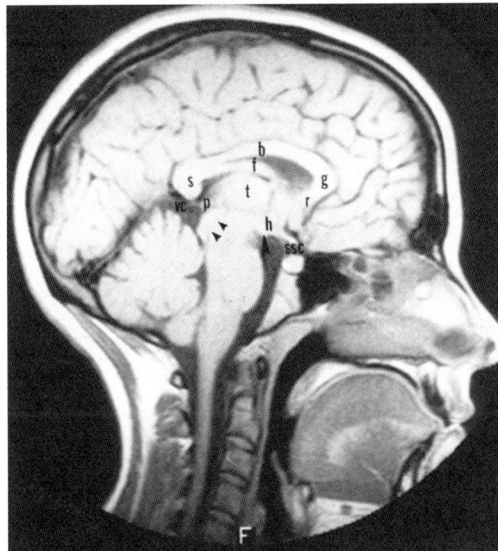

Fig. 3.20. Midline T$_1$ sagittal image. Note rostrum (r), genu (g), body (b) and splenium (s) of the corpus callosum; fornix (f); thalami (t—this actually denotes the position of the third ventricle with the paired thalami volume averaging across the midline); hypothalamus (h); suprasellar cistern (ssc); mammillary bodies *(large arrowhead)*; cerebral aqueduct *(small arrowheads)*; pineal (p); superior vermian cistern (vc).

49

4
CONGENITAL BRAIN ANOMALIES

Robin E. Osborn and Sharon E. Byrd

Congenital malformations of the brain comprise a complex spectrum of abnormalities that affect the formation and structure of brain development during intrauterine life. They can be classified into disorders of organogenesis and histogenesis (Table 4.1) (Yakovlev 1959, DeMyer 1971, Harwood-Nash and Fitz 1976). When a form of embryonic brain structure persists after birth, the abnormality is due to a fault in organogenesis. This results in structural abnormalities where parts of the brain are absent, partially developed or malformed. The majority of congenital brain malformations are of this type. Within this classification are subtypes of disorders affecting closure, diverticulation, migration, size and destructive lesions of the brain.

Histogenetic disorders result from abnormal cell differentiation, although the brain may appear grossly normal on gross examination. This group are the neurocutaneous syndromes or phakomatoses, which include neurofibromatosis, tuberous sclerosis, encephalotrigeminal angiomatosis, von Hippel–Lindau disease and ataxia–telangiectasia (Harwood-Nash and Fitz 1976).

With the advent of magnetic resonance imaging (MRI) it became possible non-invasively to obtain exquisite anatomical detail of even the most complex congenital brain malformations. Malformations due to abnormalities of organogenesis are well demonstrated by T_1-weighted images in the sagittal, axial or coronal planes. All three projections ensure complete evaluation of the brain. Intermediate and T_2-weighted images are sometimes helpful for better differentiation of gray matter abnormalities such as neuronal migrational anomalies, or to further delineate cerebrospinal fluid (CSF) spaces.

In the evaluation of disorders of histogenesis, it is important to obtain both T_1- and T_2-weighted images as well as gadolinium enhanced T_1-weighted images. T_1-weighted images demonstrate anatomic alterations and T_2-weighted images better evaluate changes involving the gray and white matter such as ischemia, neoplasia and myelination abnor-malities. The histogenetic disorders have a higher association of congenital neoplasms which are better defined on both the T_2-weighted and gadolinium enhanced T_1-weighted images. If small areas of calcification are suspected, gradient echo (GRE) acquisition images may be helpful. Computed tomography (CT) remains the best method of accurately delineating intracranial calcification.

In the evaluation of congenital brain malformations, a high resolution technique is extremely important. This involves small slice thicknesses, large matrices, large number of excitations and a small field of view (which should be tailored toward the head size). Our typical protocol is summarized in Table 4.2.

TABLE 4.1
Common congenital brain malformations

Disorders of organogenesis
    Supratentorial
        Migrational disorders
            Lissencephaly (agyria)
            Pachgyria
            Schizencephaly
            Heterotopia
            Polymicrogyria
            Hemimegalencephaly
        Holoprosencephalies
            Alobar
            Semilobar
            Lobar
        Septo-optic dysplasia
        Corpus callosal dysgenesis
    Infratentorial
        Dandy–Walker malformation
        Chiari malformations
    Other
        Cephaloceles
        Arachnoid cysts

Disorders of histogenesis
    Neurofibromatosis
    Tuberous sclerosis
    Encephalotrigeminal angiomatosis
    Von Hippel–Lindau disease
    Ataxia–telangiectasia

TABLE 4.2
MRI protocols for routine evaluation of the pediatric brain: pulse
sequences and imaging planes

Routine sequences: T_1 sagittal localizer, T_2 axial

Optional sequences: T_1 axial with gadolinium, other scan planes

	Age <2 yrs	*Age ≥ 2yrs*
Field of view	20–24 cm	24 cm
Slice thickness	3 or 5 mm	5 mm
Slice gap	0.5 or 1.0 mm	1 mm
Excitations (NEX)	2 or 4	2
Matrix	192 or 256 × 256	192 or 256 × 256

In this chapter emphasis will be placed on the primary diagnostic MRI findings of each malformation. Secondary findings which are commonly associated with the primary malformation but which are not necessary to make the diagnosis will also be discussed. In addition, the symptomatology and prognosis of the malformations will be briefly reviewed.

Neuronal migrational disorders
The neuronal migrational disorders are congenital malformations of the cerebral cortex caused by deranged migration of the subependymal neuroblast that results in abnormal gyri and sulci. These disorders are believed to arise during the sixth to 15th weeks of gestation when successive waves of neuroblasts migrate from the subependymal germinal matrix to the surface of the brain to form the standard six layered cortex. The disorder results in either a four layered cortex or a cortex with no recognizable layers. The classical forms of neuronal migrational disorder have been studied extensively in the literature and comprise the following entities: lissencephaly (agyria/pachygyria), pachy-gyria (isolated), schizencephaly, heterotopia, polymicrogyria and hemimegalencephaly. They have characteristic features which allow them to be characterized into subtypes (Zimmerman *et al.* 1983, Barth 1987, Naidich and Zimmerman 1987).

Agyria, pachygyria and polymicrogyria
In strict terminology, lissencephaly signifies a 'smooth brain' with a complete lack of gyri (agyria), whereas pachygyria signifies too few, too broad, flattened gyri. In actuality lissencephalic brains may be either completely smooth or show zones of both agyria and pachygyria (Osborn *et al.* 1988). Patients with lissencephaly commonly present with microcephaly, marked developmental delay, hypotonia which may progress to hyper-tonia, and seizures. Three clinical types of lissencephaly are recognized. Type I is characterized by microcephaly and dysmorphic facies usually associated with heritable syndromes such as Miller–Dieker, Norman–Roberts and Neu–Laxova. Type II usually lacks characteristics facies, but exhibits macrocephaly from hydrocephalus, retinal dysplasia, congenital muscular dystrophies and/or posterior fossa abnormalities such as Dandy–Walker cyst and posterior cephalocele. The Walker–Warburg and cerebro-oculo-muscular syndromes are associated with Type II lissencephaly. Type III lissencephaly encompasses isolated lissencephaly and cerebro-cerebellar lissencephaly. The isolated lissencephalies have the best prognosis and a longer survival (Stewart *et al.* 1975, Jellinger and Rett 1976, Dobyns *et al.* 1985, Dobyns 1987).

The characteristic MRI appearance of patients with lissencephaly consists of a cerebral contour which may be agyric (rare), nearly agyric or nearly equally agyric and pachygyric (Figs. 4.1–4.3). The pachygyric areas in patients with lissencephaly com-monly involve the anterior third of the cerebral hemispheres (Zimmerman *et al.* 1983; Byrd and Naidich 1988; Byrd *et al.* 1988, 1989b; Osborn *et al.* 1988).

Lissencephalic brains typically have a cerebral contour which is 'hourglass' or 'figure-of-eight' shaped due to lack of or incomplete opercularization. This lack of opercularization results in the presence of a groove, known as the sylvian groove, rather

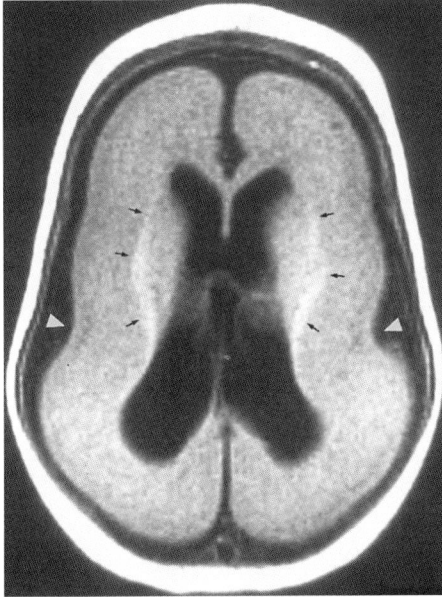

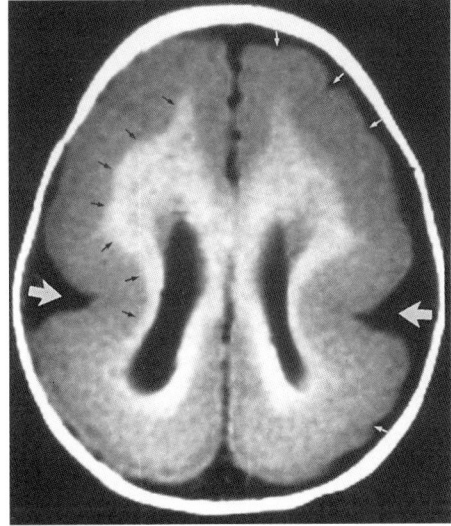

Fig. 4.1. Lissencephaly type 1. Total agyria. T_1-weighted axial image of the brain demonstrates a cortical surface which is completely smooth as no secondary sulci are present. The primary fissure or sylvian groove is identified *(arrowheads)*. The overall appearance of the brain is figure-of-eight-like. The cortex is thick, the white matter is abnormally thin and the gray–white matter interface is smooth *(small arrows)*. The ventricles are prominent in size.

Fig. 4.2. Lissencephaly type II. Near-total agyria. On this T_1-weighted axial image, the brain again has a figure-of-eight-like appearance due to the presence of a sylvian groove *(large arrows)*. The cortex is thick, the white matter is thin and their interface is smooth *(small black arrows)*. A few scattered secondary sulci are identified on the cortical surface *(small white arrows)*. There is no opercularization with lissencephaly and therefore no insula.

than the normal and more complex sylvian fissure. The middle cerebral vasculature courses superficially within this groove. When opercularization is incomplete the insulae are exposed.

The gray–white matter distribution is abnormal, with a thickened cortex and thinning of the white matter. There is either an absence (agyria) or a decreased number (agyria–pachygyria) of cortical sulci and corresponding digitations of white matter into the cortex (Zimmerman *et al.* 1983, Byrd and Naidich 1988, Byrd *et al.* 1988, Osborn *et al.* 1988).

The secondary findings in the brains of patients with lissencephaly include absent or dysgenetic corpus callosum and mild to moderate dilatation of the lateral ventricles. Colpocephaly, which is pronounced enlargement of the atria and occipital horns, occurs due to the decreased volume of white matter. Although the white matter throughout the brain is affected, the effect on the splenium of the corpus callosum produces the more noticeable result of colpocephaly. Hydrocephalus is rare and when seen usually occurs in

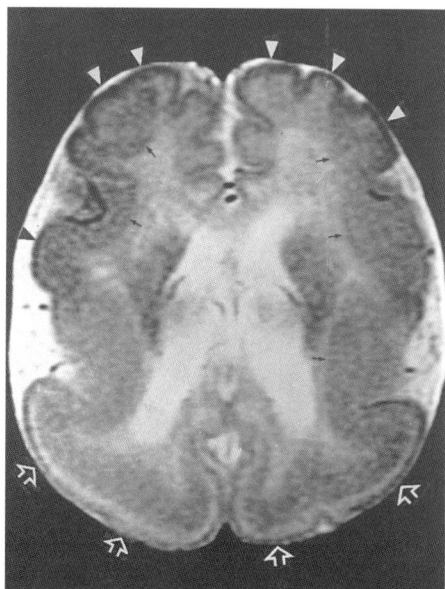

Fig. 4.3. Lissencephaly type III. Mixed agyria–pachygyria. T$_2$-weighted image demonstrates prominent areas of agyria in the parieto-occipital region *(open arrows)* and pachygria in the fronto-parietal region *(arrowheads)*. The gray–white matter interface is again noted to be smoother than normal *(small arrows)*.

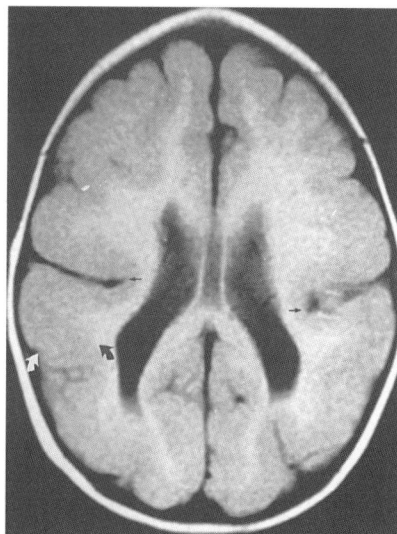

Fig. 4.4. Pachygyria. T$_1$-weighted axial image demonstrates diffusely enlarged gyri, too few in number. There are no large areas of agyria as seen in lissencephaly. The gray matter is thick *(curved arrows)*, the white matter thin, and the gray–white matter interface smoother than normal due to diminished digitations. Note also the deep sylvian grooves bilaterally *(small arrows)* without any opercularization. (Image courtesy of Donald Lash, DO, Oak Hill Hospital, Joplin, MO.)

patients with the Walker–Warburg syndrome. Heterotopias may be present as well (Zimmerman *et al.* 1983, Byrd and Naidich 1988, Byrd *et al.* 1988, Osborn *et al.* 1988).

Pachygyria may be found with no associated areas of agyria. We classify this migrational disorder as an entity separate from lissencephaly with or without areas of pachygyria. Dobyns (1987) terms isolated pachygyria as lissencephaly type 4.

Patients with isolated pachygyria present with microcephaly, seizures, delayed development, mental retardation and focal neurological deficits. These symptoms are usually milder but similar to those found in lissencephaly. They may or may not have associated dysmorphic facies. The dysmorphic facies in the majority of children with isolated pachygyria is not characteristic of any specific appearance or clinical syndrome. A very small percentage of children with isolated pachygyria have facies which resemble those associated with the Miller–Dieker syndrome. The diagnosis given to these patients is the Miller–Dieker variant syndrome. Patients with isolated pachygyria live longer than those with lissencephaly (Hanaway *et al.* 1968; Byrd *et al.* 1989*b*, 1994). Pachygyria does not preclude a productive adult life (Fig. 4.4).

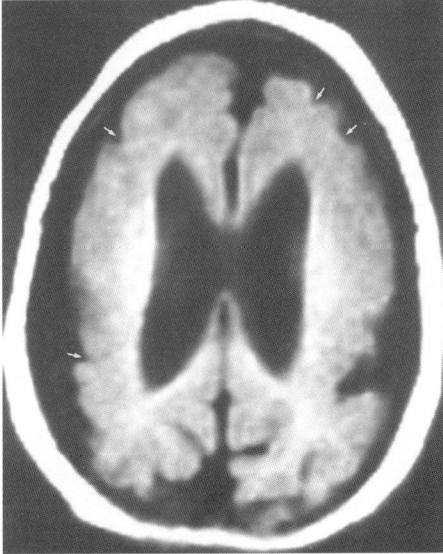

Fig. 4.5. Cytomegalovirus-induced pachygyria. T_1-weighted axial image demonstrates multiple scattered shallow sulci representing heterogeneous migrational anomaly due to congenital brain infection. Compare this appearance to the idiopathic form of pachygyria seen in Fig. 4.4.

The MRI appearance of the brains of children with isolated pachygyria consists of a cerebral surface with either focal or diffuse areas of pachygyria without areas of agyria. The pachygyric areas are commonly located in the anterior third of the cerebrum although in some children the brain may be totally pachygyric. Pachygyria consists of broad based, flat, thick and coarse gyri with shallow intervening sulci. The cerebral contour is (nearly) normal and there is normal or only mildly diminished opercularization of the brain. In the pachygyric areas the gray matter is thickened. The white matter is thinner than normal, and the white matter digitations are thickened and fewer in number corresponding to the gross appearance of the pachygyric cortex.

Pachygyria also occurs in some patients who have congenital infections of the brain, most commonly with cytomegalovirus (CMV) or *Toxoplasma gondii* (Fig. 4.5). It probably results from infection which causes ischemia and derangement of neuroblast migration. The involvement may be isolated, diffuse or unilateral. Patients who have migrational anomalies due to congenital infection often have associated microcephaly, intracranial calcification, cerebral atrophy and abnormal myelination. MRI demonstrates all of the described findings well with the exception of the calcification. These patients commonly have severe developmental delays and other neurologic sequelae. The pachygyria seen with MRI in these patients tends to be heterogeneous and irregular in appearance when compared to the classic idiopathic forms not associated with congenital brain infection.

Polymicrogyria signifies a cerebral cortex which is composed of numerous microscopic gyri. This is an abnormality of the neocortex in which there are numerous small meandering gyri with intervening sulci which may or may not be bridged by fusion of the overlying molecular layer of the neocortex. Since these gyri are microscopic the diagnosis is usually made on histologic analysis of cerebral tissue. It is not possible to make a radiologic diagnosis of polymicrogyria. On gross inspection of the brains of these patients, the involved areas resemble pachygyria or agyria and the cortical surface may be covered with small bumps. There is a high association with CMV or *T. gondii* infection (Hanaway *et al.* 1968; Byrd and Naidich 1988; Byrd *et al.* 1989*b*, 1994).

It is well recognized that polymicrogyria is associated with schizencephaly, pachygyria and agyria. Emphasis should be placed on diagnosing the radiographically apparent anomaly. The MRI appearance of the brain in children with polymicrogyria consists of localized or diffuse areas of pachygyria and agyria or schizencephaly. Large areas of the brain may be involved and it may be unilateral (Hanaway *et al.* 1968; Byrd and Naidich 1988; Byrd *et al.* 1989*b*, 1994).

Hemimegalencephaly
Hemimegalencephaly is a malformation resulting in hemihypertrophy of the brain. It may be idiopathic or result from a variety of causes including storage diseases, neurocutaneous syndromes (especially neurofibromatosis type I and tuberous sclerosis) and congenital infection such as with CMV or *T. gondii* (Osborn *et al.* 1988). These patients typically present with developmental delay and intractable seizures which may respond only to partial or complete hemispherectomy. MRI demonstrates a thickened, pachygyric or agyric cortex, a smoothed gray–white matter interface and ipsilateral ventricular enlargement (Fig. 4.6). The surface of the cortex will commonly be polymicrogyric, which is a pathologic finding and not a radiologic one. Heterotopias may also be identified (Osborn *et al.* 1988).

Heterotopia
Heterotopias are collections of gray matter in abnormal locations within the brain. They are due to arrested migration of the neuroblast anywhere from the periventricular region to the neocortex. Patients with heterotopias may be asymptomatic. Heterotopias may be an isolated entity or part of a more complex migrational disorder such as lissencephaly, schizencephaly or hemimegalencephaly. They also occur in association with other malformations such as dysgenesis of the corpus callosum and Chiari II malformation. Seizures are the most common clinical presentation of isolated heterotopias. The MRI findings consist of single or multiple masses of gray matter of variable size and shape in the subependymal layer of the lateral ventricles or subcortical white matter (Fig. 4.7). These masses maintain the same signal intensity as cortical gray matter on all pulse sequences (Zimmerman *et al.* 1983, Barth 1987, Byrd and Naidich 1988, Osborn *et al.* 1988, Byrd *et al.* 1989*a*).

Schizencephaly
Schizencephaly is a form of disordered migration that is characterized by a transcerebral cleft lined by gray matter. There is direct communication between the pia mater and ependyma (pial–ependymal seam), which is made possible by the cleft traversing the full thickness of the cerebral hemisphere (Yakovlev and Wadsworth 1946*a,b*, Page *et al.* 1975, Lazjuk *et al.* 1979, Zimmerman *et al.* 1983, Miller *et al.* 1984, Barth 1987, Bird and Gilles

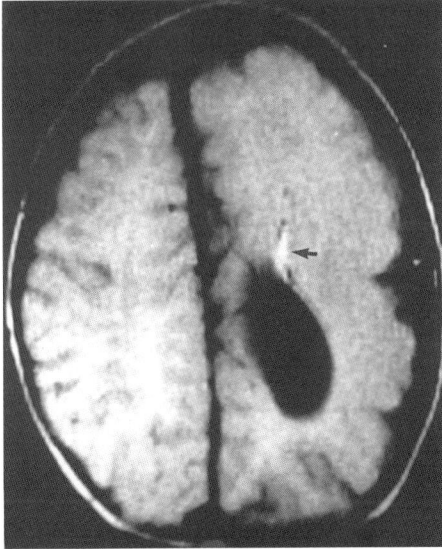

Fig. 4.6. Hemimegalencephaly. T_1-weighted axial image demonstrates enlarged left cerebral hemisphere, enlarged left lateral ventricle, and pachygyric left cerebral cortex. Note the normal gyration and sulcation of the right hemisphere. The high signal focus adjacent to the lateral ventricle was a prominent draining vein *(arrow)*.

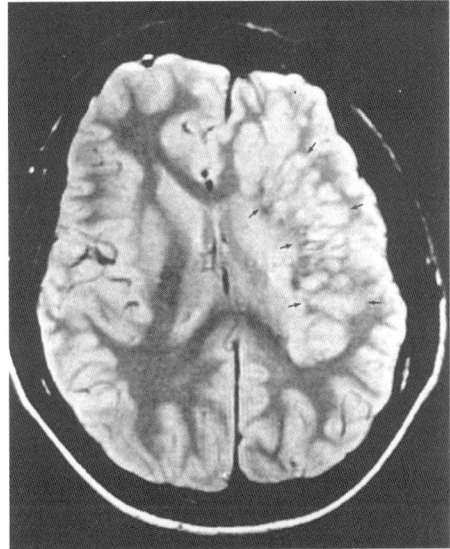

Fig. 4.7. Heterotopia. Intermediate-weighted axial MR image demonstrates multiple, left-sided, nodular collections extending from the periventricular to the subcortical regions *(arrows)*. They correspond precisely to the signal intensity of gray matter and did so on all imaging sequences. (Image courtesy of LCDR Richardo Syklawer, Naval Hospital, San Diego, CA.)

1987, Byrd and Naidich 1988).

Schizencephaly can be divided into two types depending on whether the margins of the cleft are fused or separated by a CSF cavity. Type I or fused-lip schizencephaly is characterized by a gray matter lined pial–ependymal seam without an intervening CSF cavity; the most superficial layer of cortex on either side of the cleft is fused. These patients usually present with a history of seizures, delayed development, and normal or microcephalic calvarium.

MRI demonstrates the gray matter lined cleft which commonly involves the sylvian regions of the brain (Fig. 4.8). It is usually bilateral and fairly symmetric but may be unilateral. The thickness of the gray matter lining is variable. This lining may be incomplete but there is always some gray matter within the cleft. An irregularity or dimple may be found along the ventricular surface signifying the presence of a cleft (Yakovlev and Wadsworth 1946a, Zimmerman *et al.* 1983, Barth 1987, Byrd and Naidich 1988).

In Type II or open-lip schizencephaly the gray matter lined walls of the cleft are separated by CSF. These patients commonly present with a seizure disorder, failure to thrive, developmental delay and mental retardation. Their clinical status is commonly much worse than that seen with the fused-lip form since there may be a drastic decrease

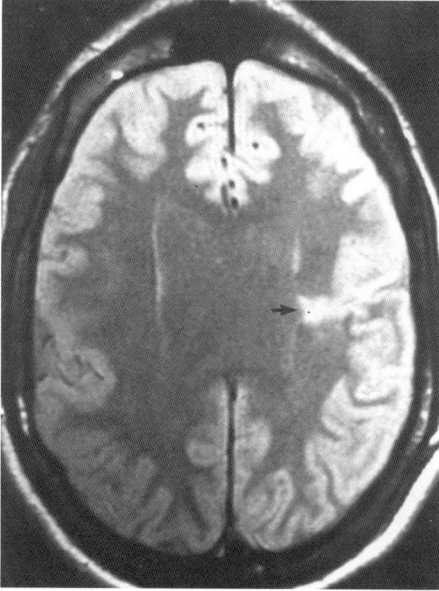

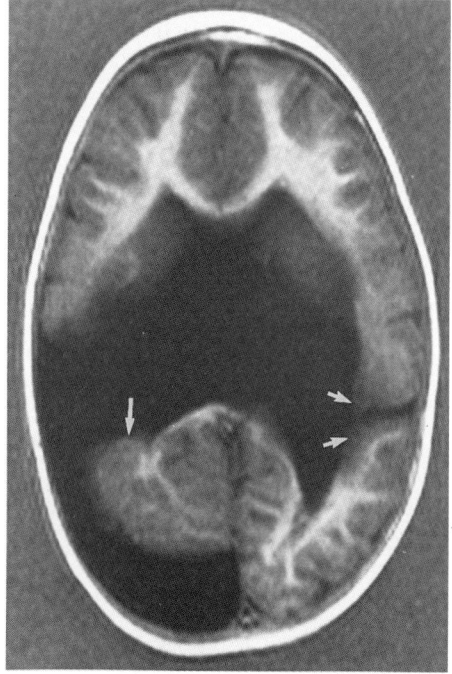

Fig. 4.8. Fused-lip or type I schizencephaly. Intermediate-weighted axial image demonstrates unilateral schizencephaly on the left. The cerebral cleft extends to the ependymal surface *(arrow)* and is lined by gray matter.

Fig. 4.9. Open-lip or type II schizencephaly. T$_1$-weighted axial image demonstrates bilateral open-lip cerebral clefts which are lined by gray matter *(arrows)*. The left-sided cleft is separated by only a small collection of cerebrospinal fluid.

in the remaining brain volume. Some of these patients will also have hydrocephalus (Yakovlev and Wadsworth 1946a).

MRI demonstrates the cleft which extends from the ventricular system to the pial surface of the brain, opened by a CSF cavity (Fig. 4.9). The CSF cavity may vary in size from small to large; it is usually bilateral and symmetric, although it may be asymmetric or even unilateral. Severe forms of open-lip schizencephaly present with massive CSF cavities. In this form of schizencephaly, there may be a relatively sparse amount of brain parenchyma involving the high convexity midline and base of the brain.

We found in our series (Osborn *et al.* 1988) that in both forms of schizencephaly the septum pellucidum is absent in about one half of cases. There is a high association with other congenital abnormalities such as heterotopia, polymicrogyria, and arachnoid cyst (Zimmerman *et al.* 1983, Barth 1987, Byrd and Naidich 1988). We have determined that there is no association between schizencephaly and septo-optic dysplasia (see below).

Holoprosencephaly

Holoprosencephaly is a congenital malformation characterized by incomplete separation

TABLE 4.3
Holoprosencephaly: classification of findings

Finding	Alobar	Semilobar	Lobar
Cyclopia	+	+	–
Ethmocephaly	+	+	–
Cebocephaly	+	+	–
Midline cleft lip and palate	+++	++	+
Trigonocephaly	+	+	+
Hypotelorism	+++	++	+
Microcephaly	++ May be normal, or macrocephalic if dorsal cyst is present	++ May be normal, or macrocephalic if dorsal cyst is present	Normal or microcephalic
Cerebral lobes	–	Occipital and/or temporal	All formed
Lateral ventricles	Monoventricle, rudimentary temporal horns	Some differentiation of atria	(Nearly) normal
Diencephalon	Fused	Partially fused	Not fused
3rd ventricle	–	+	+++
Dorsal cyst	++	+	–
Interhemispheric fissure	–	+	+++
Falx	–	+ Posterior part may be present	+++ May be hypoplastic
Corpus callosum	–	++	+++

Key: – not identified; + occasionally identified; ++ usually identified; +++ always identified.

of the primitive forebrain into the cerebral hemispheres (DeMyer *et al.*1964, Fitz 1983, Byrd and Naidich 1988). The result includes an abnormal continuation of gray and white matter across the midline. It is believed to be due to a primary disorder of the cephalic end of the notochord which leads to incomplete or defective diverticulation of the prosen-cephalon with failure to form the telencephalic vesicles during the fourth to eighth weeks of gestation.

The more severe forms of holoprosencephaly are always associated with hypo-telorism. They are also associated with dysmorphic facies, ranging from the more severe cyclopia, ethmocephaly and cebocephaly to the less severe and characteristic square-shaped cleft of the upper lip. This cleft of the midline structures is caused by absence of the intermaxillary segment which results in the absence of the middle of the upper lip, philtrum and superior alveolar ridge, central incisors, primary palate and a cleft involving the secondary palate.

These patients present clinically with micro-, normo- or macrocephaly depending upon the presence of a dorsal cyst or hydrocephalus. Clinical presentation and symptoms

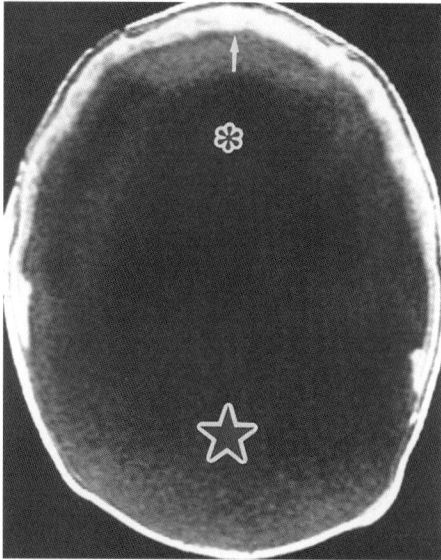

Fig. 4.10. Alobar holoprosencephaly with a dorsal cyst. T₁-weighted axial image demonstrates a marked case of this disorder. Only a minimal amount of cerebral mantle, which crosses the midline (arrow), is identified. Precise delineation between the dorsal cyst (star) and monoventricle (asterisk) cannot be made.

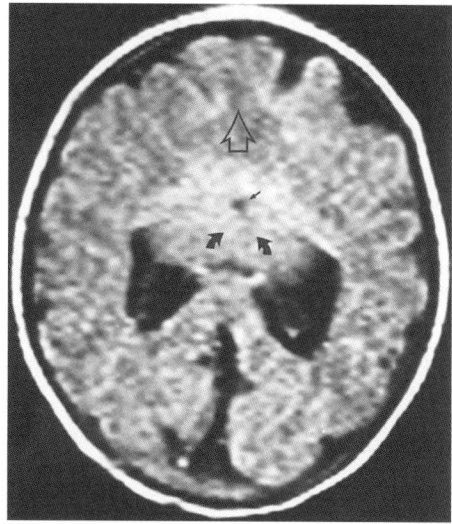

Fig. 4.11. Semilobar holoprosencephaly. T₁-weighted axial image demonstrates gray matter crossing the midline anteriorly (large open arrow). There is no falx. The thalami are fused (curved arrows) but a rudimentary third ventricle is delineated (small arrow). The bodies and atria of the lateral ventricles are partially formed but there are no frontal or occipital horns. (Image courtesy of Thomas C. Hay, DO, Denver Children's Hospital.)

include failure to thrive, developmental delay, poor temperature control, seizures, visual anomalies, and spastic quadriplegia and trigonocephaly. Patients with trisomies of chromosomes 13 and 18 may exhibit holoprosencephaly (DeMyer and Zeman 1963, DeMyer et al. 1964, Cohen et al. 1971, Fitz 1983, Byrd and Naidich 1988).

Holoprosencephaly is subdivided into three types (Table 4.3). The most severe form is alobar holoprosencephaly, in which there is complete failure to form separate cerebral hemispheres. The semilobar type is a less severe form in which the posterior portions of the hemispheres develop partially, while in the least severe form, lobar holoprosencephaly, the hemispheres are nearly normal but remain connected anteriorly and inferiorly at the level of the frontal lobes (DeMyer and Zeman 1963, DeMyer et al. 1964, Cohen et al. 1971, Fitz 1983, Byrd and Naidich 1988).

The MRI appearance of patients with alobar holoprosencephaly demonstrates a single, unlobed prosencephalon which contains an oval or U-shaped monoventricle (Fig. 4.10). Rudimentary temporal horns are nearly always identified even in the most severe cases. There is no corpus callosum, interhemispheric fissure, falx or crista galli. The diencephalon is fused so that the thalami remain as a single central mass of gray matter with no third ventricular formation. The fused diencephalon indents the monoventricle

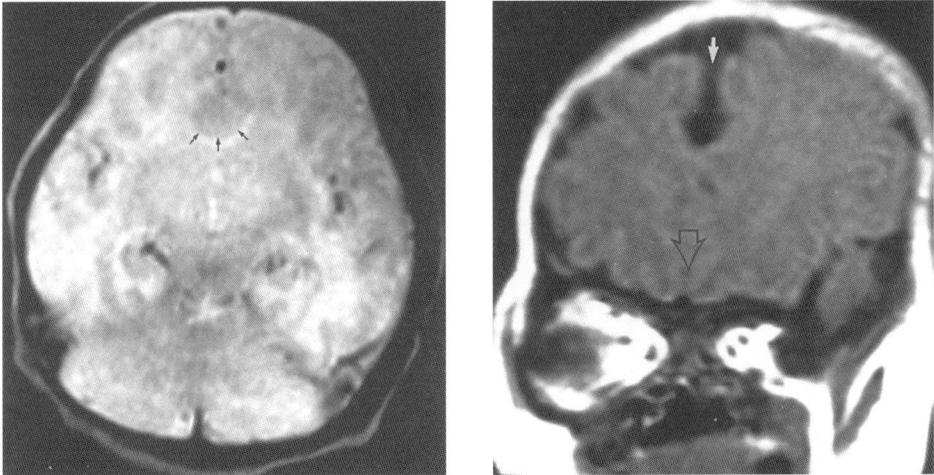

Fig. 4.12. Lobar holoprosencephaly. *(Left)* T$_2$-weighted axial image demonstrates gray matter crossing the midline *(small arrows)*. The brain is otherwise well formed. *(Right)* T$_1$-weighted (slightly oblique) coronal MR image demonstrates no evidence of an anterior interhemispheric fissure along the anterior, inferior surface of the brain *(open arrow)*. Gray matter continues uninterrupted between the cerebral hemispheres. Note the anomalously wide-appearing interhemispheric fissure superiorly *(white arrow)*. No falx was present.

giving it the U or horseshoe shape. There may be an associated dorsal cyst or sac: this is typically seen with the alobar and semilobar types. The origin of the dorsal sac is not completely understood. Theories suggest that it may be a rudimentary third ventricle or a distorted velum interpositum. When there is an associated dorsal cyst, patients may present with macrocephaly and hydrocephalus. The majority of patients with holoprosencephaly are normo- or microcephalic except for those who present with hydrocephalus secondary to an enlarged dorsal cyst. A single azygous (unpaired) anterior cerebral artery may be seen coursing in the midline frontally. The internal cerebral veins, straight sinus and superior sagittal sinus are absent (DeMyer *et al.* 1964, Fitz 1983, Byrd and Naidich 1988).

The MRI findings in patients with semilobar holoprosencephaly demonstrate an attempt at partial separation of the prosencephalon into lobes of the brain (Fig. 4.11). Early differentiation of atria and occipital horns is seen. Occipital and/or temporal lobes may also be seen, and there may be a rudimentary corpus callosum. There is partial cleavage of the diencephalon into thalami with partial formation of the third ventricle. The posterior aspect of the interhemispheric fissure, a rudimentary falx posteriorly and associated dural venous sinuses may also be delineated (DeMyer *et al.* 1964, Fitz 1983, Byrd and Naidich 1988).

Patients with the lobar form of holoprosencephaly have MRI findings that may be very subtle or go unrecognized. MRI demonstrates more normal cerebral hemispheres and thalami. However, a band of gray and white matter crosses the midline along the surface of the corpus callosum anteriorly and inferiorly. The ventricles, interhemispheric

61

fissure, arteries and veins are (nearly) normal. The falx may be incomplete. The frontal horns of the lateral ventricles have a 'squared off' appearance instead of the normal semilunar configuration, and the septum pellucidum is absent (Fig. 4.12) (DeMyer *et al.* 1964, Fitz 1983, Byrd and Naidich 1988).

Septo-optic dysplasia

Septo-optic dysplasia (SOD) signifies a syndrome which consists of optic nerve hypoplasia, hypothalamic–pituitary axis anomalies and, in 50 per cent of cases, absence of the septum pellucidum. The diagnosis of SOD is a clinical one and is based on the findings of optic nerve hypoplasia and hypothalamic–pituitary axis anomalies. The hypothalamic manifestations may lag behind the suspected clinical diagnosis by as much as 3.5 years (Arslanian *et al.* 1984). Abnormalities of growth hormone are most common, followed by adrenocorticotropic hormone, thyrotropic stimulating hormone and antidiuretic hormone. Since absence of the septum pellucidum occurs in only 50 per cent of SOD patients it should be regarded as a radiographic finding in support of the final clinical diagnosis. The diagnosis of SOD should never be made on the basis of septal absence alone.

The corpus callosum, fornix and infundibulum may also be abnormal. SOD is felt to result from an insult which occurs during the fifth to seventh weeks of fetal gestation. At this time, there is a failure in differentiation of the optic vesicle, retinal ganglionic cells and anterior wall of the diencephalon. These patients usually present early on with visual abnormalities or blindness (Hale and Rice 1970, Zaias and Becker 1978, Arslanian *et al.* 1984, Morishima and Aranoff 1986, Byrd and Naidich 1988, Osborn and Byrd 1988).

The MRI findings in these patients consist of absence of the septum pellucidum, flattening of the roofs of the frontal horns, beaking of the floors of the lateral ventricles, dilatation of the suprasellar cistern and anterior third ventricle, and small optic nerves and chiasm. The infundibulum may be absent or small, and the posterior pituitary may be absent or in an aberrant location (Fig 4.13). The corpus callosum may be dysplastic or partially absent.

Other congenital anomalies such as schizencephaly and absence of the corpus callosum may also present with absent septum pellucidum. We reported previously the findings of optic nerve hypoplasia in patients with schizencephaly (Osborn and Byrd 1988). These patients were initially incorrectly diagnosed clinically as having SOD, whereas in fact the schizencephaly resulted in a disruption of the optic pathways causing hypoplasia of the optic nerves (Fig. 4.14). Other authors have demonstrated identical findings in patients with other congenital cerebral destructive events which interrupted the optic pathways (Hoyt *et al.* 1972, Davidson *et al.* 1989). Still other authors, in a recent MRI study (Barkovich *et al.* 1989), though continuing to diagnose these schizencephaly patients with SOD, have recognized the striking dissimilarities between their patients and MRI findings. Their data indicated that none of their schizencephaly patients had hypothalamic dysfunction, and only one in five had total absence of the septum pellucidum (though it was recognized that this finding is not necessary for a clinical diagnosis of SOD).

The two static clinical criteria for diagnosis of SOD are optic nerve hypoplasia and

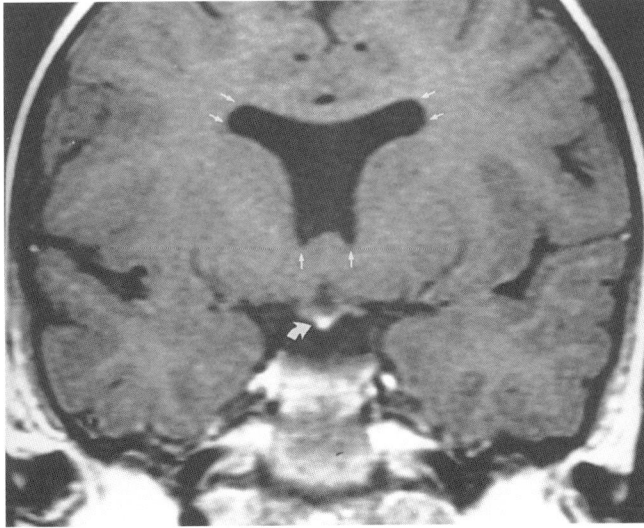

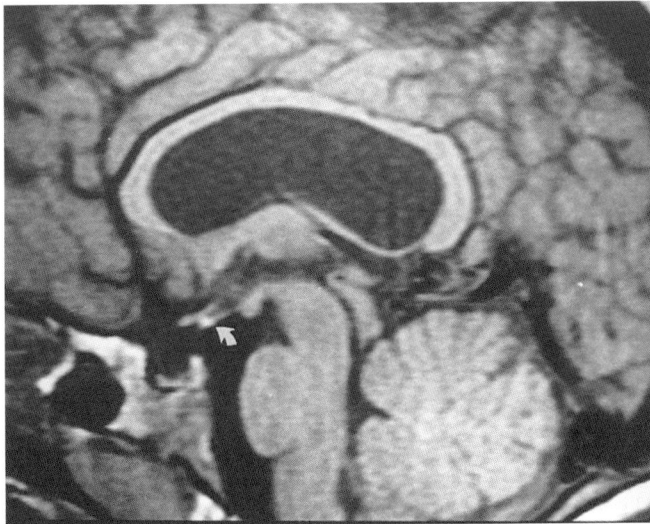

Fig. 4.13. Septo-optic dysplasia. *(Top)* Coronal and *(bottom)* sagittal T$_1$-weighted images demonstrate beaking of the floors and flattening of the upper, outer walls of the lateral ventricular frontal horns *(small arrows)*, absent septum pellucidum, absent pituitary stalk, and aberrant location of the posterior pituitary *(curved arrows)*.

hypothalamic dysfunction. We have found only one patient reported in the literature who had both schizencephaly and hypothalamic dysfunction (Zaias and Becker 1978). We conclude that SOD and schizencephaly are two distinct entities and are not closely related.

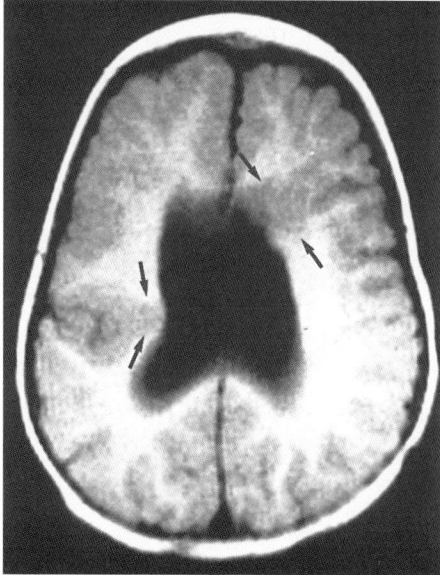

Fig. 4.14. Type I schizencephaly with optic nerve hypoplasia. T_1-weighted axial image demonstrates bilateral fused-lip schizencephaly *(arrows)* and absence of the septum pellucidum.

Corpus callosal agenesis

Dysgenesis of the corpus callosum is a general term used to designate a spectrum of abnormalities affecting the corpus callosum. The corpus callosum may be completely or partially absent due to either congenital causes or acquired intrauterine infarction (Byrd *et al.* 1990) (Table 4.4). It may be thin and hypoplastic or dysgenetic where it is partially absent, and the parts that remain appear dysplastic.

The corpus callosum begins to develop by the l0th to 12th weeks of gestation, and by 18 to 20 weeks of gestation it has attained its adult configuration. It develops in an anterior to posterior direction, with the genu forming first followed by the body and splenium. The smaller rostrum forms last (Rakic and Yakovlev 1968). Agenesis of the corpus callosum results from failure of formation of the commissural plate which allows axons to grow across the midline forming not only the corpus callosum but also the hippocampus and anterior commissure. Depending on the time of insult there may be absence of all or only portions of the corpus callosum. In cases of complete absence, there may be no hippocampal commissure. The remainder of the hippocampus is typically unaffected. The anterior commissure is nearly always present but may be thickened or hypoplastic (Kendall 1983, Atlas *et al.* 1986, Barkovich and Norman 1988). The posterior commissure may or may not be present (Kendall 1983, Byrd and Naidich 1988, Byrd *et al.* 1990). Since in true agenesis of the corpus callosum the axons from the hemispheres did not cross the midline, they instead course longitudinally and form paired callosal bundles, termed Probst bundles, which run along the medial borders of the lateral ventricles. Probst bundles are pathognomonic for true agenesis of the corpus callosum (Davidoff and Dyke 1934, Bull 1967, Wolpert *et al.* 1972, Probst 1973, Larsen and Osborn 1982, Kendall 1983, Jeret *et al.* 1985–86, Lacey 1985).

TABLE 4.4
Dysgenesis of the corpus callosum: classification of findings

Type	Primary findings	Secondary findings
Total absence	Corpus callosum not identified	Absence of part or all of the posterior and anterior commissures of the hippocampus
	Elevated 3rd ventricle	Colpocephaly
	Widely separated, parallel lateral ventricles	Interhemispheric cyst
	Probst bundles	Dandy–Walker maformation Migration disorders Cephaloceles Hydrocephalus Chiari II malformation Callosal hypoplasia Pericallosal and choroid plexus lipoma
Partial absence	Absence of variable amount of posterior corpus callosum	Other brain malformations as described above
Acquired	Absence of any part of the corpus callosum	Not associated with other brain malformations

Absence of the corpus callosum is best demonstrated with sagittal MRI. The medial hemispheric gyri and sulci have a radial or 'spoke-wheel' pattern in that they are orientated perpendicular to the narrow inferior margin of the hemisphere. The parieto-occipital and calcarine sulci fail to meet each other on the medial wall of the hemispheres. On coronal and axial images the third ventricle may be identified extending upward and becoming interposed between the bodies of the lateral ventricles. Colpocephaly may be present. The lateral ventricles are widely separated and parallel to one another. The medial borders of the frontal horns may appear concave if they are indented by Probst bundles (Bull 1967, Probst 1973, Larsen and Osborn 1982, Atlas *et al.* 1986, Byrd *et al.* 1990). The hippocampal formation and anterior commissure may be absent (Fig. 4.15).

Absence of the corpus callosum may present as an isolated abnormality but there is also a high association with other congenital malformations. Only about 10 per cent of patients with dysgenesis of the corpus callosum are asymptomatic, and most also have other associated congenital brain anomalies. Symptoms most commonly include seizures and developmental delay. Absent or dysgenetic corpus callosum is an integral component of some congenital malformations such as Aicardi syndrome, and is associated with numerous other congenital anomalies including Dandy–Walker malformation (25 per cent), Chiari II malformation (5 per cent), SOD, pericallosal lipoma (50 per cent), neuronal migrational disorders, holoprosencephaly, absence of the inferior vermis, basal cephaloceles and Apert syndrome (Bull 1967, Probst 1973, Larsen and Osborn 1982, Atlas *et al.* 1986, Byrd *et al.* 1990).

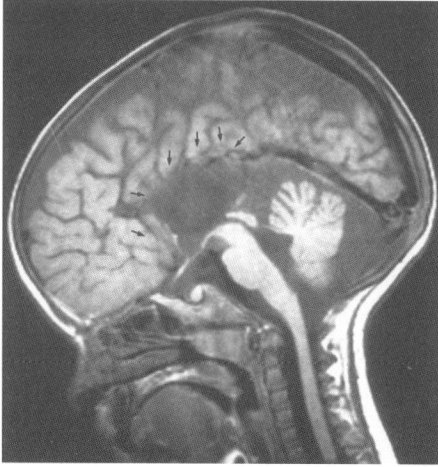

(a)

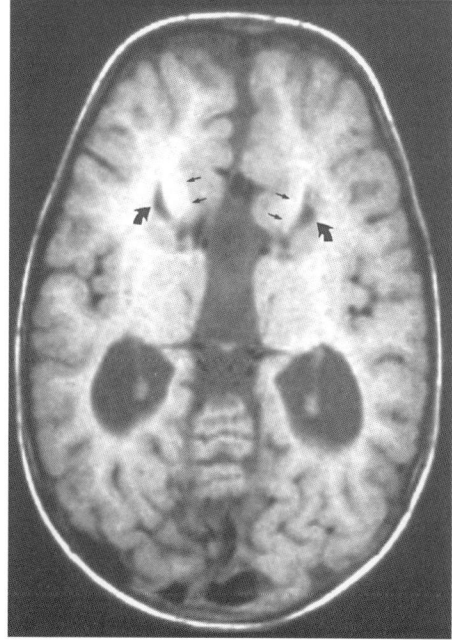

(b)

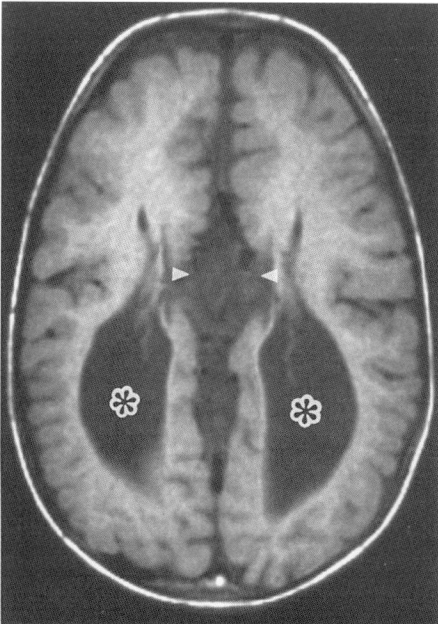

(c)

Fig. 4.15. Total absence of the corpus callosum. (a) T$_1$-weighted sagittal image demonstrates absence of corpus callosum. The medial hemispheric gyri generally course toward the inferior surface of the hemisphere *(arrows)*. (b,c) Axial images demonstrate Probst bundles *(b—small arrows)*, widely separated frontal horns *(b—curved arrows)*, parallel oriented ventricles, colpocephaly *(c—asterisks)*, and a third ventricle which extends superiorly between the lateral ventricles *(c—arrowheads)*.

Patients with dysgenesis of the corpus callosum may have an interhemispheric cyst which may communicate with all, part or none of the ventricular system. This cyst is frequently associated with hydrocephalus (Fig. 4.16). The exact origin of the cyst is not known. Some theories suggest that it is a dilated third ventricle, whereas others suggest

66

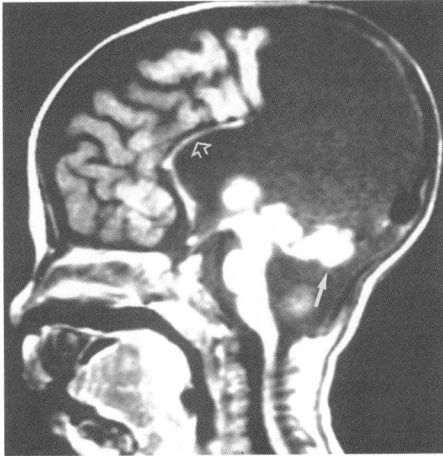

Fig. 4.16. Absent corpus callosum with inter-hemispheric cyst. T_1-weighted sagittal image demonstrates a large posterior midline cyst, partial absence of the posterior corpus callosum, and thinning of the remaining corpus callosum *(open arrow)*. There is also a Dandy–Walker variant anomaly present, represented by partial vermian agenesis and fourth ventricular enlargement *(white arrow)*.

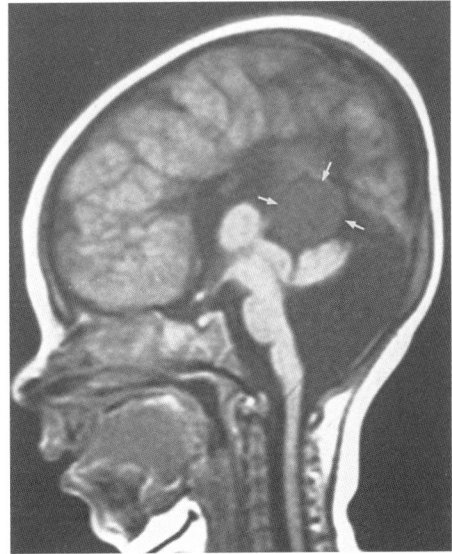

Fig. 4.17. Aicardi syndrome. T_1-weighted sagittal image demonstrates total absence of the corpus callosum, an interhemispheric cyst *(arrows)*, and Dandy–Walker malformation.

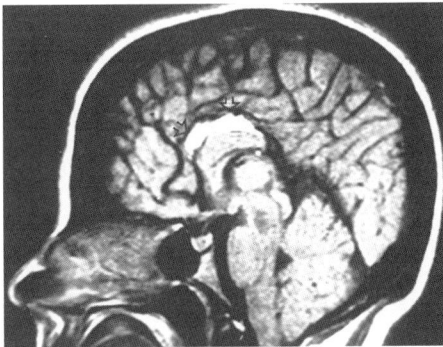

Fig. 4.18. Pericallosal lipoma with partial absence of the corpus callosum. T_1-weighted sagittal image demonstrates high signal in the pericallosal region anteriorly *(open arrows)* and absence of the splenium and posterior body of the corpus callosum. Note the spoke-wheel configuration of only the posterior, medial hemispheric gyri.

that it is a true arachnoid cyst of the interhemispheric fissure. At autopsy, the lining of these interhemispheric cysts may contain ependyma or arachnoid cells. MRI usually demonstrates similar signal intensities within the cyst and the CSF within the ventricular system (Bull 1967, Probst 1973, Larsen and Osborn 1982, Atlas *et al.* 1986, Byrd *et al.* 1990).

Aicardi syndrome occurs in females and consists of choroidoretinopathy (choroido-retinal lacunae), infantile flexion spasms, callosal agenesis and mental retardation (Fig.

4.17). Fused vertebrae and ribs, hemivertebra, scoliosis and spina bifida are common. Microphthalmia, optic nerve head colobomata and choroid plexus papillomas have a high association with Aicardi syndrome (Denslow and Robb 1979).

Pericallosal lipoma occurs in 0.06 per cent of the population and has a dysgenetic corpus callosum in about one half of cases. 13 per cent have an anterior calvarial defect, and these patients commonly have syndromic facial clefts, *i.e.* median cleft face syndrome. In a review of 164 cases of pericallosal lipomas it was found that another 13 per cent of these patients had fat extending from the pericallosal lipoma through the choroidal fissure and lying in close association with the choroid plexus of the lateral ventricles (Hughes and Osborn 1986). A recent study found this to occur in five of 16 patients (Truwit and Barkovich 1990). MRI demonstrates the high signal intensity of fat on T_1-weighted images within the pericallosal cistern and possibly hypoplasia or partial or complete absence of the corpus callosum and septum pellucidum (Fig. 4.18).

Dandy–Walker malformation
Two types of Dandy–Walker malformation (DWM) are defined: true DWM, and the Dandy–Walker variant (DWV).

DWM is believed to arise between the seventh and 10th weeks of gestation due to defective development of the roof of the fourth ventricle and adjacent meninges. These infants present at birth or in early infancy with an enlarged head or a localized bulging of the occiput. The majority (90 per cent) present with hydrocephalus (Raybaud 1982, Naidich *et al.* 1986*b*, Byrd and Naidich 1988).

The malformation is characterized by hypoplasia of the cerebellar hemispheres, agenesis of the inferior vermis, absence of the foramen of Magendie, and marked dilatation of the fourth ventricle which extends posteriorly as a cyst (Raybaud 1982, Naidich *et al.* 1986*b*, Byrd and Naidich 1988). The cyst balloons behind the cerebellum and displaces the hemispheres anterolaterally. It may also displace the superior vermis, if present, superiorly into the incisura, or it may balloon upward into the cistern of the velum interpositum. The posterior fossa is enlarged causing macrocephaly with scaphocephaly. The tentorium fails to migrate inferiorly because of the cyst's mass effect, and therefore the torcula lies superior to the lambdoid sutures. This is the classic torcular–lambdoid inversion caused by DWM. The falx cerebelli is absent.

We have not found it useful to utilize the revised classification of posterior fossa cystic lesions made by Barkovich *et al.* (1989) to further classify DWM into A and B types.

The MRI appearance of the DWM consists of a large posterior fossa cyst and a markedly dilated or non-demonstrable fourth ventricle. The inferior vermis is absent, while the superior vermis may be present, or partially or completely absent. The torcula is elevated and the occiput may be ballooned posteriorly. Hydrocephalus is nearly always present, with dilatation of the third and lateral ventricles. Other congenital malformations such as dysgenesis of the corpus callosum (25 per cent of cases), holoprosencephaly (25 per cent), migrational disorders (5–10 per cent) and posterior cephaloceles (<5 per cent) are associated with DWM (Raybaud 1982, Naidich *et al.* 1986*b*, Byrd and Naidich 1988).

DWV is characterized by partial vermian agenesis involving the inferior aspect of

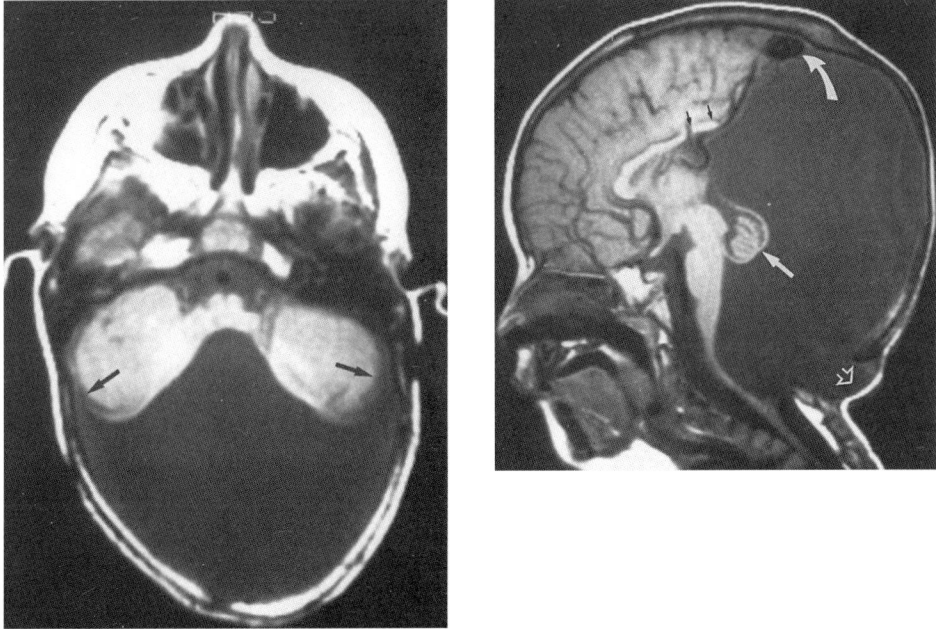

Fig. 4.19. Dandy–Walker malformation. *(Left)* T_1-weighted axial image demonstrates wide communication between the suspected region of the fourth ventricle and the large posterior fossa cyst. The cerebellar hemispheres are hypoplastic. The cyst extends laterally around the hemispheres to a point no further than their most lateral aspect *(arrows)*. *(Right)* T_1-weighted sagittal image demonstrates a large posterior fossa cyst, superiorly rotated residual superior vermis *(straight white arrow)*, lack of normal downward migration of the tentorium and torcula to its normal more inferior location *(curved white arrow)*, herniation of the cyst from a low occipital skull defect *(open arrow)*, and a thin, dysplastic callosal splenium *(small black arrows)*.

the vermis and by a less dilated and better formed fourth ventricle which communicates with the smaller retrocerebellar cyst. The posterior fossa is usually normal, although the tentorium may be elevated in up to 10 per cent of cases. The falx cerebelli may be present. Hydrocephalus may or may not be present (Raybaud 1982, Naidich *et al.* 1986*b*, Byrd and Naidich 1988).

The MRI findings in DWV consist of a large retrocerebellar cyst which is continuous with the enlarged fourth ventricle, and absence of the inferior vermis. The fourth ventricle though enlarged assumes the general shape of a normal fourth ventricle. The foramen of Magendie is present. The cerebellar hemispheres are small and may also be compressed anterolaterally by the retrocerebellar cyst (Fig. 4.19). DWV is also associated with other congenital malformations of the brain such as dysgenesis of the corpus callosum, holoprosencephaly, migrational disorders (especially lissencephaly type II) and posterior cephaloceles (Raybaud 1982, Naidich *et al.* 1986*b*, Byrd and Naidich 1988).

Chiari malformations
The Chiari malformations are four unrelated anomalies of the hindbrain which were

69

TABLE 4.5
Chiari malformations: classification of findings

Type	Primary findings	Secondary findings
Chirari I	Downward displacement of the cerebellar tonsils below the foramen magnum	Cisterna magna not visualized. Mild to moderate hydrocephalus. Syringomyelia
Chiari II	Herniation of the medulla (and at times the pons) caudally producing a cervicomedullary kink usually at C2–C4. Herniation of portions of the inferior cerebellar tonsils and vermis into the upper cervical canal. Elongation of the 4th ventricle. Downward displacement of the upper cervical cord	Hydrocephalus. 'Squared off' superolateral margins of the lateral ventricular frontal horns, 'beaking' of floors of frontal horns. Large massa intermedia. Hypoplastic falx with interdigitating medial interhemispheric gyri. Hypoplastic tentorium and wide incisura. Low insertion of the tentorium, small posterior fossa, low lying dural sinuses. Tectal beaking. Craniocaudal elongation of the cerebellum. Enlarged foramen magnum and ring of C1. Callosal dysgenesis. Syringomyelia
Chiari III	Bony defect in the infraocciput, posterior ring of the foramen magnum, posterior arch of C1, and at times C2. Herniation of the cerebellum, 4th ventricle, brainstem, upper cervical cord and meninges through defect	Herniation of venous sinuses through defect
Chiari IV	Severe cerebellar hypoplasia	Small posterior fossa. Prominent posterior fossa CSF spaces. Small brainstem

classified by Chiari in 1891 and 1895. Chiari (1891) described three types of cerebellar malformations based on pathologic studies of congenital hydrocephalus, and in 1895 added cerebellar hypoplasia as type IV. The four Chiari subtypes are classified as: type I, downward displacement of the tonsils to the foramen magnum into the upper cervical canal; type II, downward displacement of the tonsils, inferior cerebellum, fourth ventricle and medulla oblongata through the foramen magnum into the cervical canal in association with a myelomeningocele; type III, herniation of virtually all the cerebellum into an infra-occipital–high cervical cephalocele; and type IV, severe cerebellar hypoplasia (Naidich *et al.* 1986, Naidich and Zimmerman 1987, Byrd and Naidich 1988) (Table 4.5).

Chiari I malformation
The Chiari I malformation consists of protrusion of the cerebellar tonsils and, at times, adjacent parts of the inferior cerebellum through the foramen magnum into the upper cervical canal with obliteration of the cisterna magna. It is not considered an abnormality

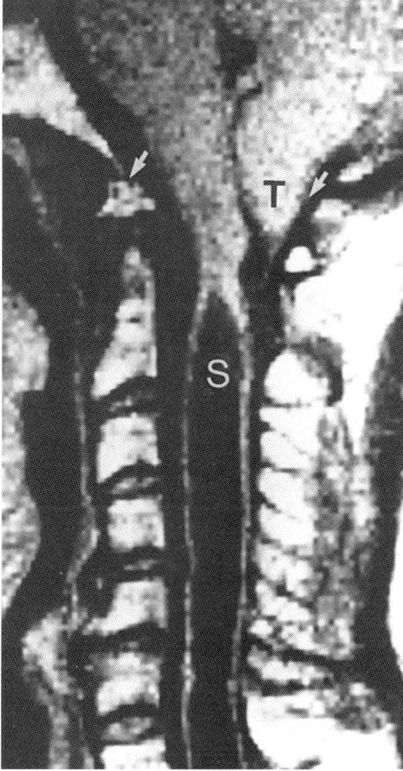

Fig. 4.20. Chiari I malformation. The cerebellar tonsils (T) extend below the margins of the foramen magnum *(arrows)*. A syrinx (S) is also present.

of closure of the neural tube, but rather a dysplasia of the base of the calvarium and cervical vertebrae (Fig. 4.20). The Chiari I malformation is associated with hydromyelia (70 per cent of cases), hydrocephalus (20–25 per cent), and segmental abnormalities of the craniovertebral junction which include basilar impression (25 per cent), assimilation of the first cervical vertebra to the occiput (10 per cent), Klippel–Feil anomaly (10 per cent), and incomplete ossification of the C1 ring (5 per cent). It is not associated with myelomeningocele (Naidich *et al.* 1986, Naidich and Zimmerman 1987, Byrd and Naidich 1988).

This condition usually affects children over 10 years of age. Clinically these patients present with headaches and occasionally raised intracranial pressure and hydrocephalus.

The MRI findings in Chiari I malformation consist of: (i) downward displacement of the tonsils and adjacent inferior portions of the cerebellum below the foramen magnum into the upper cervical canal; (ii) obliteration of the cisterna magna; (iii) mild to moderate hydrocephalus; and (iv) syringohydromyelia (Raybaud 1982, Naidich and Zimmerman 1987, Byrd and Naidich 1988). The degree of inferior displacement of the tonsils through the foramen magnum has been well categorized. Displacements greater than 5mm are adequate for the diagnosis of Chiari I malformation. Less than 2–3mm displacement is a normal finding. Intermediate displacements of greater than 3mm but less than 5mm are equivocal. If the patient is otherwise normal, an intermediate displacement should be ignored. If the patient has appropriate symptomatology or has a syrinx, a diagnosis of Chiari I malformation can be made (Barkovich *et al.* 1986).

Chiari II malformation
The Chiari II malformation is a complex anomaly affecting the calvarium, dura and hindbrain. It is virtually always associated with a myelomeningocele and is considered a disorder of closure. The embryogenesis of this malformation is complex, and current theories include: (i) traction on the hindbrain by fixation of the spinal cord at the myelo-meningocele; (ii) tissue pressure gradients between the intracranial contents and the spinal theca; and (iii) primary overgrowth of the entire CNS with persistent embryonic hydrocephalus and inferior displacement of the hindbrain (Naidich *et al.* 1983*b*, 1986*b*; Naidich and Zimmerman 1987; Byrd and Naidich 1988).

Symptoms in these patients are primarily related to the myelomeningocele and hydrocephalus. The incidence of myelomeningocele is 0.3 per cent of births in North America. Most cases are sporadic, with a female predominance of 2 to 1 over males. Most infants have sensory and motor deficits of the lower extremities apparent at birth. Intelligence should be normal or near normal in those who develop hydrocephalus provided that this is controlled by shunting and that secondary shunt infections do not occur (Naidich *et al.* 1983*b*, 1986*b*; Naidich and Zimmerman 1987; Byrd and Naidich 1988).

The MRI findings in patients with Chiari II malformation are numerous and complex. The primary findings necessary to make a diagnosis and classify this entity are as follows. (1) The upper cervical cord is displaced caudally by the downward extension of the medulla (and at times the pons) into the cervical canal posterior to the upper cervical cord producing a cervicomedullary kink, usually located between C2 and C4 but occasionally found as low as T1. This kink is found in 70 per cent of cases on MRI. In the remaining 30 per cent of cases the medulla descends into the cervical canal but remains in correct alignment and the pathognomonic kink is not seen. (2) The dysplastic cerebellum is elongated caudally so that it protrudes through the foramen magnum to rest on the upper border of C1. (3) A narrow tongue or peg of inferior cerebellar tissue (composed of parts of the dysplastic inferior vermis and cerebellar tonsils) protrudes into the upper cervical canal behind the herniated medulla (usually to the C2–C4 level). (4) The fourth ventricle is elongated craniocaudally and narrowed transversely to form a bent tube; it nearly always protrudes below the foramen magnum into the upper cervical canal. The distal aspect of the fourth ventricle may form a tear-drop diverticulum that protrudes caudal to the medulla behind the upper cord (Fig. 4.21).

Secondary findings in Chiari II malformation include: tectal beaking; hydromyelia (40 to 60 per cent of cases); hydrocephalus (98 per cent); colpocephaly (10–25 per cent); large massa intermedia; dysplasia involving the falx cerebri, allowing medial hemispheric cortical interdigitation and tentorium cerebelli; low insertion of the tentorium; small posterior fossa; enlargement of the foramen magnum and ring of C1; and dysgenesis of the corpus callosum (Naidich *et al.* 1983*b*, 1986*b*; Naidich and Zimmerman 1987; Byrd and Naidich 1988).

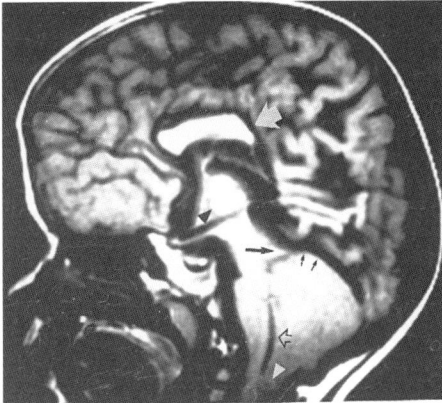

(a)

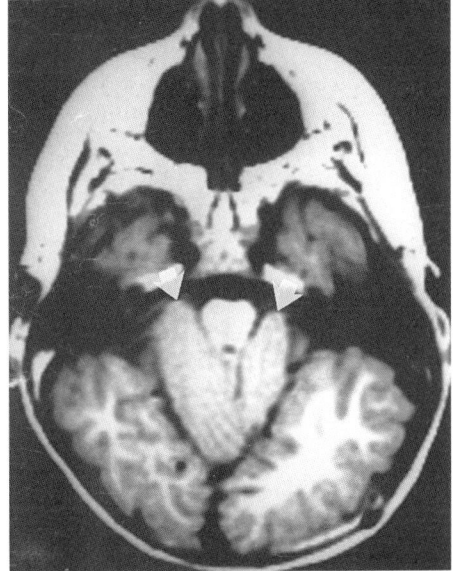

(c)

(b)

(d)

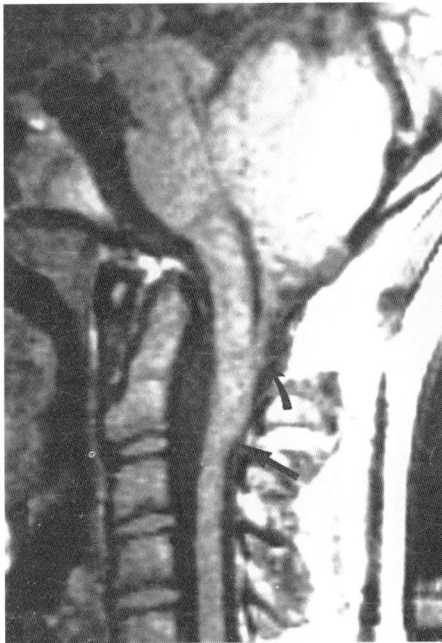

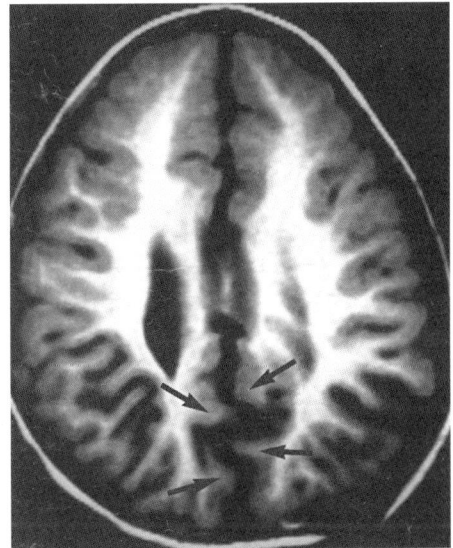

Fig. 4.21. Chiari II malformation. *(a)* T$_1$-weighted sagittal image demonstrates partial absence of the corpus callosum *(white arrow)*, large massa intermedia *(black arrowhead)*, beaked tectum *(large black arrow)*, upward extension or towering cerebellum *(small black arrows)*, elongated fourth ventricle *(open arrow)*, and inferior extent of the cerebellum into the foramen magnum *(white arrowhead)*. *(b)* T$_1$-weighted axial image demonstrates the towering cerebellum wrapping around the brainstem *(arrows)*. *(c)* Inferior displacement of the posterior fossa structures often result in the typical 'kink' at the cervicomedullary junction *(straight arrow)*. Note also the 'spur' of cerebellar tissue dorsal to the brainstem *(curved arrow)*. *(d)* The falx is often fenestrated resulting in medial interhemispheric gyral interdigitation *(arrows)*.

73

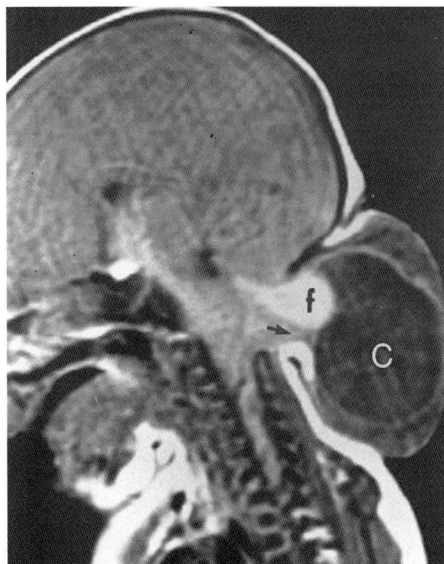

Fig. 4.22. Chiari III malformation. T_1-weighted sagittal image demonstrates a low occipital–high cervical encephalocele with a large cystic component (C), and herniation of cerebellar tissue into the defect *(arrow)*. Tissue with signal intensity of fat (f) was identified along the superior margin of the skull defect and extending into the small posterior fossa.

Chiari III malformation

The Chiari III malformation is a low occipital–high cervical cephalocele, consisting of a bony defect involving the infraocciput, the posterior rim of the foramen magnum, and the posterior arch of the first and at times the second cervical vertebrae, with herniation of cerebellar tissue as well as portions of the brainstem, fourth ventricle and upper cervical cord through the defect. It may result from defective tissue induction producing simultaneous abnormalities of the brain, spinal cord, cranial vault and upper cervical canal.

These patients are usually microcephalic and present with a posterior calvarial and cervical mass of varying size and consistency at birth. The symptoms depend on the amount and type of herniated posterior fossa–cervical tissue. Positioning is important in evaluating patients with cephaloceles. A donut-shaped or other device to prevent the head from lying on the cephalocele should be used, or the child should be placed in the lateral decubitus position in order to prevent pressure on the cephalocele. The MRI findings are quite specific and consist of: (i) bony defect in the infraocciput, the posterior rim of the foramen magnum, and the posterior arch of C1 and at times C2; (ii) herniation of an intracranial sac containing portions of the meninges, CSF, cerebellum, brainstem, fourth ventricle and upper cervical cord; and (iii) possibly also herniation of parts of the infratentorial dural venous sinuses through the bony defects (Naidich *et al.* 1986*b*, Naidich and Zimmerman 1987, Byrd and Naidich 1988) (Fig. 4.22).

Chiari IV malformation

The cerebellum develops from two lateral and one midline primordia. Complete failure to develop the primordia results in cerebellar aplasia. Lesser derangements produce variable degrees of hypoplasia of the vermis and/or the cerebellar hemispheres. The most common

74

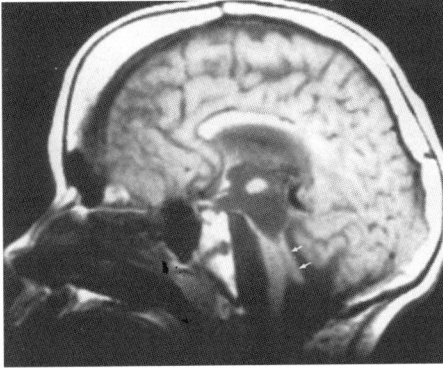

Fig. 4.23. Chiari IV malformation. T_1-weighted sagittal image demonstrates a severely hypoplastic cerebellum *(arrows)* and a small posterior fossa. There is no pontine enlargement of the brainstem, due to the lack of normal cerebellar peduncles. The CSF spaces in the posterior fossa are also prominent.

lesion is absence of part or all of the inferior vermis. This may occur as an isolated anomaly, or as part of Down syndrome (trisomy 21) or Joubert syndrome (familial vermian agenesis with episodic hyperpnea, ataxia, abnormal eye movements and mental retardation) (Raybaud 1982, Naidich *et al.* 1986*b*, Byrd and Naidich 1988).

The Chiari IV malformation is extreme cerebellar hypoplasia (Byrd and Naidich 1988). It is classified as one of the cerebellar hypoplastic anomalies. The anomalous event occurs during the eighth to 13th weeks of gestation. It is a rare condition, seen in infancy and early childhood. These children have the typical signs of cerebellar malfunction (ataxia, incoordination). The MRI findings consist of: (i) almost complete absence of the cerebellum; (ii) large posterior fossa CSF spaces without evidence of pressure or mass effect; and (iii) a small brainstem. A small pontine enlargement results from lack of formation of the cerebellar peduncles (Naidich *et al.* 1986*b*, Naidich and Zimmerman 1987, Byrd and Naidich 1988) (Fig. 4.23).

Cephaloceles
Congenital cephaloceles are considered disorders of closure. They are malformations characterized by herniation of intracranial contents through a defect in the calvarium. Specific classification depends on the type of intracranial contents within the herniated sac. A cranial meningocele is a herniation of the leptomeninges. An encephalocele is herniation of the meninges and brain tissue but not the ventricles. An encephalocysto-meningocele is herniation of meninges, brain and ventricles (Diebler and Dulac 1983, Byrd and Naidich 1988). For sake of convenience it is acceptable to refer to all of these anomalies simply as cephaloceles.

Cephaloceles are classified by location. In Europe and North America cephaloceles are more commonly found in the following order of decreasing frequency: occipital (71 per cent), parietal (10 per cent), frontal (9 per cent), nasal (9 per cent) and sphenoidal (1 per cent). In south-east Asia cephaloceles that involve the skull base (basal) are the most common (Byrd and Naidich 1988).

Congenital cephaloceles may result from defective tissular induction producing simultaneous abnormalities of the brain and cranial vault, or from defective formation of the

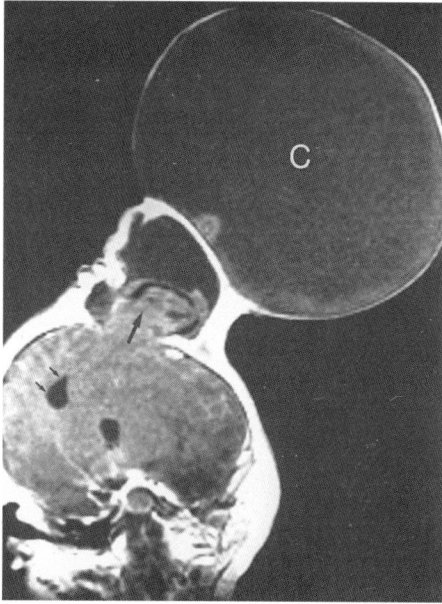

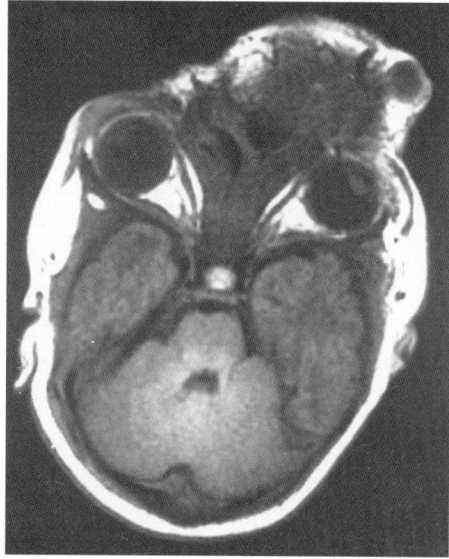

Fig. 4.24. Parietal cephalocele. T_1-weighted, gadolinium enhanced coronal image demonstrates a cephalocele with a large cystic component (C) and cerebral tissue extending outward through the skull defect *(large arrow)*. Note that the lateral ventricle *(small arrows)* appears 'pulled' toward the defect.

Fig. 4.25. Nasofrontal cephalocele. T_1-weighted axial image demonstrates a large bifrontal cranio-facial defect involving the nasofrontal region. Both frontal lobes herniate through the defect. There is also marked hypertelorism.

chondrocranium either at its junction with the membranous cranial capsule or at an isolated point (Harwood-Nash and Fitz 1976, Diebler and Dulac 1983, Byrd and Naidich 1988).

Occipital cephaloceles protrude through a defect in the occipital bone above the foramen magnum (high occipital cephalocele), through a defect in the occipital bone that extends into the foramen magnum (low occipital cephalocele), or through a cervical–occipital defect (Chiari III malformation). The occipital lobes are encountered in the herniated sac with high occipital cephalocele, whereas cerebeller tissue is found in the low occipital cephaloceles (Diebler and Dulac 1983, Byrd and Naidich 1988).

Parietal cephaloceles typically herniate in the midline just superior to the lambda near to the middle of the sagittal suture just posterior to the anterior fontanelle (Fig. 4.24). The posterior part of the interhemispheric fissures frequently enlarges and communicates with the sac. Callosal dysgenesis and DWM may commonly be associated with parietal cephaloceles (Diebler and Dulac 1983, Byrd and Naidich 1988).

Nasofrontal cephaloceles herniate between two deformed orbits through a defect in the region of the bregma, producing hypertelorism and a glabellar mass (Fig. 4.25). The herniated portions typically include the meninges, olfactory tracts and anterior parts of the frontal lobes (Diebler and Dulac 1983, Byrd and Naidich 1988).

76

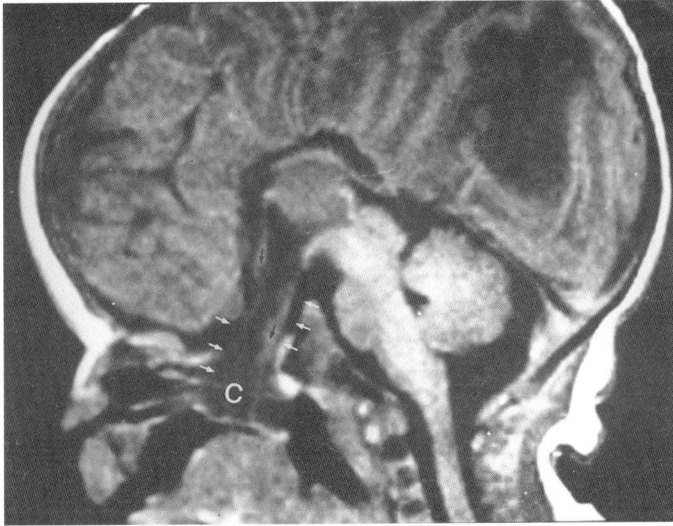

Fig. 4.26. Sphenoidal cephalocele. T$_1$-weighted sagittal image demonstrates a defect in the body of the sphenoid bone *(white arrows)* with a cephalocele (C) extending into the oral cavity. Vertically oriented linear neural or vascular structures *(black arrows)* extend toward or into the cephalocele. Note that the corpus caliosum is absent. This patient also had a true midline cleft upper lip.

Naso-orbital cephaloceles extend through a defect in the lamina papyracea of the ethmoids to enter the medial parts of one or both orbits. Interfrontal cephaloceles usually herniate through a defect in the lower portions of the metopic suture, in the nasal process of the two frontal bones and the nasal frontal suture. Frontal cephaloceles may extend through the frontal bones more superiorly, and may coexist with a frontal subcutaneous lipoma or a lipoma in the interhemispheric fissure (Diebler and Dulac 1983, Byrd and Naidich 1988).

Basal cephaloceles involve the skull base typically in the inferior frontal, ethmoidal, nasal, orbital and sphenoidal regions. These cephaloceles are named for the various areas they may involve, *i.e.* nasofrontal, spheno-ethmoidal, etc. The larger the cephalocele the more of these terms one can string together to describe it. Basal cephaloceles have a higher incidence of associated absence or dysgenesis of the corpus callosum, interhemispheric lipomas and hypertelorism. These patients also have a true midline cleft upper lip (Naidich *et al.* 1983*a*).

MRI of cephaloceles demonstrates the site of herniation, the contents of the sac, and the structures from which the sac contents arise. Portions of the ventricles contained within the sac are usually more dilated than those that remain intracranially. Typically the head is microcephalic. The residual intracranial structures appear distorted and drawn toward the site of herniation. Not only are brain parenchyma, meninges and ventricular parts herniated in the sac, but at times components of the cerebral vasculature, pituitary gland and optic pathways may be there as well. With basal cephalocele, the arteries may exhibit a variable branching, sometimes with an azygous anterior cerebral artery. Large veins and dural sinuses return through the cranial defect to drain into the intracranial structures (Diebler and Dulac 1983, Byrd and Naidich 1988).

The sphenoidal and sphenoido-ethmoidal cephaloceles constitute a special group and may be considered as occult cephaloceles. They present with signs of hypertelorism, nasal stuffiness, endocrine dysfunction and mental retardation. Nearly two-thirds of these have true midline clefts of the nose, upper lip or both. Approximately 40 per cent have some form of optic nerve dysplasia such as optic pit or coloboma.

MRI demonstrates herniation of intracranial contents through the body of the sphenoid bone just anterior to the dorsum sella and medial to the two cavernous sinuses (Fig. 4.26). The anterior edge of the herniated defect is variable, accounting for both pure sphenoidal and sphenoido-ethmoidal types. The cephalocele thus protrudes inferiorly to occupy the nasal fossa or herniate further downward through a cleft palate into the oral cavity. The sac nearly always contains the third ventricle and hypothalamus. The pituitary gland is variable in location within this cephalocele. The optic chiasm and nerves usually extend inferiorly. Callosal dysgenesis is present in around 40 per cent of cases (Diebler and Dulac 1983, Byrd and Naidich 1988).

Arachnoid cysts

True arachnoid cysts are congenital CSF cavities contained within the single layer of arachnoid. They are felt to arise from aberrations in the formation of the subarachnoid space. They may or may not communicate with the normal CSF spaces of the brain. Symptoms vary depending on the size and location of the cysts. Small cysts are usually asymptomatic. Half of these cysts are situated within the middle cranial fossa. If the cysts are large or in an area where they are adjacent to vital brain structures the patient may present with headaches, seizures, psychomotor retardation, and raised intracranial pressure secondary to the cysts themselves and/or to hydrocephalus. There may also be calvarial asymmetry with ballooning of part of the calvarium adjacent to the large arachnoid cysts.

Arachnoid cysts are more common in males. They may be found in any location where arachnoid mater is found, but are more common in the anterior temporal fossa (50 per cent of cases), the posterior fossa (33 per cent) and the suprasellar cistern region (10 per cent). Those occurring in the midline tend most often to cause symptoms due to mass effect and hydrocephalus. Arachnoid cysts of the middle cranial fossa have a higher tendency to bleed within the cysts or to produce subdural hematomas because of associated cortical venous anomalies (Naidich *et al.* 1986*a*). There is also an association of arachnoid cysts with neoplasms (astrocytomas, meningiomas), and with trauma or surgery of the brain, meninges or calvarium.

In the MRI evaluation of arachnoid cysts, diagnosis is based on the identification of an extra-axial mass which exhibits signal intensities (nearly) equal to CSF on all pulse sequences (Fig. 4.27). However, arachnoid cysts may have a high protein content or they may bleed within their cavity, in which case the signal intensity will be different from the normal CSF of the ventricular system (Naidich *et al.* 1986*a*). MRI of middle cranial fossa

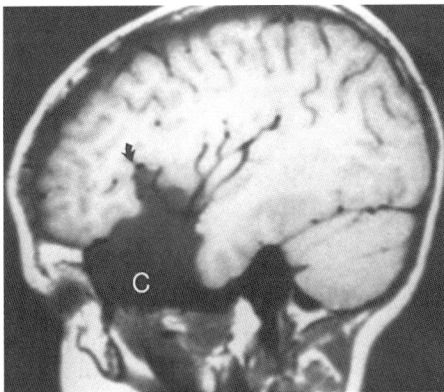

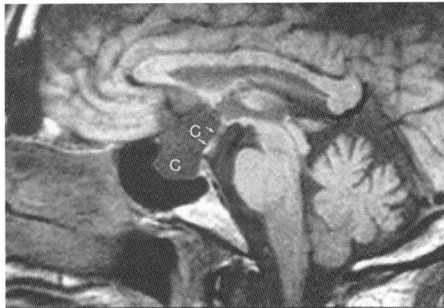

Fig. 4.28. Suprasellar arachnoid cyst. T_1-weighted sagittal image demonstrates a cystic mass (C) extending out of the moderately enlarged sella. Pituitary tissue is not readily delineated. The infundibulum is displaced posteriorly by the cyst *(arrows)*.

Fig. 4.27. Middle cranial fossa arachnoid cyst. T_1-weighted parasagittal image demonstrates an extra-axial, temporal fossa fluid collection (C). The temporal fossa is enlarged. The cyst extends upward into the sylvian fissure *(curved arrow)*. Little or no mass effect is present.

and sylvian fissure arachnoid cysts demonstrates a cystic mass in the area of the antero-inferior region of the middle cranial fossa with apparent posterior and superior displacement of the inferior aspect of the temporal lobe. The temporal fossa is commonly enlarged with thinning of the calvarium. In a previous study the authors suggested that the temporal lobe was hypogenetic and that the formation of the arachnoid cyst and the temporal lobe anomaly were associated.

When the cyst extends into the sylvian fissure the middle cerebral vessels are displaced posteriorly and medially. Anomalous venous drainage may be seen at times coursing over the cyst, and the superficial middle cerebral vein and sphenoparietal sinus may be absent (Naidich *et al.* 1986*a*).

Suprasellar cysts extend superiorly to compress the floor of the third ventricle with compression of the pituitary stalk (Fig. 4.28). They also commonly extend into the sella turcica as well as behind the dorsum sella and into the anterior cranial fossa (if it is large). High convexity area arachnoid cysts may produce effacement, displacement and compression of the gyri and sulci adjacent to the cysts (Naidich *et al.* 1986*a*).

Posterior fossa cysts may cause scalloping of the petrous bone along the cerebello-pontine angle with displacement of adjacent structures (Fig. 4.29). Clival arachnoid cysts may displace the brainstem and basilar artery posteriorly. Superior vermian arachnoid cysts may displace the superior aspect of the vermis downward, and they may extend up into the quadrigeminal cistern with compression of the colliculi and producing aqueductal stenosis. Arachnoid cysts in the region of the cisterna magna may or may not cause mass effect. If they do, they are easily diagnosed as arachnoid cysts and appropriate therapy can be instituted. If there is no mass effect then differentiation between an arachnoid cyst

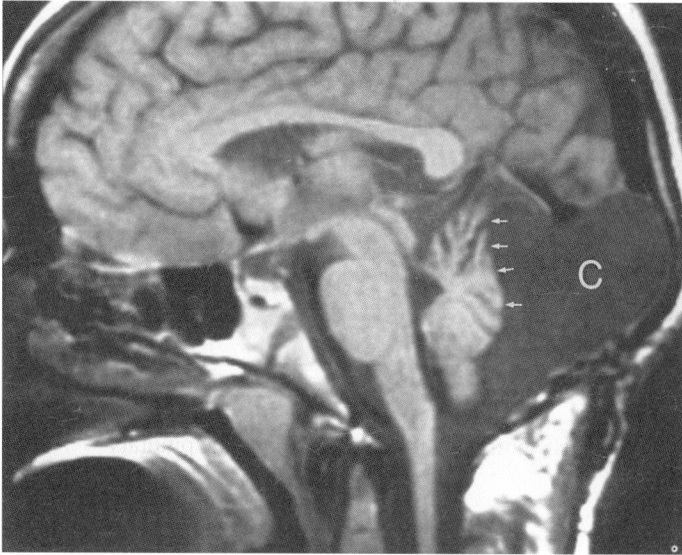

Fig. 4.29. Posterior fossa arachnoid cyst. T_1-weighted midline sagittal image demonstrates a retrocerebellar cyst (C) which does not widely communicate with the fourth ventricle. The vermis is displaced anteriorly by the cyst *(arrows)*.

and a so-called megacisterna magna cannot be made. In such a case, accurate differentiation of the cyst/cistern is clinically meaningless.

Neurocutaneous syndromes

The term neurocutaneous syndromes is used in general to describe a group of congenital malformations that share neurologic and cutaneous manifestations (Yakovlev and Guthrie 1931, Harwood-Nash and Fitz 1976, Diebler and Dulac 1987). The classification used in this discussion will consist of the classic entities as originally described by Van de Hoeve (1921, 1923, 1933) as the phakomatoses—neurofibromatosis, tuberous sclerosis, Sturge–Weber syndrome and von Hippel–Lindau disease—plus the more recently added ataxia–telangiectasia (AT) (Sedgwick and Boder 1972, Adams and Victor 1985).

The manifestations of neurocutaneous syndromes are predominantly dysplastic and/or neoplastic and involve the ectodermal structures (skin, eye, central and peripheral nervous systems), the mesoderm (bone and blood vessels) and to a lesser degree the endoderm (body organs). Most neurocutaneous syndromes are inherited as autosomal dominant or recessive disorders with the exception of Sturge–Weber syndrome which is sporadic, although familial cases have been reported (Diebler and Dulac 1987).

MRI of the neurocutaneous syndromes should consist of T_1-, intermediate and T_2-weighted sequences, with gadolinium enhancement where necessary to evaluate for neoplasms. Gradient echo (GRE) sequences may be helpful for the evaluation of calcification (Atlas *et al.* 1987, Braffman *et al.* 1988, Huk *et al.* 1990).

Neurofibromatosis

Neurofibromatosis (NF) is the most common of the neurocutaneous syndromes. The National Institutes of Health Consensus Development Conference (1988) has classified NF into two main types, NF1 and NF2.

NEUROFIBROMATOSIS TYPE 1

NF1 is inherited as an autosomal dominant disease with the genetic defect being related to the long arm of chromosome 17. It occurs in 1 in 3000 persons and is commonly referred to as the childhood, peripheral or von Recklinghausen form of NF.

The most reliable diagnostic criteria consist of the demonstration of six or more 'café-au-lait' spots of 1.5 cm or more in size, Lisch spots (pigmented iris hamartomas) and a familial history. Other diagnostic criteria include the demonstration of optic nerve glioma, osseous dysplasia (*e.g.* sphenoidal, orbital), two or more neurofibromas, plexiform neurofibroma, and hyperpigmentation of the axilla or inguinal areas (Eldridge 1981, Riccardi 1981). Patients with NF1 may also have seizures, kyphoscoliosis, pseudoarthrosis, and gastrointestinal, endocrine, genitourinary and pulmonary abnormalities (Riccardi 1981, Diebler and Dulac 1987, Braffman *et al.* 1988). The CNS and calvarial manifestations of NF1 consist of the following: gliomas (optic nerves, chiasm, hypothalamus, thalamus, basal ganglia, brainstem and cerebral hemispheres); neuromas, neurofibromas or schwannomas of the cranial, spinal and peripheral nerves; dysplasia of sphenoid bone and orbit; buphthalmos; plexiform neurofibroma of the scalp; macrocephaly secondary to megalencephaly or hemimegalencephaly; hydrocephalus secondary to aqueductal stenosis; kyphoscoliosis and miscellaneous hyperintense brain lesions demonstrated on MRI with long TR sequences (Casselman *et al.* 1977, Holt 1978, Stern *et al.* 1980, Lott and Richardson 1981, Daniels *et al.* 1984, Holman *et al.* 1985, Brown *et al.* 1987, Burk *et al.* 1987, Bognanno *et al.* 1988, Braffman *et al.* 1988, Russell *et al.* 1989).

The MRI evaluation of NF1 should consist of short and long TR sequences to evaluate for anatomic detail of lesions and abnormal signal intensities, and with gadolinium enhancement to evaluate for neoplasms.

Optic nerve glioma (ONG) is frequently seen in patients with NF1 (Diebler and Dulac 1987), usually presenting at between 3 and 7 years of age. 10 to 20 per cent are bilateral. The enlargement and anatomic detail of the optic nerves is best demonstrated with fat suppression pulse sequences of the orbits. The ONG enlarges the optic nerve and is fusiform in appearance. It demonstrates isointensity with gray matter of the brain on inversion recovery and spin echo sequences with short TR and hyperintensity on spin echo sequences with long TR (Fig. 4.30). It may enhance with gadolinium and the enhancement may be peripheral, with a central area of decreased contrast due to central necrosis, or diffuse. The optic nerves in NF1 may demonstrate an irregularity in outline without enlargement. This irregularity is thought to represent the dural ectasia which can be seen in NF1. The optic nerves are normally no larger than 5 mm in diameter in children. In patients with bilateral ONG, hyperintensity of the optic pathways, especially the optic tracts and radiations, can be seen on long TR sequences. If there is no enhancement of these areas of hyperintensity with gadolinium then they may represent edema, atypical

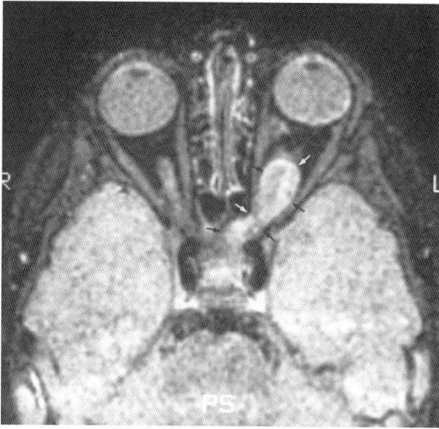

(a)

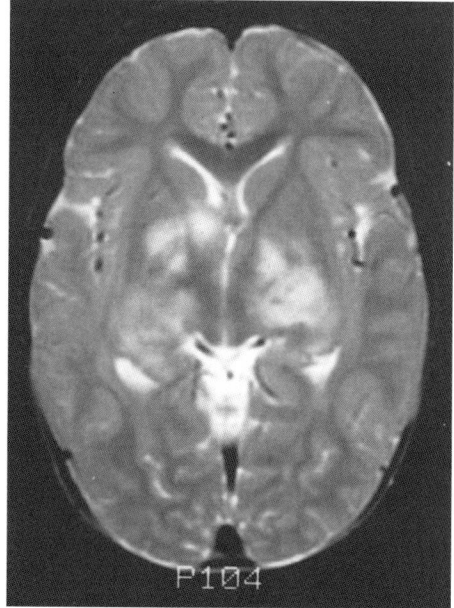

(b)

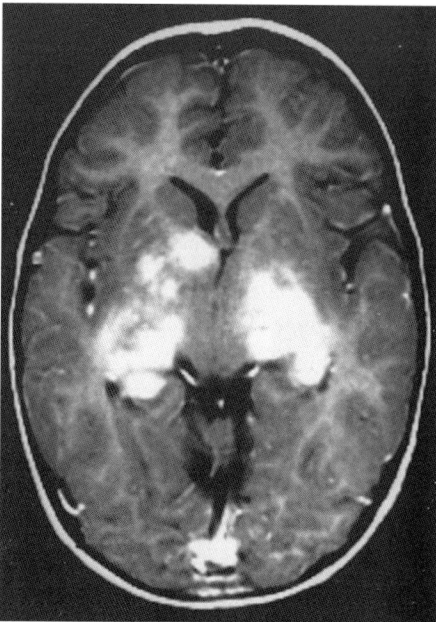

(c)

Fig. 4.30. Optic nerve glioma in NF1. *(a)* Axial, inversion recovery sequence with long inversion time for fat suppression demonstrates a fusiform high signal intense glioma of the optic nerve *(arrows)*. The tumor extended through the optic canal to the chiasm (not depicted). *(b)* T₂-weighted axial image demonstrates high signal in the basal ganglia regions bilaterally due to direct tumor extension. *(c)* Gadolinium enhanced, T₁-weighted axial image demonstrates enhancement of all the involved areas.

glial cells or infiltrating glioma. An ONG commonly extends to the optic chiasm and may infiltrate the optic chiasm, hypothalamus, thalamus, basal ganglia, brainstem and occipital lobe. These infiltrating gliomas demonstrate iso- or hypointensity to white matter on short TR sequences, hyperintensity on long TR sequences and enhancement with gadolinium (Fig. 4.30) (Stern *et al.* 1980, Daniels *et al.* 1984, Holman *et al.* 1985, Brown *et al.* 1987, Bognanno *et al.* 1988).

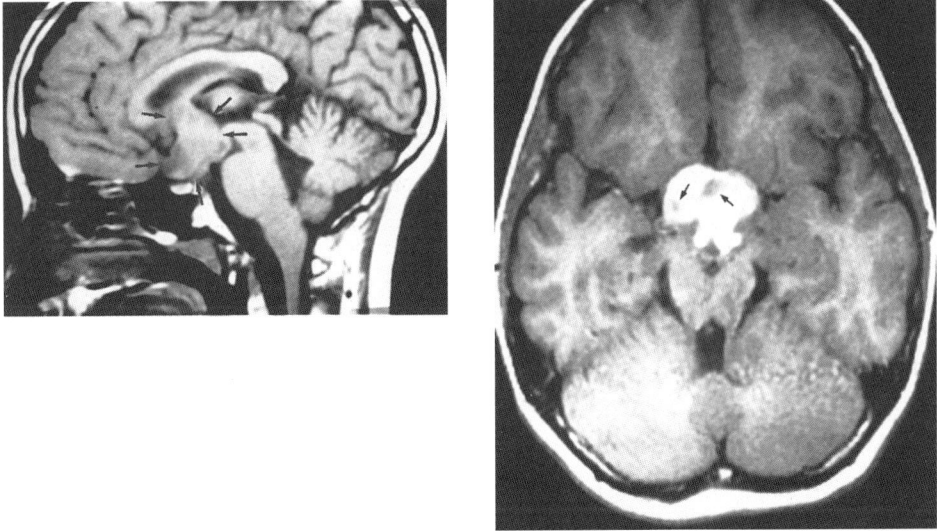

Fig. 4.31. Chiasmatic glioma in NF1. *(Left)* T₁-weighted sagittal image demonstrates an intermediate signal chiasmatic region mass *(arrows)* extending upward to efface the third ventricle. *(Right)* Gadolinium enhanced, T₁-weighted axial image demonstrates an enhancing chiasmatic region mass with small internal foci that do not enhance *(arrows)*. These foci probable represent areas of previous necrosis.

Ten to 15 per cent of patients with NF1 have a primary glioma of the chiasm, hypothalamus, thalamus, basal ganglia, occipital lobe or brainstem without extension from an ONG. These gliomas have mass effect and demonstrate the classic MRI appearance of iso- or hypointensity on short TR and hyperintensity on long TR sequences and enhancement with gadolinium (Fig. 4.31) (Diebler and Dulac 1987, Bognanno *et al.* 1988).

Meningiomas and acoustic neuromas are rare in NF1 and occur predominantly in NF2 (see below) (Eldridge 1981, Lott and Richardson 1981).

The most common neuromas associated with NF1 are Vth nerve neuromas. The MRI appearance is the same for neuromas or schwannomas in patients without NF. They are isointense to brain on short TR sequences and hyperintense on long TR sequences. Neuromas tend to be inhomogeneous due to foci of necrosis, and this may assist in distinguishing them from other extra-axial masses such as meningiomas. Neuromas enhance with gadolinium (Russell *et al.* 1989).

Dysplasia of the sphenoid bone (mainly the greater wing) with enlargement of the middle cranial fossa and possible herniation of the temporal lobe into the orbit is sometimes found with NF1. MRI demonstrates partial absence of the dysplastic greater wing of the sphenoid with enlargement of the middle cranial fossa and herniation of CSF or temporal lobe into the orbit.

The orbital involvement in NF1 consist of buphthalmos (enlargement of the globe due to congenital glaucoma) with or without bony orbital enlargement. Osseous dysplasia frequently involves the bony orbit with enlargement (Fig. 4.32) (Diebler and Dulac 1987).

83

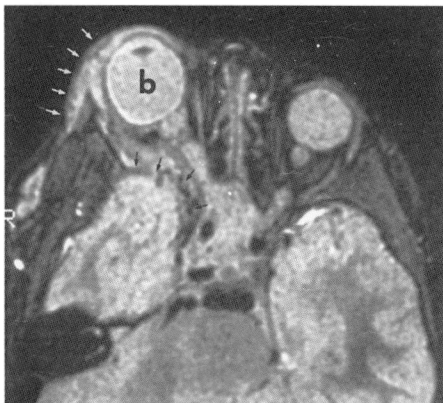

Fig. 4.32. Orbital anomalies in NF1. Inversion recovery image with long inversion time demonstrates buphthalmos (b), sphenoid wing dysplasia with herniation of the temporal lobe into the orbit *(black arrows)*, and cutaneous plexiform neurofibroma lateral to the orbital globe *(white arrows)*.

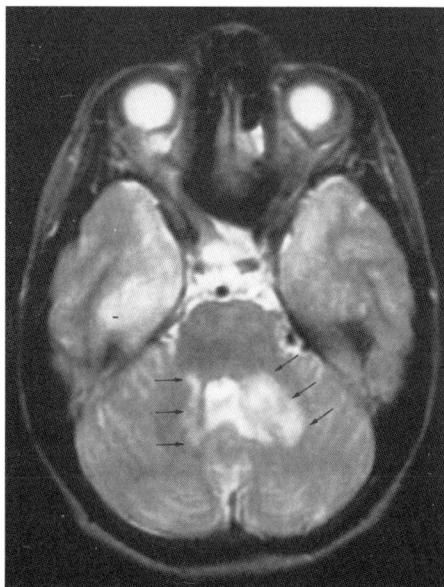

Fig. 4.33. Hyperintense lesion in NF1. Axial T_2-weighted image through the posterior fossa demonstrates white matter high intensity commonly seen in NF1 patients *(arrows)*.

Plexiform neurofibromas frequently involve the scalp. On MRI they demonstrate iso- or hypointensity to muscle on short TR sequences, hyperintensity on long TR sequences and enhancement with gadolinium. When the plexiform neurofibroma involves the temporal area of the scalp with extension into the frontal area and eyelid, it is often associated with ipsilateral dysplasia of the bony orbit and sphenoid bone with enlargement of the bony orbit and buphthalmos (Diebler and Dulac 1987, Bognanno *et al.* 1988).

Macrocephaly can be seen in NF1 patients and is due to megalencephaly or hemi-megalencephaly. The brain is enlarged, with mild to moderate enlargement of the lateral ventricles in megalencephaly and ipsilateral enlargement of the lateral ventricle with hemimegalencephaly. There may or may not be an increase in gray matter and a decrease in white matter in the affected hemisphere(s).

Hydrocephalus may be seen secondary either to obstruction of CSF from associated neoplasm or to aqueductal stenosis.

In 50 per cent or more of patients with NF1 there are abnormal areas of hyperintensity on long TR sequences in the basal ganglia, especially the medial aspect of the globus pallidus, cerebellum, brainstem (Fig. 4.33), thalamus, hypothalamus, centrum semiovale and corpus callosum. These areas of hyperintensity are usually multiple and bilateral, although they can be single or unilateral. They are mostly isointense to gray or white

84

matter on short TR sequences and have no mass effect, but occasionally are hyperintense, and typically they do not enhance with gadolinium, although again a small proportion may do so. A very small percentage of the basal ganglia lesions may demonstrate hyperintensity on T_1-weighted sequences. The exact etiology of these abnormal hyperintense lesions is not known. They may represent atypical glial cells, hamartomas or multiple gliomas (Brown *et al.* 1987, Bognanno *et al.* 1988, Braffman *et al.* 1988). Mirowitz *et al.* (1990) have suggested that the hyperintensity may be due to melanin deposits within heterotopic lesions containing Schwann cells.

The common spinal abnormalities seen in NF1 consist of scoliosis (kyphoscoliosis), bony dysplasia, dural ectasia, neurofibromas, schwannomas of the spinal and paraspinal nerves, extensive plexiform neurofibromatosis of the spinal and paraspinal nerves, neurofibrosarcoma and lateral thoracic meningocele (Casselman *et al.* 1977, Holt 1978).

The bony abnormalities consist of dysplastic and abnormal development of the vertebral bodies, hypoplasia of the posterior elements (pedicles, transverse and spinous processes), and scalloping of the posterior aspect of the vertebral bodies. About one-third of children with NF1 have a scoliosis or kyphoscoliosis of the thoracic–lumbosacral spine (Casselman *et al.* 1977, Holt 1978, Burk *et al.* 1987). Although CT and conventional pluridirectional tomography are better imaging modalities to evaluate bony detail, MRI can adequately evaluate most bony abnormalities (Burk *et al.* 1987).

Neurofibromas and schwannomas of the spinal and paraspinal nerves are commonly seen in NF1. These lesions can be single or multiple. It is not possible to differentiate neurofibroma from schwannoma with MRI or any other imaging modality. The MRI appearance consists of a circular or oval enlargement of the involved intervertebral foramen with the lesion extending outward forming the typical 'dumb-bell shaped' lesion. If the nerve sheath tumor is completely intracanalicular, differentiation from meningioma may be difficult. It is iso- or slightly hyperintense to skeletal muscle on short T_1-weighted images and hyperintense on intermediate and T_2-weighted images. Some neurofibromas may demonstrate a central area of hypointensity on long T_2-weighted images. This is due to a central collagenous core of the tumor with myxoid tissue peripherally (Burk *et al.* 1987) or areas of necrosis. Enhancement with gadolinium may or may not be homogeneous depending on whether necrosis is present. Meningiomas tend to be isointense on all imaging sequences, enhance homogeneously, and be broad based unlike nerve sheath tumors.

Children with NF1 may have extensive neurofibromas (bilateral and multiple) involving the paraspinal, peripheral and spinal nerves, plexiform NF. These lesions appear the same as solitary neurofibromas on MRI (Burk *et al.* 1987). Neurofibrosarcomas can be seen in patients with neurofibromatosis and may be difficult to differentiate from benign neurofibromas while still small. Once these invasive, infiltrating tumors become large their malignant nature becomes obvious.

Lateral meningoceles are common in the thoracic region, associated with dural ectasia and a defect in the lateral aspect of the vertebra with lateral herniation of the thecal sac. They contain CSF and have the same signal intensities as CSF on short and long TR sequences.

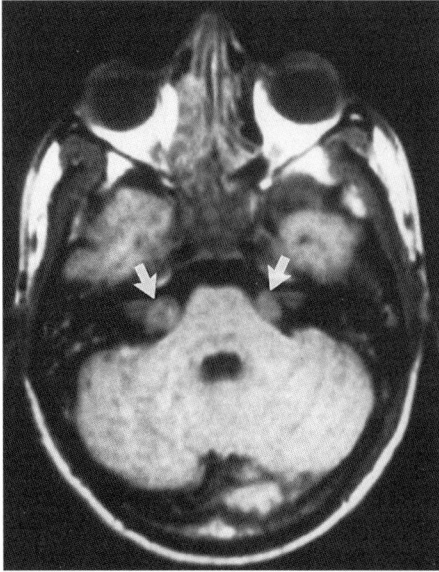

Fig. 4.34. Bilateral acoustic neuromas in NF2. Axial, unenhanced T$_1$-weighted image demonstrates bilateral cerebellopontine angle intermediate signal masses adjacent to the porus acoustici *(arrows)*.

NEUROFIBROMATOSIS TYPE 2

NF2 normally first manifests in late adolescence or early adulthood and is rare in childhood. It is an autosomal dominant disease with the abnormality located on chromosome 22. NF2 is also known as central NF (Lott and Richardson 1981, Seizinger *et al.* 1986, Brown *et al.* 1987, National Institutes of Health 1988). The diagnostic criteria for NF2 consist of bilateral VIIIth cranial nerve schwannomas (Fig. 4.34) or unilateral VIIIth nerve schwannoma with two of the following additional findings: (i) other neurofibroma or schwannoma, (ii) meningioma, (iii) glioma, or (iv) a relative with NF2.

NF2 is distinct from NF1. These patients may have café-au-lait spots but Lisch nodules, cutaneous neurofibromas, ONG and skeletal dysplasias are rare. NF2 is commonly associated with other cranial nerve schwannomas, cranial and spinal meningiomas, paraspinal neurofibromas and spinal cord ependymomas. The MRI appearance of these neoplasms is the same as that described in the literature in patients without NF (Bognanno *et al.* 1988, Russell *et al.* 1989). Meningiomas occur in the typical cranial locations and are commonly seen in intradural locations in the thoracic spine. Ependymomas most frequently involve the conus medullaris but may be found anywhere in the spinal cord. The neoplasm is usually isointense to spinal cord on T$_1$-weighted images and mildly to moderately hyperintense on intermediate and T$_2$-weighted images. There is usually contrast enhancement with gadolinium. An associated area of syringomyelia may be present, and there may be foci of hemorrhage within the tumor. Ependymomas are relatively slow growing tumors and often result in enlargement of the spinal canal.

Tuberous sclerosis

Tuberous sclerosis (TS) is an autosomal dominant disease which occurs with a frequency of 1 in 20,000 of the general population (Diebler and Dulac 1987). It is a disorder of cellular differentiation in which the clinical manifestations are secondary to hamartomatous malformations of the skin, brain, heart and kidneys. TS is more commonly seen in children with the classic symptoms of mental retardation, epilepsy, sebaceous adenomas of the face (especially the nasolabial region), depigmented nevi and various tumors. The most common and earliest cutaneous sign of TS is the depigmented nevi (flat, well-delineated, round or oval vitiliginous lesions of the skin) (Monaghan *et al.* 1981, Nagib *et al.* 1984, McLaurin and Towbin 1985–86, Diebler and Dulac 1987).

The main site of CNS involvement is the brain. Features include hamartomas (tubers) involving the cortex, white matter and the subependymal region of the lateral ventricles. Linear abnormalities within the white matter extending from the ventricular surface toward the cortex may be seen. Malignant degeneration of a periventricular tuber results in a giant cell astrocytoma, usually occurring in the region of the foramina of Monro, which is histologically benign (Monaghan *et al.* 1981, Nagib *et al.* 1984, McLaurin and Towbin 1985–86, Diebler and Dulac 1987, Braffman *et al.* 1988). Histopathology of the hamartomas in TS shows an increase in the number of fibrillary astrocytes and large, plump, oval cells with two or three nuclei some of which may resemble astrocytes or neurons. There is also dense fibrillary gliosis, abnormal myelination and at times foci of calcification (Monaghan *et al.* 1981).

The MRI evaluation of TS should consist of T_1- and T_2-weighted images as well as gadolinium enhanced sequences to evaluate for neoplasm (giant cell astrocytoma) (Atlas *et al.* 1987, Roach *et al.* 1987, Terwey and Doose 1987). CT criteria dictate that an enhancing tuber represented malignant degeneration. Even periventricular tubers without degeneration may enhance with MRI due to the high sensitivity of this imaging technique.

On gross pathology the cortical hamartomas in TS have a firm, hardened appearance. On MRI they flatten the gyri giving them a more pachygyric appearance. The cortical hamartomas can occur in any location but they are predominantly frontal and parietal. Gross calcification within these hamartomas is extremely rare in infants but can be seen in children of 2 years and older. These cortical hamartomas involve the cortex and at times the adjacent subcortical white matter. On MRI the cortical and subcortical hamartomas can have different signal intensities in infants and young children when compared to older children and adults. They can be solitary but are usually multiple. They are usually isointense to gray matter on T_1-weighted images and hyperintense on T_2-weighted images. In infants and young children these cortical–subcortical hamartomas usually demonstrate a thin isointense rim of flattened cortex (gyri) with a large cortical–subcortical area of hypointensity on T_1-weighted images. On T_2-weighted images almost all parts of these lesions demonstrate hyperintensity (Monaghan *et al.* 1981, Altman *et al.* 1987, McMurdo *et al.* 1987, Roach *et al.* 1987, Terwey and Doose 1987, Braffman *et al.* 1988).

The subependymal hamartomas commonly occur at the head of the caudate nucleus just posterior to the foramen of Monro, at the lateral borders of the bodies of the lateral ventricles, and at the anterior aspect of the atria of the lateral ventricles. They are usually multiple and bilateral, and vary in size up to about 10mm. These lesions may be better

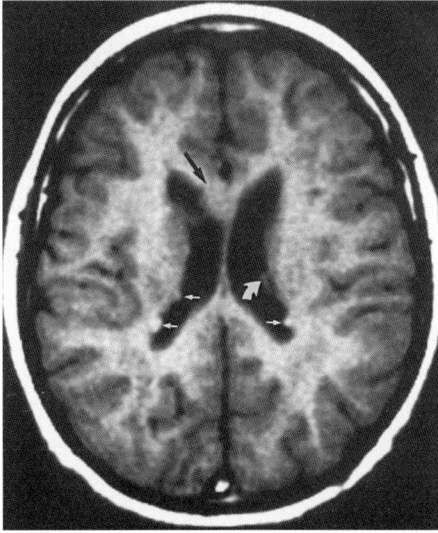

(a)

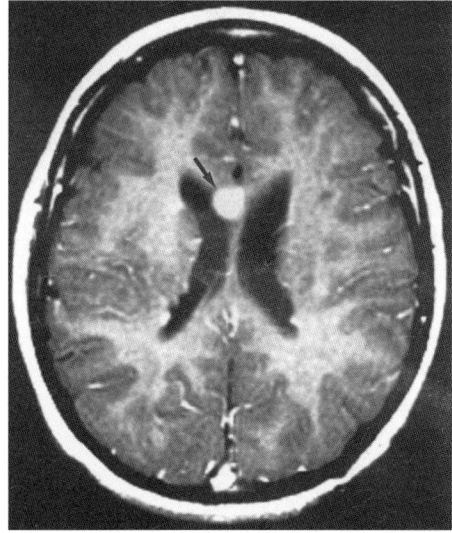

(b)

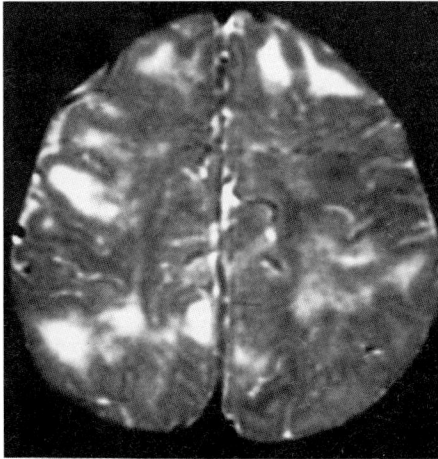

(c)

Fig. 4.35. Tuberous sclerosis. *(a)* Axial T$_1$-weighted image demonstrates subependymal hamartomas along the lateral aspect of both lateral ventricles. Most of the hamartomas in this case are similar in intensity to white matter *(small white arrows)*, while others have intensities similar to gray matter *(curved arrow)*. *(b)* Gadolinium enhanced, T$_1$-weighted, axial image demonstrates a giant cell astrocytoma in the region of the foramen of Monro *(arrow)*; this was also present on the unenhanced image *(a—black arrow)*. *(c)* T$_2$-weighted axial image in an unrelated patient demonstrates multiple subcortical white matter foci of high intensity representing parenchymal hamartomas.

demonstrated with long TR/short TE sequences (Atlas *et al.* 1987, McMurdo *et al.* 1987, Roach *et al.* 1987, Terwey and Doose 1987, Altman *et al.* 1988). Hamartomas located near the foramen of Monro are usually the largest and commonly contain calcification. Subependymal hamartomas show calcification more frequently than either the cortical or white matter lesions. They are usually isointense or slightly hyperintense to gray or white matter on T$_1$-weighted images and may demonstrate some additional slight increase in signal on T$_2$-weighted images. If the calcification is large, it may be seen as hypointensity on both sequences. If identification of the periventricular calcification is important, GRE sequences may be helpful; where this is inconclusive, CT scanning should be performed.

Hamartomas can occur in the white matter of the cerebral hemispheres and to a lesser extent the cerebellar hemispheres. These lesions demonstrate hyperintensity on T_2-weighted images (Fig. 4.35c) (Diebler and Dulac 1987, McMurdo *et al.* 1987, Roach *et al.* 1987, Terwey and Doose 1987, Altman *et al.* 1988, Braffman *et al.* 1988).

The hamartoma can degenerate into a giant cell astrocytoma or astroblastoma. The most common location is adjacent to the head of the caudate nucleus at the foramen of Monro. Giant cell astrocytomas generally grow faster than benign hamartomas and frequently contain calcification. They show contrast enhancement with gadolinium (Fig. 4.35) (Diebler and Dulac 1987, McMurdo *et al.* 1987, Roach *et al.* 1987, Terwey and Doose 1987, Altman *et al.* 1988, Braffman *et al.* 1988).

On MRI with T_2-weighted images, linear areas of hyperintensity can be seen within the white matter extending from the region of the lateral borders toward the cortex in TS. These areas are felt to represent regions of fibrillary gliosis and/or disturbances in myelination (Monaghan *et al.* 1981, Diebler and Dulac 1987, Braffman *et al.* 1988).

The MRI appearance of the hamartoma is one of iso- or hypointensity to gray or white matter with T_1-weighted images and mild to marked hyperintensity with T_2-weighted images. The appearance depends on the composition of fibrillary astrocytes, and on the presence of gliosis, of hypertrophied, heterotopic giant cells, or of abnormal myelination. The benign hamartoma may occasionally enhance with intravenous gadolinium. If marked homogeneous or inhomogeneous enhancement does occur with gadolinium this is considered evidence of degeneration of the hamartoma into a giant cell astrocytoma (McMurdo *et al.* 1987, Roach *et al.* 1987, Terwey and Doose 1987, Altman *et al.* 1988).

Sturge–Weber syndrome
Sturge–Weber syndrome (SWS) (encephalotrigeminal angiomatosis) is considered to be a sporadic non-inherited abnormality, although familial cases have been reported. Its primary abnormalities consist of a port wine nevus (capillary hemangioma) involving the skin of the face in the distribution of the first division of the Vth nerve (region of the eye-lid, forehead and cheek), venous angiomatosis of the pia mater typically in the temporo-parieto-occipital region and retinal angiomas. Over 90 per cent of these patients have seizures with additional symptomatology such as hemiparesis, hemianopia, mental retardation and glaucoma (Diebler and Dulac 1987). 15 per cent of cases are bilateral.

Other than the pial angiomatosis, the brain findings include gyriform cortical calcification, cerebral hemiatrophy, and ipsilateral choroid plexus angiomatosis. The deep venous system may be prominent due to lack of cortical veins in the involved area. Calvarial findings include hemiatrophy with enlarged paranasal sinuses secondary to the cerebral hemiatrophy (Bentson *et al.* 1971, Enzmann *et al.* 1977, Wasenko *et al.* 1990).

MRI demonstrates cerebral hemiatrophy, gyral enhancement, enlarged choroid plexus, possibly gyriform calcification and advanced myelination in the involved areas (Wasenko *et al.* 1990) (Fig. 4.36). Focal areas of high signal may also be seen within the white matter on T_2-weighted images. This is believed most likely to represent infarction or demyelination. The gyral enhancement is thought to be due to the ischemic changes

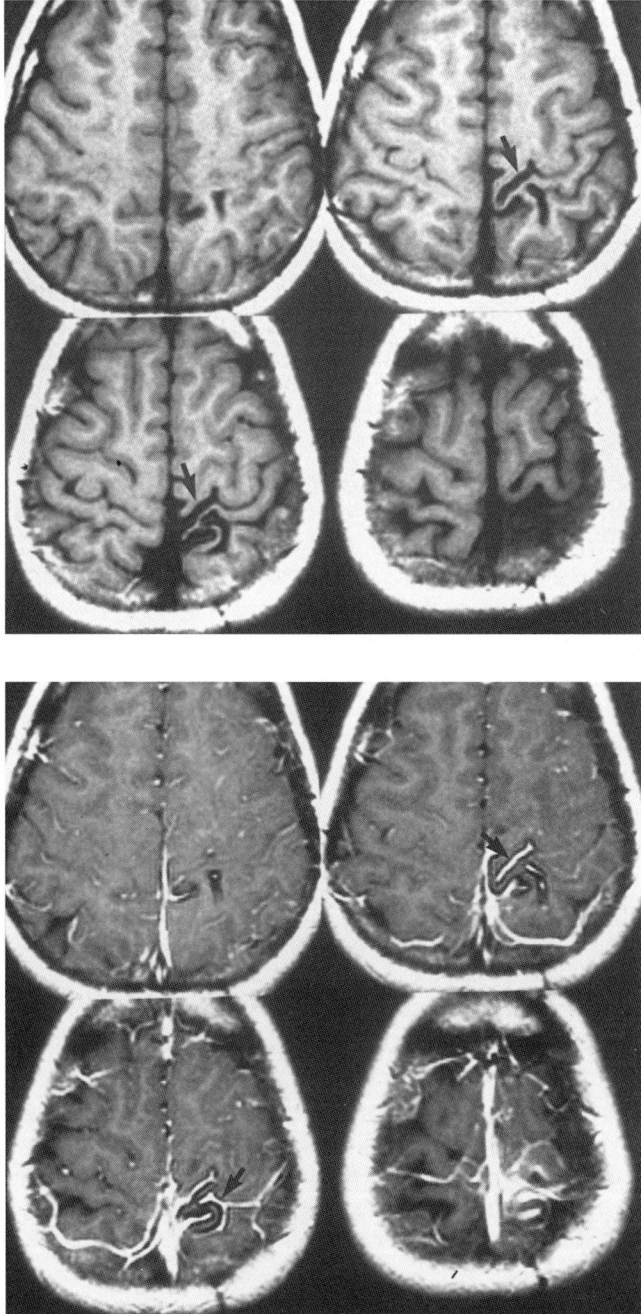

Fig. 4.36. Sturge–Weber syndrome. *(Top)* Axial, T_1-weighted images demonstrate gyriform signal void due to calcification involving the parietal cortex *(arrows)*. *(Bottom)* After administration of gadolinium, gyriform enhancement was identified *(arrows)*.

90

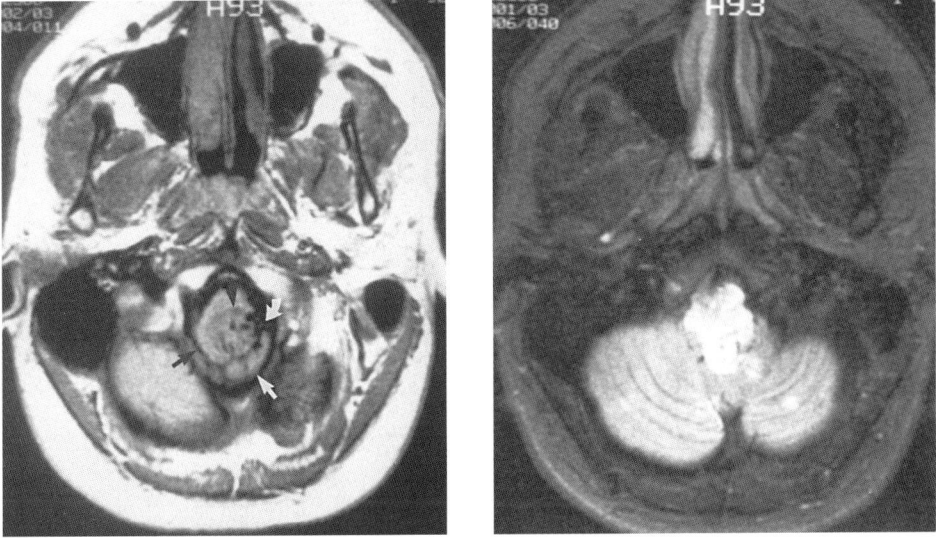

Fig. 4.37. Solid medullary hemangioblastoma. *(Left)* Axial T$_1$-weighted image demonstrates a solid, vascular, brainstem mass *(arrows)*. Note the prominent feeding arteries and/or draining veins *(curved arrow)*. *(Right)* T$_2$-weighted axial image demonstrates high intensity signal throughout the tumor.

that occur within the cortex underlying the angiomatous malformation of the pia mater. Ipsilateral calvarium findings may include enlarged paranasal sinus and mastoid air cells and an elevated petrous ridge.

CT remains the most sensitive modality for evaluating calcification in SWS (Wasenko *et al.* 1990).

In young children (usually 2 years or under) an infantile form of SWS can be seen on MRI. Calcification is not present. On the involved side, the sulci are smaller, the cortical gray matter is hypointense on short TR/TE sequences in relation to the normal side, and the choroid plexus is enlarged. On long TR/TE sequences there may be slight hyperintensity of the involved cortex. If gadolinium is given there may be cortical enhancement on the involved side.

Von Hippel–Lindau syndrome
The von Hippel–Lindau syndrome (VHL) is an autosomal dominant disease consisting of CNS and retinal angiomatosis (Huson *et al.* 1986, Jones 1988). Common manifestations include cerebellar hemispheric (40–60 per cent) and retinal (50–70 per cent) hemangioblastomas (Fig. 4.37), cysts and angiomas of the liver and kidney, renal cell carcinoma (20–40 per cent) and pheochromocytoma (10 per cent) (Horton *et al.* 1976, Jones 1988). The diagnosis is based on one of the following: hemangioblastomas of the CNS; one hemangioblastoma of the CNS with a visceral manifestation; or one hemangioblastoma of the CNS or a visceral manifestation with a known family history.

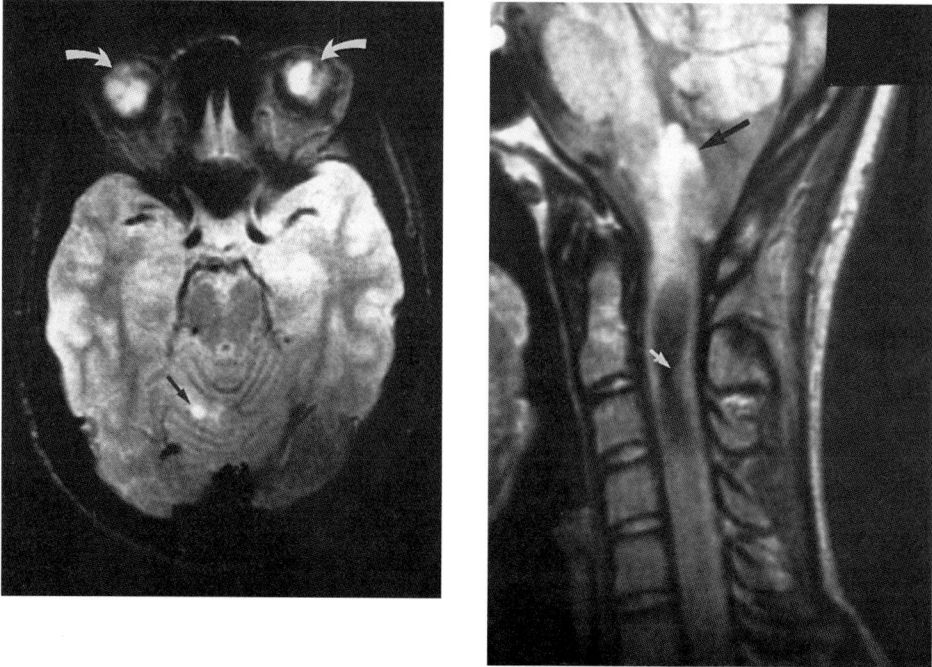

Fig. 4.38. Von Hippel–Lindau disease. *(Left)* Axial T$_2$-weighted image demonstrates an angiographically proven, high signal, 4mm hemangioblastoma in the superior aspect of the right cerebellar hemisphere *(black arrow)*. Retinal angiomas with repeated intraocular hemorrhages also result in high signal *(white arrows)*. *(Right)* Sagittal, midline, intermediate-weighted image of the craniocervical junction region demonstrates an hemangioblastoma *(white arrow)* with a cyst or syrinx. Another hemangioblastoma involved the medulla *(black arrow)*.

The primary CNS finding in VHL is hemangioblastoma—usually unifocal but occasionally multiple—generally involving the cerebellum, medulla or spinal cord. Cerebral involvement has also been reported (Loftus *et al.* 1984). The hemangioblastoma may be cystic with a small mural nodule (50 per cent), mixed cystic and solid (25 per cent), or solid (25 per cent). The cystic fluid may have an increased protein or blood content.

The MRI findings include prominent feeding arteries of draining veins within and around the tumor mass. The nodule itself is relatively isointense on T$_1$-weighted images and hyperintense on T$_2$-weighted images. It enhances brightly with gadolinium (Fig. 4.38). There is commonly a mild degree of peritumoral white matter edema due to associated mass effect. The cystic fluid is usually clear yellow grossly and has mildly to moderately higher signal than CSF on T$_1$-weighted images and higher signal on intermediate and T$_2$-weighted images (Elster and Arthur 1988, Sato *et al.* 1988).

Ataxia–telangiectasia
Ataxia–telangiectasia (AT) is an autosomal recessive inherited disorder described by

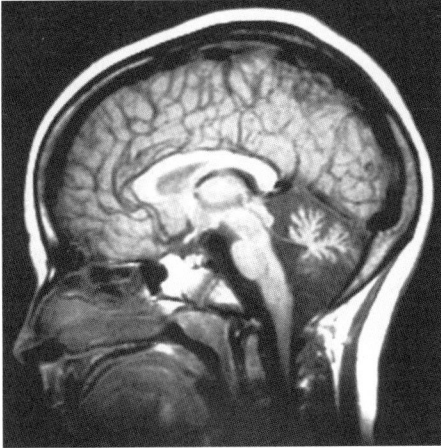

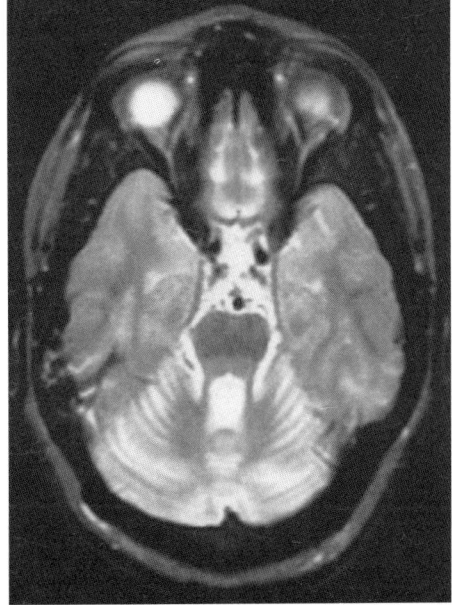

Fig. 4.39. Ataxia–telangiectasia. *(Above)* Midline sagittal T_1-weighted image demonstrates vermian atrophy. *(Right)* Axial T_2-weighted image demonstrates prominent cerebellar hemispheric atrophy as well.

Louis-Bar in 1941 (Jeret *et al.* 1985–86). It is a progressive disorder with involvement of the CNS, skin, and respiratory and immune systems. It is characterized by telangiectasias involving the skin (face) and eyes, with progressive cerebellar ataxia, immunodeficiencies, and infections of the paranasal sinuses and lungs. It may occur at any time from birth to 14 years of age but is most common from 2 to 4 years. The telangiectasia commonly involves the pia mater and white matter of the brain, predominantly of the cerebellum. MRI demonstrates severe cerebellar atrophy with enlarged cerebellar sulci, enlarged fourth ventricle and enlarged CSF cisterns of the posterior fossa (Fig. 4.39) (McFarlin *et al.* 1972, Paller 1987).

REFERENCES

Adams, R.D., Victor, M. (1985) *Principles of Neurology, 3rd Edn.* New York: McGraw–Hill.

Altman, N.R., Purser, R.K., Post, M.J.D. (1988) 'Tuberous sclerosis: characteristics at CT and MR imaging.' *Radiology,* **167**, 527–532.

Arslanian, S.A., Rothfus, W.E., Foley, T.P., Becker, D.J. (1984) 'Hormonal, metabolic, and neuroradiologic abnormalities associated with septo-optic dysplasia.' *Acta Endocrinologica,* **107**, 282–288.

Atlas, S.W., Zimmerman, R.A., Bilaniuk, L.T., Rorke, L., Hackney, D.B., Goldberg, H.I., Grossman, R.I. (1986) 'Corpus callosum and limbic system: neuroanatomic MR evaluation of developmental anomalies.' *Radiology,* **160**, 355–362.

—— Grossman, R.I., Hackney, D.B., Gomori, J.M., Goldberg, H.I., Bilaniuk, L.T., Zimmerman, R.A. (1987) 'Calcified intracranial lesions: detection with gradient echo acquisition rapid MR imaging.' *American Journal of Neuroradiology,* **8**, 932–933. *(Abstract.)*

Barkovich, A.J., Wippold, F.J., Sherman, J.L., Citrin, C.M. (1986) 'Significance of cerebellar tonsillar position on MR.' *American Journal of Neuroradiology,* **7**, 795–799.

—— Kjos, B.O., Norman, D., Edwards, M.S. (1989) 'Revised classification of posterior fossa cysts and cystlike malformations based on the results of multiplanar MR imaging.' *American Journal of Neuroradiology*, **10**, 977–988.

Barth, P.G. (1987) 'Disorders of neuronal migration.' *Canadian Journal of Neurological Sciences*, **14**, 1–16.

Bentson, J.R., Wilson, G.H., Newton, T.H. (1971) 'Cerebral venous drainage pattern of the Sturge–Weber syndrome.' *Radiology*, **101**, 111–118.

Bird, C.R., Gilles, F.H. (1987) 'Type I schizencephaly: CT and neuropathologic findings.' *American Journal of Neuroradiology*, **8**, 451–454.

Bognanno, J.R., Edwards, M.K., Lee, T.A., Dunn, D.W., Roos, K.L., Klatte, E.C. (1988) 'Cranial MR imaging in neurofibromatosis.' *American Journal of Neuroradiology*, **9**, 461–468.

Braffman, B.H., Bilaniuk, L.T., Zimmerman, R.A. (1988) 'The central nervous system manifestations of the phakomatoses on MR.' *Radiologic Clinics of North America*, **26**, 773–800

Brown, E.W., Riccardi, V.M., Mawad, M., Handel, S., Goldman, A., Bryan, R.N. (1987) 'MR imaging of optic pathways in patients with neurofibromatosis.' *American Journal of Neuroradiology*, **8**, 1031–1036.

Bruyer, R., Dupuis, M., Ophoven, E., Rectem, D., Reynaert, C. (1985) 'Anatomical and behavioral study of a case of asymptomatic callosal agenesis.' *Cortex*, **21**, 417–430.

Bull, J. (1967) 'The corpus callosum.' *Clinical Radiology*, **18**, 2–18.

Burk, D.L., Brunberg, J.A., Kanal, E., Latchaw, R.E., Wolf, G.L. (1987) 'Spinal and paraspinal neurofibromatosis: surface coil MR imaging at 1.5 T.' *Radiology*, **162**, 797–801.

Byrd, S.E., Naidich, T.P. (1988) 'Common congenital brain anomalies.' *Radiologic Clinics of North America*, **26**, 755–772.

—— Bohan, T.P., Osborn, R.E., Naidich, T.P. (1988) 'The CT and MR evaluation of lissencephaly.' *American Journal of Neuroradiology*, **9**, 923–927.

—— Osborn, R.E., Bohan, T.P., Naidich, T.P. (1989*a*) 'The CT and MR evaluation of migrational disorders of the brain. Part I. Lissencephaly and pachygyria.' *Pediatric Radiology*, **19**, 151–156.

—— —— —— (1989*b*) 'The CT and MR evaluation of migrational disorders of the brain. Part II. Schizencephaly, heterotopia and polymicrogyria' *Pediatric Radiology*, **19**, 219–222.

—— Radkowski, M.A., Flannery, A., McLone, D.G. (1990) 'The clinical and radiological evaluation of absence of the corpus callosum.' *European Journal of Radiology*, **10**, 65–73.

—— Osborn, R.E., Radkowski, M.A. (1991) 'The MR evaluation of pachygyria and associated syndromes.' *European Journal of Radiology*, **12**, 53–59.

Casselman, E.S., Miller, W.T., Lin, S.R., Mandell, G.A. (1977) 'Von Recklinghausen's disease: incidence of roentgenographic findings with a clinical review of the literature.' *CRC Critical Reviews in Diagnostic Imaging*, **9**, 387–419.

Chiari, H. (1891) 'Über Veranderungen des Kleinhirns Infolge von Hydrocephalie des Groshirns.' *Deutche Medizinischer Wochenschrift*, **17**, 1172.

—— (1895) 'Über des Veranderungen des Kleinhirns, des Pons und der Medulla Oblongata Infolge von congenitaler Hydrocephalie des Groshirns.' *Deukschrifter der Akademie der Wissenschafen*, **63**, 71.

Cohen, M.M., Jirasek, J.E., Guzman, R.T., Gorlin, R.J., Peterson, M.Q. (1971) 'Holoprosencephaly and facial dysmorphia: nosology, etiology and pathogenesis.' *Birth Defects Original Article Series*, **7** (XI), 125–135.

Curnes, J.T., Laster, D.W., Koubek, T.D., Moody, D.M., Ball, M.R.,Witcofski, R.L. (1986) 'MRI of corpus callosal syndromes.' *American Journal of Neuroradiology*, **7**, 617–622.

Daniels, D.L., Herfkins, R., Gager, W.E., Meyer, G.A., Koehler, P.R., Williams, A.L., Haughton, V.M. (1984) 'Magnetic resonance imaging of the optic nerves and chiasm.' *Radiology*, **152**, 79–83.

Davidoff, L.M., Dyke, C.G. (1934) 'Agenesis of the corpus callosum. Its diagnosis by encephalography. Report of three cases.' *American Journal of Roengenology*, **32**, 1–10.

Davidson, J.E., McWilliam, R.C., Evans, T.J., Stephenson, J.B.P. (1989) 'Porencephaly and optic hypoplasia in neonatal isoimmune thrombocytopenia.' *Archives of Disease in Childhood*, **64**, 858–860.

DeMyer, W. (1971) 'Classification of cerebral malformations.' *Birth Defects Original Article Series*, **7** (VI), 78–93.

—— Zeman, W. (1963) 'Alobar holoprosencephaly (arhinencephaly) with median cleft lip and palate: clinical, electroencephalographic and nosologic considerations.' *Confinia Neurologica*, **23**, 1–36.

—— —— Palmer, C.G. (1964) 'The face predicts the brain: diagnostic significance of median facial anomalies for holoprosencephaly (arhinencephaly).' *Pediatrics*, **34**, 256–263.

Denslow, G.T., Robb, R.M. (1979) 'Aicardi's syndrome: a report of four cases and review of the literature.' *Journal of Pediatric Ophthalmology and Strabismus*, **16**, 10–15.

Diebler, C., Dulac, O. (1983) 'Cephaloceles: clinical and neuroradiological appearance. Associated cerebral malformations.' *Neuroradiology*, **25**, 199–216.

—— —— (1987) *Pediatric Neurology and Neuroradiology*. New York: Springer–Verlag.

Dobyns, W.B. (1987) 'Developmental aspects of lissencephaly and the lissencephaly syndromes.' *Birth Defects Original Article Series*, **23**, 225–241.

—— Gilbert, E.F., Opitz, J.M. (1985) 'Further comments on the lissencephaly syndromes.' *American Journal of Medical Genetics*, **22**, 197–211. *(Letter.)*

Eldridge, R. (1981) 'Central neurofibromatosis with bilateral acoustic neuroma.' *Advances in Neurology*, **29**, 57–65.

Elster, A.D., Arthur, D.W. (1988) 'Intracranial hemangioblastomas: CT and MR findings.' *Journal of Computer Assisted Tomography*, **12**, 736–739.

Enzmann, D.R., Hayward, R.W., Norman, D., Dunn, R.P. (1977) 'Cranial computed tomographic scan appearance of Sturge–Weber disease: unusual presentation.' *Radiology*, **122**, 721–724.

Ettlinger, G., Blakemore, C.B., Milner, A.D., Wilson, J. (1974) 'Agenesis of the corpus callosum: a further behavioural investigation.' *Brain*, **97**, 225–234.

Fitz, C.R. 'Holoprosencephaly and related entities.' *Neuroradiology*, **25**, 225–238.

François, J., Eggermont, E., Evens, L., Nogghe, N., De Bock, F. (1973) 'Agenesis of the corpus callosum in the median facial cleft syndrome and associated ocular malformations.' *American Journal of Ophthalmology*, **76**, 241–245.

Hale, B.R., Rice, P. (1970) 'Septo-optic dysplasia: clinical and embryological aspects.' *Developmental Medicine and Child Neurology*, **16**, 812–817.

Hanaway, J., Lee, S.I., Netsky, M.G. (1968) 'Pachygyria: relation of findings to modern embryologic concepts.' *Neurology*, **18**, 791–799.

Harwood-Nash, D.C., Fitz, C.R. (1976) 'Congenital malformations of the brain.' *In: Neuroradiology in Infants and Children*. Saint Louis, MI: C.V. Mosby, pp. 998–1053.

Holman, R.E., Grimson, B.S., Drayer, B.P., Buckley, E.G., Brennan, M.W. (1985) 'Magnetic resonance imaging of optic gliomas.' *American Journal of Ophthalmology*, **100**, 596–601.

Holt, J.F. (1978) 'Neurofibromatosis in children.' *American Journal of Radiology*, **130**, 615–639.

Horton, W.A., Wong, V., Eldridge, R. (1976) 'Von Hippel–Lindau disease. Clinical and pathological manifestations in nine families with 50 affected members.' *Archives of Internal Medicine*, **136**, 769–777.

Hoyt, W.F., Rios-Montenegro, E.N., Behrens, M.M., Eckelhoff, R.J. (1972) 'Homonymous hemioptic hypoplasia. Fundoscopic features in standard and red-free illumination in three patients with congenital hemiplegia.' *British Journal of Ophthalmology*, **56**, 537–545.

Hughes, D.S., Osborn, R.E. (1986) 'Corpus callosal lipoma: report of 2 cases and review of the literature.' *Journal of the American Osteopathic Association*, **86**, 564–567.

Huk, W.J., Gademann, G., Friedmann, G. (1990) *MRI of Central Nervous System Diseases*. New York: Springer–Verlag.

Huson, S.M., Harper, P.S., Hourihan, M.D., Cole, G., Weeks, R.D., Compston, D.A.S. (1986) 'Cerebellar haemangioblastoma and von Hippel–Lindau disease.' *Brain*, **109**, 1297–1310.

Jellinger, K., Rett, A. (1976) 'Agyria–pachygyria (lissencephaly syndrome).' *Neuropädiatrie*, **7**, 66–91.

Jeret, J.S., Serur, D., Wisniewski, K., Fisch, C. (1985–86) 'Frequency of agenesis of the corpus callosum in the developmentally disabled population as determined by computerized tomography.' *Pediatric Neuro-science*, **12**, 101–103.

Jones, K.L. (1988) *Smith's Recognizable Patterns of Human Malformation, 4th Edn*. Philadelphia: W.B. Saunders.

Kendall, B.E. (1983) 'Dysgenesis of the corpus callosum.' *Neuroradiology*, **25**, 239–256.

Lacey, D.J. (1985) 'Agenesis of the corpus callosum. Clinical features in 40 children.' *American Journal of Diseases of Children*, **139**, 953–955.

Larsen, P.D., Osborn, A.G. (1982) 'Computed tomographic evaluation of corpus callosum agenesis and associated malformations.' *Journal of Computer Assisted Tomography*, **6**, 225–230.

Lazjuk, G.I., Lurie, I.W., Ostrowskaja, T.I., Cherstvoy, E.D., Kirillova, I.A., Nedzved, M.K., Usoev, S.S. (1979) 'The Neu–Laxova syndrome—a distinct entity.' *American Journal of Medical Genetics*, **3**, 261–267.

Loftus, C.M., Marquardt, M.D., Stein, B.M. (1984) 'Hemangioblastoma of the third ventricle.' *Neurosurgery*, **15**, 67–72.

Lott, I.T., Richardson, E.P. (1981) 'Neuropathological findings and the biology of neurofibromatosis.' *Advances in Neurology*, **29**, 23–32.

95

Louis-Bar, D. (1941) 'Sur un syndrome progressif comprenant des telangectasis capillaries cutanées et conjonctivales symetriques à disposition naevoide et des troubles cérébellaux.' *Confinia Neurologica*, **4**, 32.

McFarlin, D.E., Strober, W., Waldmann, T.A. (1972) 'Ataxia–telangiectasia.' *Medicine*, **51**, 281–314.

McLaurin, R.L., Towbin, R.B. (1985–86) 'Tuberous sclerosis: diagnostic and surgical considerations.' *Pediatric Neuroscience*, **12**, 43–48.

McMurdo, S.K., Moore, S.G., Brant-Zawadzki, M., Berg, B.O., Koch, T., Newton, T.H., Edwards, M.S.B. (1987) 'MR imaging of intracranial tuberous sclerosis.' *American Journal of Roentgenology*, **148**, 791–796.

Miller, G.M., Stears, J.C., Guggenheim, M.A., Wilkening, G.N. (1984) 'Schizencephaly: a clinical and CT study.' *Neurology*, **34**, 997–1001.

Mirowitz, S.A., Sartor, K., Gado, M. (1990) 'High-intensity basal ganglia lesions on T_1-weighted MR images in neurofibromatosis.' *American Journal of Roentgenology*, **154**, 369–373.

Monaghan, H.P., Krafchik, B.R., MacGregor, D.L., Fitz, C.R. (1981) 'Tuberous sclerosis complex in children.' *American Journal of Diseases of Children*, **135**, 912–917.

Morishima, A., Aranoff, G.S. (1986) 'Syndrome of septo-optic-pituitary dysplasia: the clinical spectrum.' *Brain and Development*, **8**, 233–239.

Nagib, M.G., Haines, S.J., Erickson, D.L., Mastri, A.R. (1984) 'Tuberous sclerosis. a review for the neurosurgeon.' *Neurosurgery*, **14**, 93–98.

Naidich, T.P., Zimmerman, R.A. (1987) 'Common congenital malformations of the brain.' *In:* Brandt-Zawadzki, M., Normal, D. (Eds.) *Magnetic Resonance Imaging of the Central Nervous System.* New York: Raven Press, pp. 131–150.

—— McClone, D.G., Bauer, B.S., Kernohan, D.A., Zaparackas, Z.G. (1983*a*) 'Midline craniofacial dysraphism: midline cleft upper lip, basal encephalocele, callosal agenesis, and optic nerve dysplasia.' *Concepts in Pediatric Neurosurgery*, **17**, 961–971.

—— —— Fulling, K.H. (1983*b*) The Chiari II malformation. Part IV. The hindbrain deformity.' *Neuroradiology*, **25**, 179–197.

—— —— Radkowski, M.A. (1986*a*) 'Intracranial arachnoid cysts.' *Pediatric Neuroscience*, **12**, 112–122.

—— Radkowski, M.A., Bernstein, R.A., Tan, W.S. (1986*b*) 'Congenital malformation of the posterior fossa.' *In:* Taveras, J.M., Ferucci, J.T. (Eds.) *Radiology.* Philadelphia: J.B. Lippincott, pp 1–17.

National Institutes of Health Consensus Development Conference. (1988) 'Neurofibromatosis. Conference Statement.' *Archives of Neurology*, **45**, 575–578.

Osborn, R.E., Byrd, S.E. (1988) 'Schizencephaly with optic nerve hypoplasia simulating septo-optic dysplasia and other syndromes.' *Journal of Medical Imaging*, **2**, 240–244.

—— —— Naidich, T.P., Bohan, T.P., Friedman, H. (1988) 'MR imaging of neuronal migrational disorders.' *American Journal of Neuroradiology*, **9**, 1101–1106.

Page, L.K., Brown, S.B., Fargano, P., Shortz, R.W. (1975) 'Schizencephaly: a clinical study and review.' *Child's Brain*, **1**, 348–358.

Paller, A.S. (1987) 'Ataxia–telangiectasia.' *Neurologic Clinics*, **5**, 447–449.

Probst, F.P. (1973) 'Congenital defects of the corpus callosum: morphology and encephalographic appearances.' *Acta Radiologica*, Suppl. 331, 1–152.

Raybaud, C. (1982) 'Cystic malformations of the posterior fossa: abnormalities associated with the development of the roof of the fourth ventricle and adjacent meningeal structures.' *Journal of Neuroradiology*, **9**, 103–133. *(In French.)*

Riccardi, V.M., 'Von Recklinghausen neurofibromatosis.' *New England Journal of Medicine*, **305**, 1617–1627.

Roach, E.S., Williams, D.P., Laster, D.W. (1987) 'Magnetic resonance imaging in tuberous sclerosis.' *Archives of Neurology*, **44**, 301–303.

Russell, E.J., Schaible, T.F., Dillon, W., Drayer, B., LiPuma, J., Mancuso, A., Maravilla, K., Goldstein, H.A. (1989) 'Multicenter double-blind placebo-controlled study of gadopentetate dimeglumine as an MR contrast agent: evaluation in patients with cerebral lesions.' *American Journal of Neuroradiology*, **10**, 53–63.

Sato, Y., Waziri, M., Smith, W., Frey, E., Yuh, W.T.C., Hanson, J., Franken, E.A. (1988) 'Hippel–Lindau disease: MR imaging.' *Radiology*, **166**, 241–246.

Sedgwick, R.P., Boder, E. (1972) 'Ataxia–telangiectasia.' *In:* Vinken, P.J., Bruyn, G.W., (Eds.) *Handbook of Clinical Neurology. Vol 14. The Phakomatoses.* Amsterdam: North Holland, pp. 267–334.

Seizinger, B.R., Martuza, R.L., Gusella, J.F. (1986) 'Loss of genes on chromosome 22 in tumorigenesis of human acoustic neuroma.' *Nature*, **322**, 644–647.

96

Stern, J., Jacobiec, F.A., Housepian, E.M. (1980) 'The architecture of optic nerve gliomas with and without neurofibromatosis.' *Archives of Ophthalmology*, **98**, 505–511.

Stewart, R.M., Richman, D.P., Caviness, V.S.(1975) 'Lissencephaly and pachygyria. An architectonic and topographical analysis.' *Acta Neuropathologica*, **31**, 1–12

Terwey, B., Doose, H. (1987) 'Tuberous sclerosis: magnetic imaging of the brain.' *Neuropediatrics*, **18**, 67–69.

Van der Hoeve, J. (1921) 'Augengeschwülste bei der tuberösen Hirnsklerose (Bourneville)' *Albrecht von Graefe's Archiv für Ophthalmologie*, **105**, 880–898.

—— (1923) 'Augengeschwülste bei der tuberösen Hirnsklerose (Bourneville) und verwandten Krankheiten.' *Albrecht von Graefe's Archiv für Ophthalmologie*, **111**, 1–16.

—— (1933) 'Les phakomatoses de Bourneville, de Recklinghausen et de von Hippel–Lindau.' *Journal Belge de Neurologie et de Psychiatrie*, **33**, 752–762.

Wasenko, J.J., Rosenbloom, S.A., Duchesneau, P.M., Lanzieri, C.F., Weinstein, M.A. (1990) 'The Sturge–Weber syndrome: comparison of MR and CT characteristics.' *American Journal of Neuroradiology*, **11**, 131–134.

Wolpert, S.M., Carter, B.L., Ferris, E.J. (1972) 'Lipomas of the corpus callosum. An angiographic analysis.' *American Journal of Roentgenology*, **115**, 92–99.

Yakovlev, P.I. (1959) 'Pathoarchitectonic studies of cerebral malformations. III. Arrhinencephalies (holotelen-cephalies).' *Journal of Neuropathology and Experimental Neurology*, **18**, 22–55.

—— Guthrie, R.H. 'Congenital ectodermoses (neurocutaneous syndromes) in epileptic patients.' *Archives of Neurology and Psychiatry*, **26**, 1145–1194.

—— Wadsworth, R.C. (1946*a*) 'Schizencephalies. A study of the congenital clefts in the cerebral mantle. I. Clefts with fused lips.' *Journal of Neuropathology and Experimental Neurology*, **5**, 116–130.

—— —— (1946*b*) 'Schizencephalies. A study of the congenital clefts in the cerebral mantle. II. Clefts with hydrocephalus and lips separated.' *Journal of Neuropathology and Experimental Neurology*, **5**, 169–206.

Zaias, B., Becker, D. (1978) 'Septo-optic dysplasia: developmental or acquired abnormality? A case report.' *Transactions of the American Neurological Association*, **103**, 273–277.

Zimmerman, R.A., Bilaniuk, L.T., Grossman, R.I. (1983) 'Computed tomography in migratory disorders of human brain development.' *Neuroradiology*, **25**, 257–263.

5
TRAUMA

Michele H. Johnson and Eric N. Faerber

Trauma is the leading cause of death in children over 1 year of age. The incidence of injury related fatalities is twice that of deaths from childhood cancer and congenital malformations combined (Baker *et al.* 1984). Head trauma in infants and children may occur in the neonatal period due to birth trauma or result from accidental injuries or abuse (non-accidental trauma). Early surgical and medical intervention, facilitated by early intracranial imaging, has resulted in significant improvement in patient outcome (Saul and Ducker 1980, McCort 1987).

Ultrasound and computed tomography (CT) are the preferred imaging modalities for the evaluation of birth trauma, and CT for the immediate post-injury period because the scans can be rapidly obtained and life support systems and monitors can be safely used (Barkovich 1990).

The advent of CT revolutionized the care of patients with acute craniocerebral trauma, providing rapid, non-invasive evaluation of critically ill patients. Zimmerman *et al.* (1978c) reported lowered morbidity and mortality in their patients studied by CT, as compared to patients evaluated in the pre-CT period. They found the need for skull X-ray was reduced by 24 per cent, for angiography by 84 per cent, and for surgical intervention by 58 per cent.

CT facilitates earlier detection of many extracerebral hematomas, often while patients are still conscious. This is the period during which surgical evacuation results in the least morbidity and mortality (Miller *et al.* 1988, Servadei *et al.* 1988).

Magnetic resonance imaging (MRI) is particularly useful in the evaluation of head injury during the subacute and chronic phases of recovery. At this time, demonstration of hemorrhagic and non-hemorrhagic contusions, diffuse axonal injury and small extra-axial hematomas may correlate with clinical symptomatology better than CT (Zimmerman *et al.* 1986, Gentry *et al.* 1988a,b, Hesselink *et al.* 1988). The multiplanar capability of MRI is particularly useful in the anatomic localization of lesions. For example, subdural hematomas in subtemporal locations that may be missed on CT may be readily detected by MRI in the coronal plane. MRI also has special advantages over CT in cases of child abuse, as discussed below.

Technical considerations

Magnetic resonance images should be obtained in at least two imaging planes using T_1- and T_2-weighted imaging sequences, with or without gradient echo (GRE) imaging. This allows for accurate lesion detection and temporal staging of hemorrhagic lesions (Gomori *et al.* 1985, Gentry *et al.* 1988a). A standard protocol includes sagittal and axial T_1-

weighted images and axial T_2-weighted images (Mark 1989). The sagittal images are particularly useful in demonstrating injuries to the corpus callosum, suprasellar region and craniocerebral junction, while the T_2-weighted images are extremely sensitive for the majority of traumatic lesions. Coronal images are ideal for detection of abnormalities in the temporal and subfrontal regions. Short flip angle GRE images may be included in the protocol, because of the increased sensitivity to magnetic susceptibility effects, thus enhancing the detection of hemorrhagic lesions (Atlas *et al.* 1988, Mark 1989).

Mechanisms of head trauma

Blunt cerebral injury results from a direct blow to the head as in a motor vehicle accident, an assault, or a fall to a hard surface. Such injuries frequently result in skull fractures, sometimes depressed, with or without associated skin laceration. Contusions, intraparenchymal hematomas, and/or extra-axial collections may occur intracranially near the site of injury. In addition, extra-axial sequelae may occur on the side of the head contralateral to the point of impact (contrecoup injuries).

Closed head injury implies cerebral injury without skull fracture. Rotational forces, particularly those involving rapid acceleration and deceleration, have been proposed as mechanisms for significant cerebral injury in many of these cases. When the brain suffers extreme acceleration/deceleration or other severe rotational forces, the brain lags behind the skull in its motion. Based on an experimental model, Gennarelli and Thibault (1982) proposed such a mechanism for subdural hematoma development. Diffuse axonal injury (axonal disruption, shearing injury) results from these forces, and manifests as petechial hemorrhages and diffuse cerebral swelling. The junctures between grey and white matter are stressed and stretched, causing disruption of axons. Axonal disruption also occurs in the deep white matter where long axonal fibers are subject to injury, *e.g.* the corpus callosum (Gurdjian 1972, Zimmerman *et al.* 1978*a,b*).

Extra-axial processes

Epidural hematomas

Epidural hematomas (EDHs) occur within the potential space existing between the inner table of the skull and the dura. These two structures are normally tightly adherent from suture to suture, thus epidural collections have a lenticular configuration. EDH in children most commonly results from tears in dural veins, rather than from laceration of the middle meningeal artery, which is more frequently seen in adults (Zimmerman and Danziger 1982, Menkes 1985). The acute arterial EDH creates a sharply marginated, biconvex collection with mass effect upon the underlying brain parenchyma. In children, the clinical course often takes longer to evolve than in adults. The child may appear stunned without manifesting the adult pattern of rapid neurologic deterioration (Menkes 1985).

EDHs in the posterior fossa constitute only 4–13 per cent of all EDHs, and are seen more commonly in children. They may produce critical mass effect upon posterior fossa structures (Garza-Mercado 1983, Ammirati and Tomita 1984). Despite their relative rarity, they represent 25–38 per cent of posterior fossa traumatic injuries. In the majority

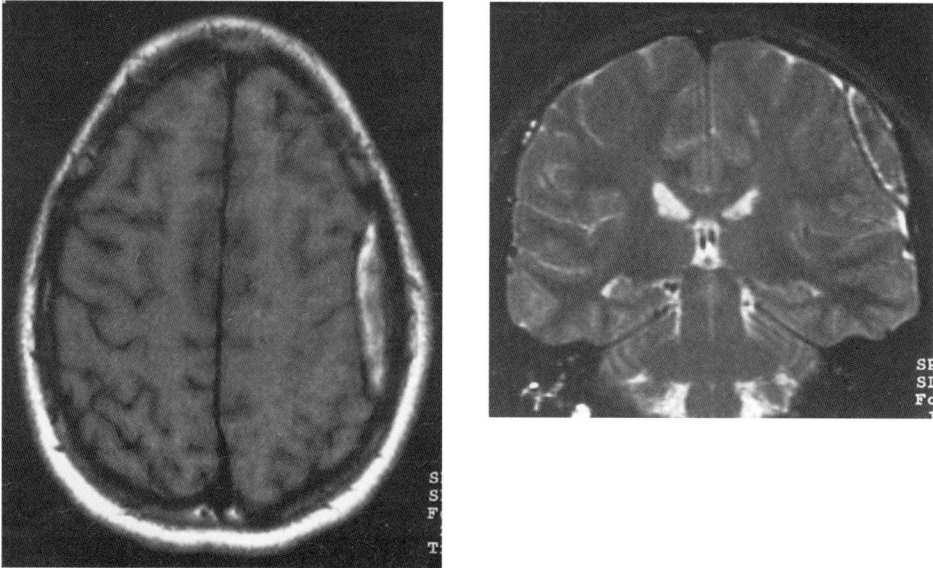

Fig. 5.1. Epidural hematoma. *(Left)* Axial T_1-weighted MRI shows a high signal epidural hematoma with mild mass effect on the subjacent brain. *(Right)* Coronal T_2-weighted image shows a low signal intensity acute epidural hematoma with low signal medially in the expected location of a dural membrane.

of cases, a typical lenticular-shaped EDH is seen, usually associated with occipital fracture (Garza-Mercado 1983, Ammirati and Tomita 1984). Garza-Mercado (1983) divided posterior fossa EDH into three categories: acute (less than 24 hours); subacute (majority); and chronic (more than 10 days). The source of bleeding in posterior fossa EDH may be emissary veins or dural venous sinuses. Bleeding directly from the diploic space has also been implicated. Venous EDHs usually result from a tear in a dural venous sinus. EDH arising from a laceration of the superior sagittal sinus appears as a bi-lentiform hematoma, lying between the falx and the calvarium at the vertex. Transverse sinus rupture may result in both supra- and infratentorial venous EDH. Asymptomatic children, as well as those with minimal symptoms, may sometimes be managed expectantly (without surgery). Complete resolution of the hematoma may occur over time.

EDHs may, less commonly, present hours to days after head injury (delayed EDH) (Cooper *et al.* 1979, Fukamachi *et al.* 1984, Reale and Biancotti 1985). In a series of 22 cases of EDH, Fukamachi *et al.* (1984) found that 18 patients had skull fractures at the site of the delayed EDH. In 16 of these 22 patients, the development of delayed EDH was preceded by surgery for decompression of another intra- or extra-axial process. The reduction in the tamponade effect caused by removal of the initial surgical lesion has been suggested as the etiology of these delayed EDHs (Cooper and Ho 1983, Fukamachi *et al.* 1984).

The imaging appearance of EDHs is identical in both children and adults. On non-contrast CT, the typical EDH is a biconvex, extra-axial mass of increased density which

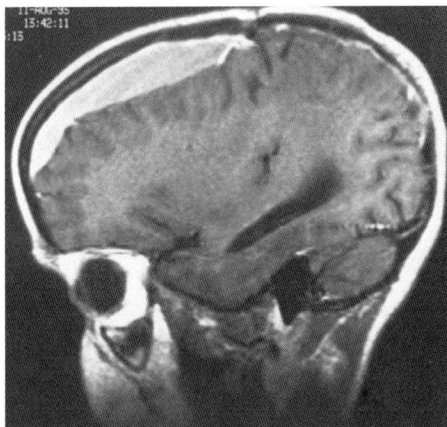

Fig. 5.2. Subdural hematoma. Sagittal T_1-weighted MRI to the left of midline reveals a hyperintense subdural collection causing effacement of the cortical sulci and mass effect upon the brain.

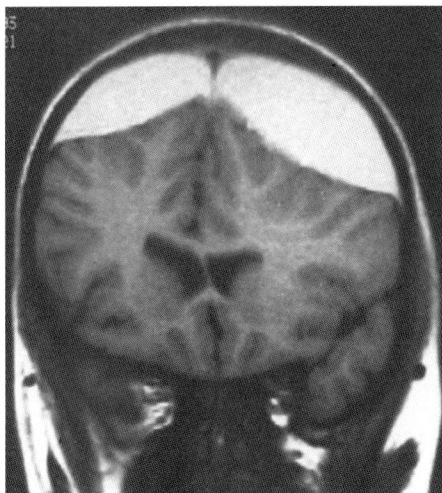

Fig. 5.3. Bilateral parafalcine subdural hematoma. Coronal T_1-weighted MRI illustrates bilateral subacute parafalcine subdural collections. Note the prominent mass effect upon both cerebral hemispheres.

displaces the gray–white matter interface away from the overlying calvarium. There is uniform high density in two-thirds of acute EDHs; the remaining one-third of EDHs are mixed density lesions, related to the presence of acute unclotted blood (Osborne 1994).

On MRI, the acute EDH may be isointense on T_1-weighted images and hypointense on T_2-weighted images (Fig. 5.1). In the early subacute stage, EDHs are hyperintense on T_1-weighted images and hyperintense with central hypointensity on T_2-weighted images. Hematomas between two and four weeks old are hyperintense on both T_1- and T_2-weighted images. Chronic hematomas are iso- to hypointense on T_1-weighted images and hyperintense on T_2-weighted images. The dural membrane may be apparent as a line of low signal intensity between the hematoma and the brain (Fig. 5.1).

Subdural hematomas
Subdural hematomas (SDHs) occur within the potential space between the dura and arachnoid membranes (Fig. 5.2). SDH most commonly extends over the cerebral convexity and may extend into the interhemispheric fissure on the ipsilateral side of the falx. This subdural potential space also exists on both sides of the tentorium. One third of acute and subacute SDHs occur as contracoup lesions (contralateral to the site of the injury) (Lanksch *et al.* 1979). In adults, traumatic SDH is usually unilateral, while SDHs in infants are bilateral in 80–85 per cent (Barkovich 1990).

SDH usually results from venous bleeding secondary to laceration of bridging veins or the wall of a dural venous sinus. Rarely, it may originate from rupture of a paren-

101

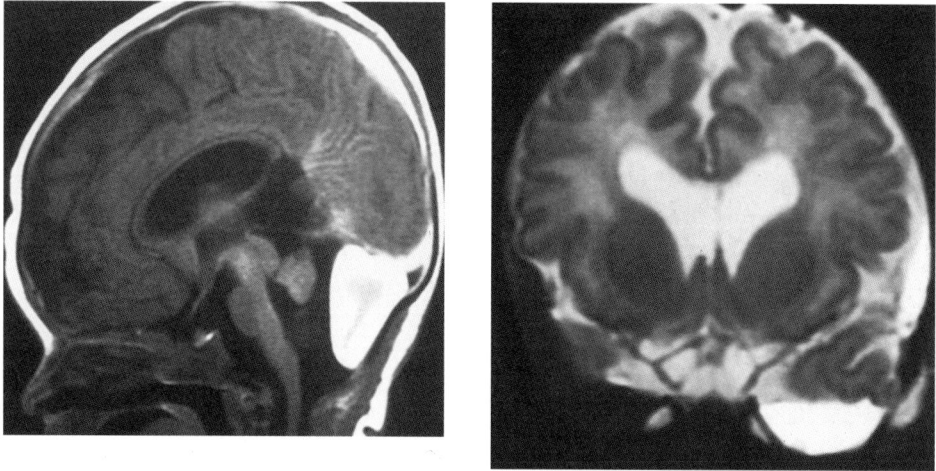

Fig. 5.4. Birth trauma with subdural hematoma (SDH). Sagittal *(left)* and coronal *(right)* T$_1$-weighted images depict a large posterior fossa SDH which extends into the subdural space under the left temporal lobe and over the left cerebral convexity.

chymal artery. 95 per cent of acute SDHs in the series of Forbes *et al.* (1978) were associated with significant mass effect upon the lateral ventricles. The patient with bilateral 'balanced' SDH is an exception to this usual pattern of ventricular compression and midline shift. Unilateral SDH may cause lesser degrees of mass effect when there is underlying parenchymal volume loss (Tomaszek *et al.* 1983).

Interhemispheric SDHs are usually unilateral and are produced by bleeding from bridging veins between the superior sagittal sinus and the parieto-occipital cortex. This is the most common site for SDH in children, in whom the morbidity is greater than that in adults (Cronin and Shippey 1987). The bridging parieto-occipital veins are particularly subject to damage associated with the shaking injury, typically occurring in non-accidental trauma. The interhemispheric SDH has a straight medial border and a convex lateral border, and displaces the brain parenchyma away from the midline (Ho *et al.* 1977). The two interhemispheric subdural spaces do not communicate across the midline due to the firm attachment of the falx to the inferior sagittal sinus; however, bilateral interhemispheric SDH may occur in children (Fig. 5.3). Thus, bilateral interhemispheric collections are rare in adults, usually occurring only following penetrating trauma with falx laceration (Cronin and Shippey 1987). Inferior extension of SDH along the tentorium is not uncommon. Interhemispheric and convexity SDHs may co-exist (Zimmerman and Danziger 1982) (Fig. 5.4).

The CT and MRI appearances of SDHs depend on the age and the subsequent organization of the hematoma.

On CT, although the typical acute SDH is uniformly hyperdense at the time of presentation, variations in appearance can be seen (Scotti *et al.* 1977, Zimmerman and

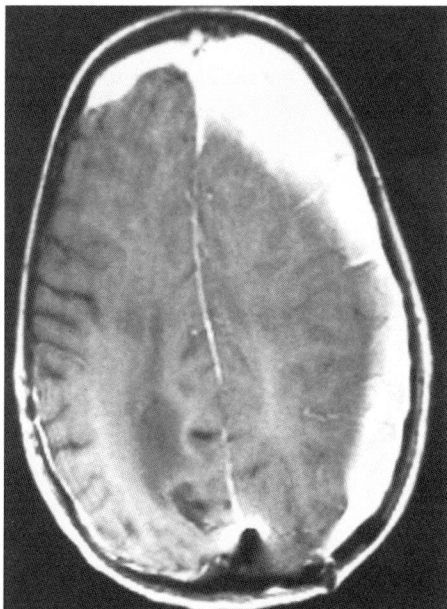

Fig. 5.5. Bilateral subacute subdural hematoma (SDH). Axial T_1-weighted image demonstrates bilateral subacute SDH. Note the greater mass effect from the larger left SDH.

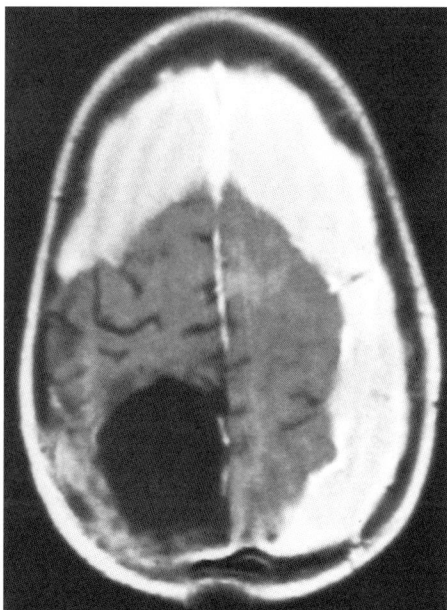

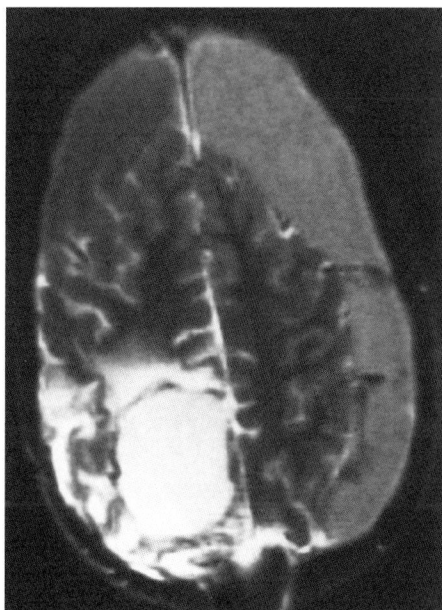

Fig. 5.6. Bilateral subdural hematoma (SDH) following removal of a parafalcine meningioma. *(Left)* Axial T_1-weighted image demonstrates the large frontoparietal left SDH and the similar right frontal SDH. A post-surgical cavity is seen. *(Right)* Axial T_2-weighted image demonstrates a large left SDH, intermediate in signal intensity. A low signal intensity right SDH is identified. High signal, similar to that of CSF, is seen within the postoperative cavity.

Danziger 1982). Inhomogeneity within acute SDHs, similar to that described for acute EDHs, may be seen in the presence of whole unclotted blood (Zimmerman and Bilaniuk 1981). Layering of clot within an acute SDH may be associated with rebleeding into a chronic SDH, usually producing a marginal (laminar) pattern of layering. When there are variations in the time of clot formation within a hematoma, gravitational layering may occur. With gravitational layering, the more dense portions of the collection rest at the bottom, with those of lesser density resting on top.

During the first several days post-injury, the SDH initially becomes hyperdense, due to loss of water within the clot and clot retraction. Subsequently, the SDH becomes increasingly hypodense. The density of the hematoma correlates with its hematocrit. An acute SDH may be almost isodense with adjacent brain when the hemoglobin concentration approaches 8–10g/dL (Boyko et al. 1991, Stein et al. 1992).

In the subacute phase, the SDH becomes isodense with surrounding brain within days to weeks after injury (Wilms et al. 1992). Following contrast administration, displacement of cortical vessels or a subdural membrane may be demonstrated. Features that assist in the diagnosis of isodense SDH are failure of surface sulci to reach the inner calvarial table, displacement of the gray–white matter interface, and comparison of the extra-axial fluid collection to the density of underlying gray and white matter (Osborne 1994). Chronic SDHs are hypodense, approaching CSF density, and may be either crescentic or lentiform in shape.

On MRI, SDHs are usually crescentic in shape, although unusual configurations may occur in patients with previous injury or infection, due to the presence of fibrous bands or septation. The appearance of SDH on MRI changes over time depending upon the stage of the hematoma. The evolution of SDH is somewhat similar to that of intracerebral hemorrhage, although hemosiderin is rarely found within a chronic SDH. This is due to two factors, the absence of a blood–brain barrier and the rapid clearance of blood products by dilution (Fobben et al. 1989). In the hyperacute stage, the collection is isointense on T_1-weighted images and iso- to hyperintense on T_2-weighted images. Thereafter, in the acute stage (<2 weeks), the collection is either iso- or moderately hyperintense on T_2-weighted images. The subacute (2–4 weeks) collection is hyperintense on both T_1- and T_2-weighted images (Fig. 5.5). In the chronic stage (>4 weeks), one third of cases are iso- or hypointense on T_1-weighted images and mostly hyperintense on T_2-weighted images (Hosoda et al. 1987, Osborne 1994) (Fig. 5.6).

Subarachnoid hemorrhage

The most common cause of subarachnoid hemorrhage (SAH) is craniocerebral trauma. SAH is ubiquitous in trauma, even if it is not a prominent feature clinically or on CT (Johnson and Lee 1992). CT is more sensitive than MRI in the demonstration of acute SAH (Bradley and Schmidt 1985) (Fig. 5.7). SAH on non-contrast CT manifests as high density fluid within the cisterns, sulci and interhemispheric fissure. A low signal intensity area corresponding to pial or subpial hemosiderin may occasionally be seen at the site of previous SAH on follow-up MRI scans after trauma (Gomori et al. 1985). Subacute SAH may occasionally be identified as hyperintensity on T_1-weighted images.

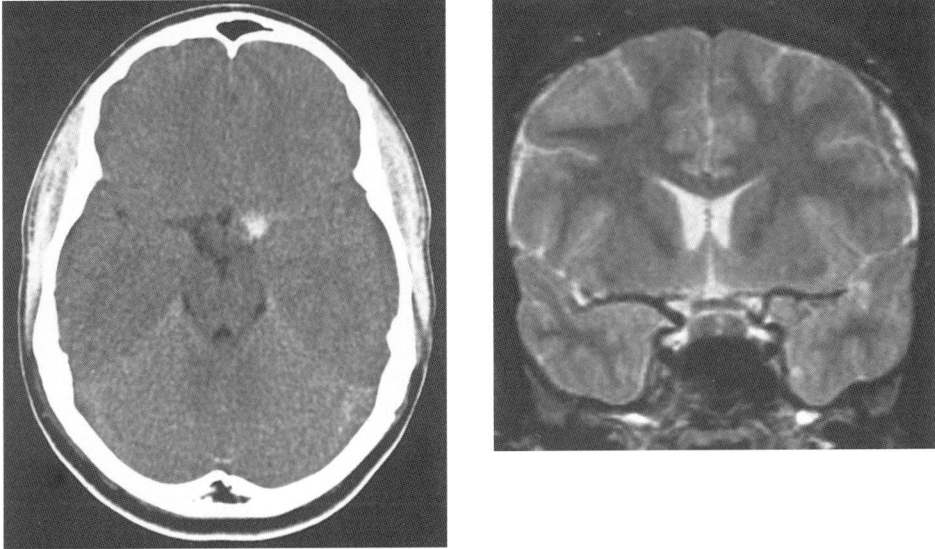

Fig. 5.7. Subarachnoid hemorrhage (SAH). Axial non-contrast enhanced CT *(left)* reveals focal SAH in the suprasellar cistern, not visible on T$_2$-weighted image *(right)*.

Intra-axial processes
Edema and mass effect
Diffuse cerebral edema occurs in 10–20 per cent of serious brain injuries, and is twice as common in children as in adults (Aldrich *et al.* 1992). By definition, the presence of edema connotes increased brain water. Edema within a single hemisphere may result from brain compression secondary to an extra-axial collection. Focal patterns of edema may accompany intraparenchymal hematomas, brain contusions and shear injury. The primary parenchymal or extra-axial lesions, and the associated edema and mass effect, lead to elevations in intracranial pressure (Kishore *et al.* 1981).

On both CT and MRI, edema results in decreased differentiation between gray and white matter, effacement of cortical sulci, and compression of brain parenchyma and/or cerebral ventricles (Barkovich 1990). Partial or complete obliteration of the basal cisterns on initial CT scans positively correlates with increased intracranial pressure, and thus is a potent predictor of outcome in patients with severe closed head injury (Toutant *et al.* 1984). In Toutant's series, a poor outcome was experienced in 44 per cent of patients with normal cisterns, 64 per cent of those with partially obliterated cisterns, and 85 per cent of those with completely obliterated cisterns (Tomaszek *et al.* 1983).

Contusions
Brain contusions are parenchymal lacerations with hemorrhage, which may occur by direct impact or by contrecoup mechanisms (Lindenberg and Freytag 1960). On CT, 'bland contusions' generally have a lower Hounsfield number than normal brain (Koo

105

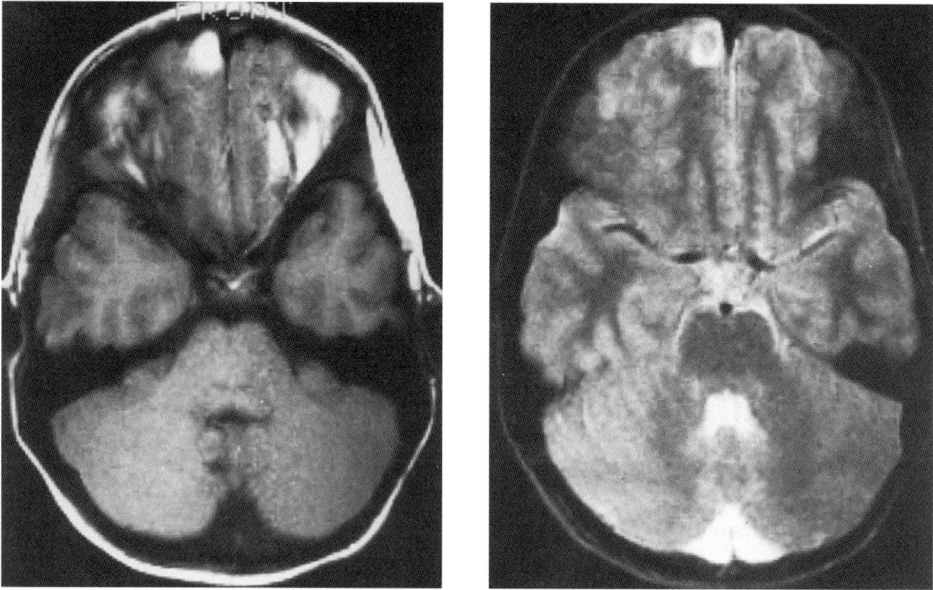

Fig. 5.8. Cerebral contusion. This typical contusion of the right frontal pole demonstrates high signal intensity on the T$_1$-weighted image *(left)* and high signal intensity with central low intensity on the T$_2$-weighted image *(right)*.

and Laroque 1977). These areas are often irregular, patchy, or may be only vaguely coalescent at the time of the initial examination. Contusions may also be associated with diffuse brain edema. The edema associated with parenchymal contusions typically begins about 24 hours after injury, steadily increases over the next seven days, and subsequently slowly resolves (Ito *et al.* 1986). Lesions are usually cortical or near the grey–white matter junction, occurring where a concussive force has impacted the brain parenchyma against the skull. A contusion is particularly likely to result from a depressed skull fracture (Weisberg 1979). Contusions are most commonly located at the frontal or temporal poles, or the inferior frontal lobes (Hryshko and Deeb 1983, Hesselink *et al.* 1988). The temporal lobe is involved in almost 50 per cent of cases, most frequently at the temporal tip (Osborne 1994).

The imaging appearance of cerebral contusions evolves with time (Osborne 1994). As previously indicated, the initial CT findings may be normal or subtly abnormal, with the subsequent appearance of patchy, ill-defined frontal or temporal low density lesions (Hesselink *et al.* 1988, Osborne 1994). Delayed hemorrhages may develop in previously non-hemorrhagic hypodense regions (Gentry *et al.* 1988*b*).

MRI is considerably more sensitive than CT for the detection of cerebral contusions, especially in the subacute stage (Gentry *et al.* 1988*a*, Kelly *et al.* 1988) (Fig. 5.8). The lesions are often of mixed signal intensity on T$_1$- and T$_2$-weighted images because of hemorrhagic components, and appear hyperintense on T$_2$-weighted images.

106

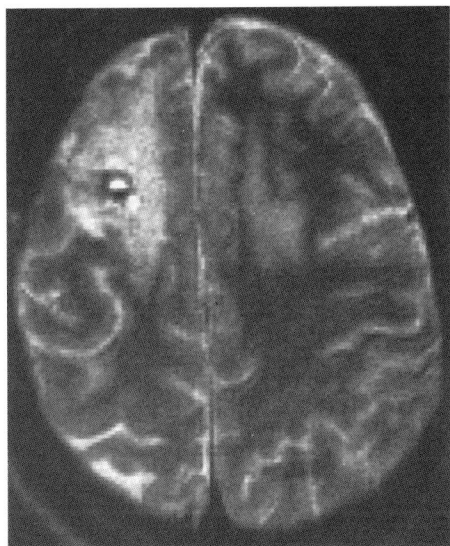

Fig. 5.9. Parenchymal hematoma. Axial T$_2$-weighted MRI reveals a right parenchymal hematoma of high signal intensity with a peripheral rim of low signal intensity. Focal edema is present in the left frontal lobe.

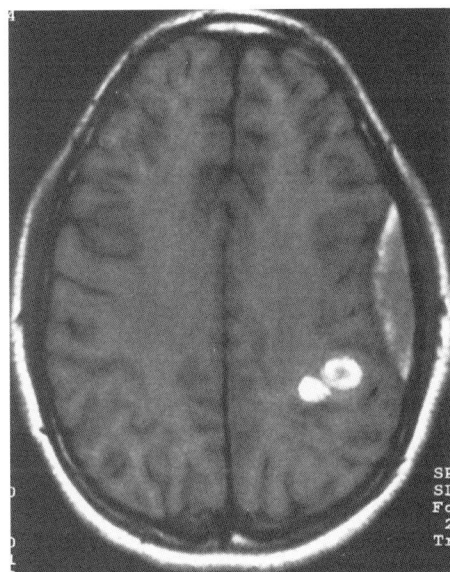

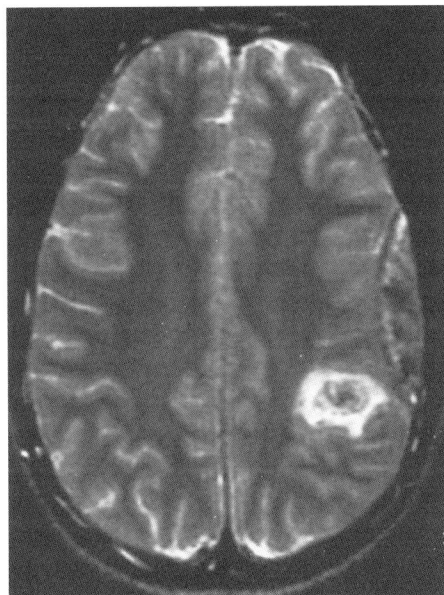

Fig. 5.10. Parenchymal hematoma and extradural hematoma (EDH). *(Left)* Axial T$_1$-weighted image shows the low signal EDH with medial high signal and the parenchymal hemorrhage with high peripheral signal and central hypodensity. *(Right)* Axial T$_2$-weighted image shows the EDH as low signal intensity. The parenchymal hematoma is of low signal intensity centrally with surrounding high signal intensity.

Intraparenchymal hematomas

Intraparenchymal hematomas are uncommon complications of trauma in infants and children, and occur three times more frequently in adults (Zimmerman and Bilaniuk 1981). Temporal and frontal hematomas are most common (Fig. 5.9). Hematomas in neonates are frequently located subcortically and are less common than surface contusions at this stage (McLaurin and Towbin 1989). The signal intensity of intracerebral hematomas is similar to that of extracerebral hematomas, with the exception that hemosiderin deposits may be identified in chronic hematomas (Hesselink *et al.* 1988) (Fig. 5.10).

Cerebral infarction

Cerebral infarction is a well-recognized complication of craniocerebral trauma. The exact frequency with which infarction occurs in children following craniocerebral trauma has not been well documented, but Mirvis *et al.* (1990) found it in 1.9 per cent of neurotrauma patients of all ages. Infarction may ensue directly from vascular injury, or may occur secondary to vascular compression resulting from herniation. Occlusion and dissection are the most common vascular injuries resulting from head trauma. In the majority of cases in this series, gross mechanical shift of the brain with subfalcine or transtentorial herniation accounted for the infarctions, which were mostly in the anterior or posterior cerebral vascular territories. Occipital lobe infarction is the most common, caused by compression of the posterior cerebral artery against the rigid tentorial edge by the herniating medial temporal lobe (Sato *et al.* 1986). The CT and MRI appearances of infarction are identical to those of infarction from any other etiology. These appearances are described in Chapter 7.

Diffuse axonal injury

Diffuse axonal injury (DAI), or shear injury, represents a significant part of the spectrum of brain injury in infants and children, particularly in the patient presenting with coma following head injury. Acute axonal injury results from rapid acceleration/deceleration forces which pull white matter fibers apart, resulting in petechial hemorrhages. These are identified as tiny focal areas of hemorrhage in a field of edema. DAI is found predominately in three areas, the corpus callosum, the lobar white matter (especially at the gray–white matter interface), and the contralateral aspect of the upper brainstem (Gentry 1991).

Frequently the initial CT scan is normal in comatose patients following severe head trauma (Zimmerman 1978*c*). Subsequent CT scans may demonstrate bilateral cerebral edema with cisternal and ventricular compression, without identifiable mass lesion to explain the presence of the edema (Zimmerman 1978*a*). SAH and hemorrhages within the corpus callosum and/or other periventricular white matter zones may be seen (Zimmerman *et al.* 1978*b*, Gentry 1992). The identification of DAI in the acute trauma patient portends a grim prognosis (Zimmerman 1987*a,b,c*). Non-hemorrhagic shear injury is almost impossible to identify on CT, although a follow-up CT may occasionally demonstrate low density lesions in areas of injured parenchyma.

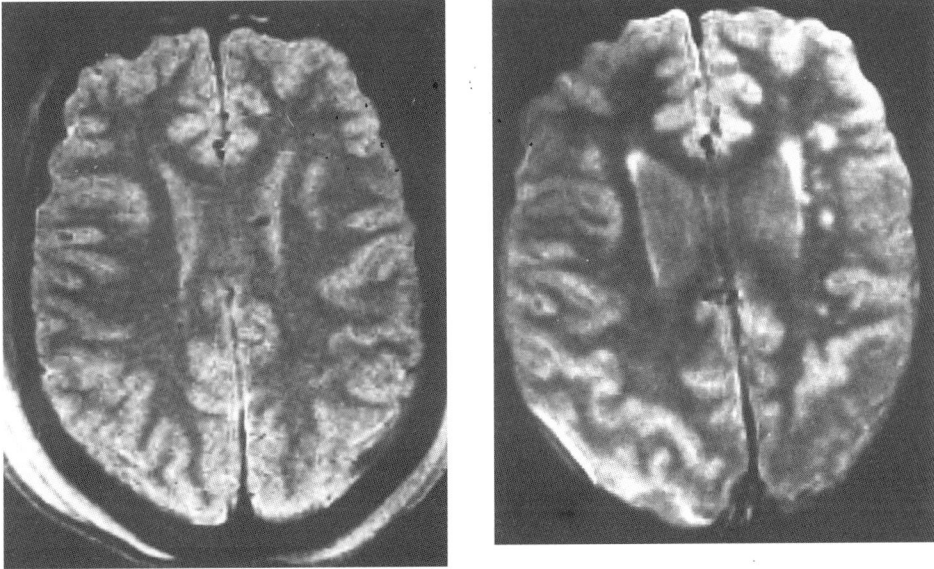

Fig. 5.11. Shear injury. *(a)* Initial axial T$_2$-weighted image demonstrates normal sized ventricles and normal brain parenchyma in this patient with closed head injury. *(b)* Follow-up axial T$_2$-weighted image, three weeks later, demonstrates multiple lesions typical of shear injury.

MRI is superior to CT for the diagnosis of non-hemorrhagic shear injury (Gentry 1988*a,b*, 1989). T$_1$-weighted images often appear normal. The most common abnormality on T$_2$-weighted images is the presence of multiple hyperintense foci at the gray–white matter interface or within the corpus callosum (Osborne 1994). MRI is especially valuable when there is significant disparity between the patient's clinical state and the CT image. MRI may demonstrate lesions not visible on CT. MRI is also useful for follow-up of DAI as a part of the assessment of patient prognosis (Levin *et al.* 1985, 1987; Gentry 1988*a,b*; Kelly *et al.* 1988). Occasionally, the initial MRI may be normal, yet the follow-up scan demonstrates multiple lesions resulting from DAI (Fig. 5.11).

Non-accidental craniocerebral trauma (child abuse)
Child abuse and neglect is an ever increasing problem with profound medical, moral and legal implications. Over half a million pediatric cases of physical abuse per annum have been reported (American Humane Association 1982). Although this condition was first recognized by Tardier in 1860, the pioneering radiologic findings by Caffey (1946), Silverman (1953), who introduced the term 'battered child', and Kempe *et al.* (1961), have produced a marked medical and social impact.

Head trauma constitutes the leading cause of morbidity and mortality in the abused child. In a review of infants under 1 year of age hospitalized for head trauma, 64 per cent of all head injuries and 95 per cent of significant intracranial injuries were due to abuse (Billmire and Myers 1985).

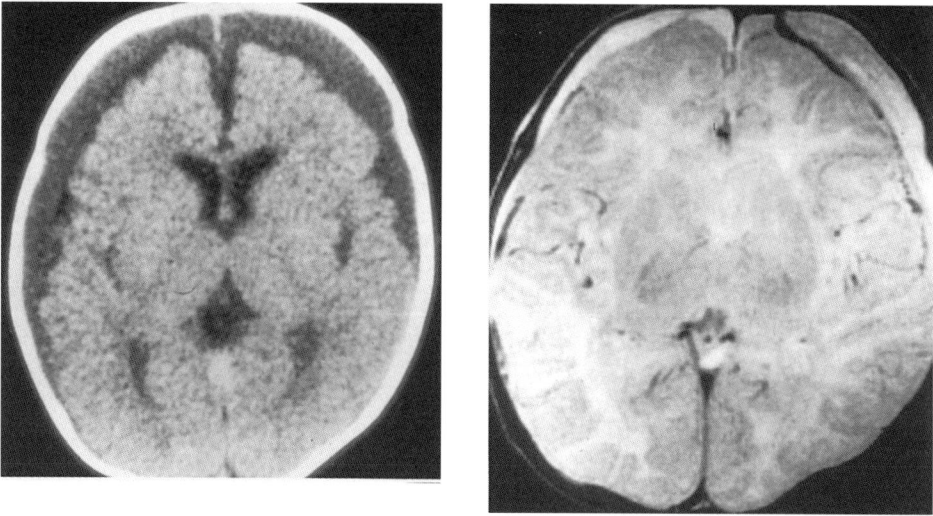

Fig. 5.12. Non-accidental craniocerebral trauma. *(a)* Axial non-contrast-enhanced CT demonstrates bilateral chronic subdural collections. *(b)* Axial T$_1$-weighted image reveals these collections to be in differing stages of hemoglobin degradation, indicating recurrent injury.

Imaging plays a most important role in the diagnosis of this condition. Unsuspected post-traumatic abnormalities, incidental to the clinical history, should alert the radiologist to the underlying cause. In the original 1946 description by Caffey, subdural hematomas, intraocular hemorrhages and evidence of multiple long fractures were the main features identified. The major craniocerebral abnormalities include skull fractures, extracranial hematomas and intra-axial injuries. Extradural, subdural and intracerebral hematomas are common in violent child abuse and may often coexist (Harwood-Nash 1992). Subdural hematoma is the most common intracranial abnormality in the abused child (Ball 1989, Sato *et al.* 1989). CT can detect most acute and chronic subdural hematomas; however, MRI is superior for identifying subdural collections of varying ages, and for demonstrating small or inferiorly located (subfrontal, subtemporal, tentorial or infratentorial) hematomas (Sato *et al.* 1989) (Fig. 5.12).

DAI may be caused by vigorous shaking as described above. Cerebral contusions are usually accompanied by external bruising or skull fracture and result from a direct blow to the head (Duhaime *et al.* 1987). CT demonstrates these intra-axial injuries, but MRI is superior for characterizing lesions of varying ages and defining their precise locations (Sato *et al.* 1989).

Cerebral ischemia may be unilateral or bilateral, focal or diffuse, and may accompany any of the other manifestations of child abuse.

CT and MRI are both excellent modalities for demonstration of these injuries, although each has specific advantages. The following algorithm has been proposed by Ball (1989).

110

(1) CT is the initial modality of choice for the evaluation of acute head injury in suspected child abuse. It permits superior detection of intracranial hemorrhage and is useful in the evaluation of calvarial injuries. The ease of performance in the unstable child, and the ability to also examine the chest, abdomen and pelvis if clinically warranted, makes CT the optimal choice.

(2) MRI is most valuable when there is a high index of suspicion of child abuse, despite a normal or equivocal CT, or when clinical findings on fluoroscopy or neurologic examination suggest intracranial injury secondary to abuse. The ability to image hematomas in various stages, indicating multiple traumatic incidents, is unique to MRI.

Vascular lesions

A wide spectrum of vascular lesions may follow craniocerebral trauma. These include arterial dissection, laceration, occlusion, arterial pseudoaneurysm, carotid cavernous fistula, and abnormalities of the dural sinuses including laceration and occlusion (Davis and Zimmerman 1983, Goldberg *et al.* 1986).

The role of MRI and magnetic resonance angiography (MRA) in craniocerebral trauma is evolving. MRI shows alterations in the normal luminal flow voids on spin echo sequences in cases of arterial dissection and/or occlusion (Bernardi *et al.* 1993). MRA may demonstrate limited residual or collateral flow in this clinical setting. MRA is potentially useful in the initial assessment of vascular injury, particularly as it can be performed with little additional time commitment during normal imaging.

Brain death

Brain death is the term used for irreversible cessation of global brain function as determined by EEG, with or without arteriography or other imaging correlation (Bernat 1992). The current imaging study of choice is a radionuclide scan using 99^{m}Tc HMPAO.

Brain death has been demonstrated by MRI when there is absence of cerebral blood flow (lack of flow voids) on images obtained using standard and flow-sensitive pulse sequences (Jones and Barnes 1992). Expense and the lack of portability limit the usefulness of MRI in the diagnosis of brain death. Patients on life support systems require MRI compatible equipment and may be difficult to transport to the MRI site. A major limitation of MRI in the diagnosis of brain death is that slow blood flow may simulate complete occlusion, leading to a false-positive diagnosis (Brant-Zawadzki 1990). MRA may prove useful in the future, although similar difficulties may be found (Osborne 1994).

Sequelae of trauma

Clinical and radiographic sequelae of craniocerebral trauma sustained in infancy and childhood are influenced both by brain maturation and plasticity, and by the type of trauma (Bernardi *et al.* 1993).

A wide spectrum of sequelae may ensue, including encephalomalacia, atrophy, hydrocephalus, extracranial collections (hygromas), pneumocephalus and/or pneumatocele formation, CSF leaks and acquired cephalocele or leptomeningeal cyst, cranial nerve injury and diabetes insipidus (Bernardi *et al.* 1993, Osborne 1994). MRI is most useful

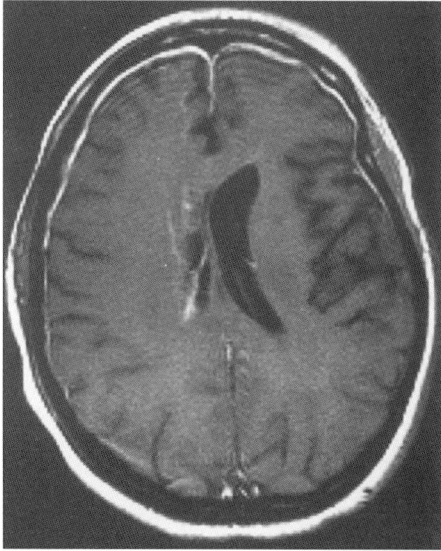

Fig. 5.13. Atrophy following head trauma. Axial, contrast enhanced T₁-weighted image demonstrates small bilateral subdural collections. There is *ex vacuo* dilatation of the left lateral ventricle and atrophy in the sylvian region, two months after head injury and evacuation of the subdural hematoma.

for imaging the wide range of post-traumatic sequelae and has a better correlation with clinical patient status than does CT (Levin *et al.* 1987) (Fig. 5.13).

Conclusion

MRI is important in the evaluation of children with traumatic cerebral injury. In acute injury, and in the case of suspected non-accidental trauma, assessment of extracerebral and parenchymal hemorrhages is facilitated by the unique imaging features of hematomas on MRI. MRI may provide diagnostic and prognostic information when employed for the evaluation of post-traumatic brain injury, thus facilitating patient management.

REFERENCES

Aldrich, E.F., Eisenberg, H.M., Saydjari, C., Luerssen, T.G., Foulkes, M.A., Jane, J.A., Marshall, L.F., Marmarov, A., Young, H.E. (1992) 'Diffuse brain swelling: severely head injured children. A report from the NIH Traumatic Coma Data Bank.' *Journal of Neurosurgery*, **76**, 450–454.

American Humane Association, Child Protection Division (1982) *National Analysis of Official Child Neglect and Abuse Reporting 1982.* Denver: American Humane Association.

Ammirati, M., Tomita, T. (1984) 'Posterior fossa epidural hematoma during childhood.' *Neurosurgery*, **14**, 541–544.

Atlas, S.W., Mark, A.S., Grossman, R.I., Gomori, J.M. (1988) 'Intracranial hemorrhage: gradient-echo MR imaging at 1.5T: comparison with spin-echo imaging and clinical applications.' *Radiology*, **168**, 803–807.

Baker, S.P., O'Neill, B., Karpf, R.S. (1984) *The Injury Fact Book.* Lexington, KY: Lexington Books.

Barkovich, A.J. (1990) *Pediatric Neuroimaging.* New York: Raven Press.

Ball, W.S. (1989) 'Nonaccidental craniocerebral trauma (child abuse): MR imaging.' *Radiology*, **173**, 609–610.

Bernardi, B., Zimmerman, R.A., Bilaniuk, L.T. (1993) 'Neuroradiologic evaluation of pediatric craniocerebral trauma.' *Topics in Magnetic Resonance Imaging*, **5**, 161–173.

Bernat, J.L. (1992) 'Brain death. Occurs only with destruction of the cerebral hemispheres and the brain stem.' *Archives of Neurology*, **49**, 569–570.

Billmire, M.E., Myers, P.A. (1985) 'Serious head injury in infants: accident or abuse?' *Pediatrics*, **75**, 340–342.

Boyko, O.B., Cooper, D.F., Grossman, C.B. (1991) 'Contrast-enhanced CT of acute isodense subdural hematoma.' *American Journal of Neuroradiology*, **12**, 341–343.

Bradley, W.G., Schmidt, P.G. (1985) 'Effect of methemoglobin formation on the MR appearance of subarachnoid hemorrhage.' *Radiology*, **156**, 99–103.

Brant-Zawadzki, M. (1990) 'Routine MR imaging of the internal carotid artery siphon: angiographic correlation with cervical carotid lesions.' *American Journal of Neuroradiology*, **11**, 467–471.

Caffey, J. (1946) 'Multiple fractures in the long bones of infants suffering from chronic subdural hematoma.' *American Journal of Roentgenology*, **56**, 163–173.

Cooper, P.R., Ho, V. (1983) 'Role of emergency skull x-ray films in the evaluation of the head-injured patient: a retrospective study.' *Neurosurgery*, **13**, 136–140.

—— Maravilla, K., Moody, S., Clark, W.K. (1979) 'Serial computerized tomographic scanning and the prognosis of severe head injury.' *Neurosurgery*, **5**, 566–569.

Cronin, T.G., Shippey, D.U. (1987) 'Bilateral interhemispheric subdural hematoma: a case report.' *American Journal of Neuroradialogy*, **8**, 909–910.

Davis, J.M., Zimmerman, R.A. (1983) 'Injury of the carotid and vertebral arteries.' *Neuroradiology*, **25**, 55–69.

Duhaime, A-C., Gennarelli, T.A., Thibault, L.E., Bruce, D.A., Margulies, S.S., Wiser, R. (1987) 'The shaken baby syndrome. A clinical, pathological and biomechanical study.' *Journal of Neurosurgery*, **66**, 409–415.

Fobben, E.S., Grossman, R.I., Atlas, S.W., Hackney, D.B., Goldberg, H.I., Zimmerman, R.A., Bilaniuk, L.T. (1989) 'MR characteristics of subdural hematomas and hygromas at 1.5 T.' *American Journal of Neuroradiology*, **10**, 687–693.

Forbes, G.S., Sheedy, P.F., Piepgras, D.G., Houser, O.W. (1978) 'Computed tomography in the evaluation of subdural hematomas.' *Radiology*, **126**, 143–148.

Fukamachi, A., Misumi, S., Kaneko, M., Wakao, T. (1984) 'Traumatic extradural hematomas with delayed development.' *Computerized Radiology*, **8**, 197–201.

Garza-Mercado, R. (1983) 'Extradural hematoma of the posterior cranial fossa: report of seven cases with survival.' *Journal of Neurosurgery*, **59**, 664–672.

Gennarelli, T.A., Thibault, L.E. (1982) 'Biomechanics of acute subdural hematoma.' *Journal of Trauma*, **22**, 680–686.

Gentry, L.R. (1992) 'Head trauma.' *In:* Atlas, S.W. (Ed.) *Magnetic Resonance Imaging of the Brain and Spine.* New York: Raven Press, pp. 439–456.

—— Godersky, J.C., Thompson, B. (1988*a*) 'MR imaging of head trauma: review of the distribution and radiopathologic features of traumatic lesions.' *American Journal of Neuroradiology*, **9**, 101–110.

—— —— —— Dunn, V.D. (1988*b*) 'Prospective comparative study of intermediate field MR and CT in the evaluation of closed head trauma.' *American Journal of Neuroradiology*, **9**, 91–100.

—— Thompson B., Godersky, J.C. (1988*c*) 'Trauma to the corpus callosum: MR features.' *American Journal of Neuroradiology*, **9**, 1129–1138.

—— Godersky, J.C., Thompson, B. (1989) 'Traumatic brain stem injury: MR imaging.' *Radiology*, **171**, 177–187.

Goldberg, H.I., Grossman, R.I., Gomori, J.M., Asbury, A.K., Bilaniuk, L.T., Zimmerman, R.A. (1986) 'Cervical internal carotid dissecting hemorrhage: diagnosis using MR.' *Radiology*, **158**, 157–161.

Gomori, J.M., Grossman, R.I., Goldberg, H.I., Zimmerman, R.A., Bilaniuk, L.T. (1985) 'Intracranial hematomas: imaging by high-field MR.' *Radiology*, **157**, 87–93.

Gurdjian, E.S. (1972) 'Recent advances in the study of the mechanism of impact injury of the head—a summary.' *Clinical Neurosurgery*, **19**, 1–42.

Harwood-Nash, D.C. (1992) 'Abuse to the pediatric central nervous system.' *American Journal of Neuroradiology*, **13**, 569–575.

Hesselink, J.R., Dowd, C.F., Healy, M.E., Hajek, P., Baker, L.L., Luerssen, T.G. (1988) 'MR imaging of brain contusions: a comparative study with CT.' *American Journal of Neuroradiology*, **9**, 269–278.

Ho, S.U., Spehlmann, R., Ho, H.T. (1977) 'CT scan in interhemispheric subdural hematoma. Clinical and pathological correlation.' *Neurology*, **27**, 1097–1098.

Hosoda, K., Tamaki, N., Masumura, M., Matsumoto, S., Maeda, F. (1987) 'Magnetic resonance images of chronic subdural hematomas.' *Journal of Neurosurgery*, **67**, 677–683.

Hryshko, F.G., Deeb, Z.L. (1983) 'Computed tomography in acute head injuries.' *Journal of Computed Tomography*, **7**, 331–344.

Ito, U., Tomita, H., Yamazaki, S., Takada, Y., Inaba, Y. (1986) 'Brain swelling and brain oedema in acute head injury.' *Acta Neurochirurgica*, **79**, 120–124.

Johnson, M.H., Lee, S.H. (1992) 'Computed tomography of acute cerebral trauma.' *Radiologic Clinics of North America*, **30**, 325–352.

Jones, K.M., Barnes, P.D. (1992) 'MR diagnosis of brain death.' *American Journal of Neuroradiology*, **13**, 65–66.

Kelly, A.B., Zimmerman, R.D., Snow, R.B., Gandy, S.E., Heier, L.A., Deck, M.D.F. (1988) 'Head trauma: comparison of MR and CT—experience in 100 patients.' *American Journal of Neuroradiology*, **9**, 699–708.

Kempe, C.H., Silverman, F.N., Steele, B.F., Droegemueller, W., Silver, H.K. (1961) 'The battered child syndrome.' *Journal of the American Medical Association*, **181**, 17–24.

Kishore, P.R.S., Lipper, M.H., Becker, D.P., Domingues da Silva, A.A., Narayan, R.K. (1981) 'Significance of CT in head injury: correlation with intracranial pressure.' *American Journal of Roentgenology*, **137**, 829–833.

Koo, A.H., LaRoque, R.L. (1977) 'Evaluation of head trauma by computed tomography.' *Radiology*, **123**, 345–350.

Lanksch, W., Grumme, T.H., Kazner, E. (1979) *Computed Tomography in Head Injuries.* New York: Springer Verlag.

Levin, H.S., Kalisky, Z., Handel, S.F., *et al.* (1985) 'Magnetic resonance imaging in relation to the sequelae and rehabilitation of diffuse closed head injury: preliminary findings.' *Seminars in Neurology*, **5**, 221–232.

—— Amparo, E., Eisenberg, H.M., Williams, D.H., High, W.M., McArdle, C.B., Weiner, R.L. (1987) 'Magnetic resonance imaging and computerized tomography in relation to the neurobehavioral sequelae of mild and moderate head injuries.' *Journal of Neurosurgery*, **66**, 706–713.

Lindenberg, R., Freytag, E. (1960) 'The mechanism of cerebral contusions. A pathologic–anatomic study.' *Archives of Pathology*, **69**, 440–469.

Mark, A.S. (1989) 'MRI in evaluation of cerebral trauma.' *MRI Decisions*, **3**, 26–33.

McCort, J.J. (1987) 'Caring for the major trauma victim: the role for radiology.' *Radiology*, **163**, 1–9.

McLaurin, R.L., Towbin, R. (1989) 'Posttraumatic hematomas.' *In:* McLaurin, R.L., Venes, J.L., Schut, L. (Eds.) *Pediatric Neurosurgery. 2nd Edn.* Philadelphia: WB Saunders, pp. 277–289.

Menkes, J.H. (1985) *Textbook of Child Neurology.* Philadelphia: Lea & Febiger.

Miller, J.D., Tocher, J.L., Jones, P.A. (1988) 'Extradural hematoma—earlier detection, better results.' *Brain Injury*, **2**, 83–86. *(Editorial.)*

Mirvis, S.E., Wolf, A.L., Numaguchi, Y., Corradino, G., Joslyn, J.N. (1990) 'Posttraumatic cerebral infarction diagnosed by CT: prevalence, origin, and outcome.' *American Journal of Neuroradiology*, **11**, 355–360.

Osborne, A.G. (1994) *Diagnostic Radiology.* St Louis: C.V. Mosby.

Reale, F., Biancotti, R. (1985) 'Acute bilateral epidural hematoma.' *Surgical Neurology*, **24**, 260–262.

Sato, M., Tanaka, S., Kohama, A., Fujii, C. (1986) 'Occipital lobe infarction caused by tentorial herniation.' *Neurosurgery*, **18**, 300–305.

Sato, Y, Yuh, W.T.C., Smith, W.L., Alexander, R.C., Kao, S.C.S., Ellerbroek, C.J. (1989) 'Head injury in child abuse: evaluation with MR imaging.' *Radiology*, **173**, 653–657.

Saul, T.G., Ducker, T.B. (1980) 'The role of computed tomography in acute head injury.' *Journal of Computed Tomography*, **4**, 296–308.

Scotti, G., Terbrugge, K., Melançon, D., Bélanger, D. (1977) 'Evaluation of the age of subdural hematomas by computerized tomography.' *Journal of Neurosurgery*, **47**, 311–315.

Servadei, F., Piazza, G., Seracchioli, A., Acciarri, N., Pozzati, E., Gaist, G. (1988) 'Extradural haematomas: an analysis of the changing characteristics of patients admitted from 1980 to 1986. Diagnostic and therapeutic implications in 158 cases.' *Brain Injury*, **2**, 87–100.

Silverman, F.N. (1953) 'The roentgen manifestations of unrecognized skeletal trauma in infants.' *American Journal of Roentgenology*, **69**, 413–427.

Stein, S.C., Young, G.S., Talucci, R.C., Greenbaum, B.H., Ross, S.E. (1992) 'Delayed brain injury after head trauma. Significance of coagulopathy.' *Neurosurgery*, **30**, 160–165.

Tomaszek, D.E., Tyson, G.W., Mahaley, M.S. (1983) 'Unilateral subdural hematoma without midline shift.' *Surgical Neurology*, **20**, 71–73.

Toutant, S.M., Klauber, M.R., Marshall, L.F., Toole, B.M., Bowers, S.A., Seelig, J.M., Varnell, J.B. (1984) 'Absent or compressed basal cisterns on first CT scan: ominous predictors of outcome in severe head injury.' *Journal of Neurosurgery*, **61**, 691–694.

Weisberg, L.A. (1979) 'CT and acute head trauma.' *Computerized Tomography*, **3**, 15–28.

Wilms, G., Marchal, G., Geusens, E., Raaijmakers, C., van Calenbergh, F., Goffin, J., Plets, C. (1992) 'Isodense subdurals on CT: MRI findings.' *Neuroradiology*, **34**, 497–499.

114

Zimmerman, R.A., Bilaniuk, L.T. (1981) 'Computed tomography in pediatric head trauma.' *Journal of Neuroradiology*, **8**, 257–271.
—— Danziger, A. (1982) 'Extracerebral trauma.' *Radiologic Clinics of North America*, **20**, 105–121.
—— Bilaniuk, L.T., Bruce, D., Dolinskas, C., Obrist, W., Kuhl, D. (1978*a*) 'Computed tomography of pediatric head trauma: acute general cerebral swelling.' *Radiology*, **126**, 403–408.
—— —— Gennarelli, T. (1978*b*) 'Computed tomography of shearing injuries of the cerebral white matter.' *Radiology*, **127**, 393–396.
—— —— —— Bruce, D., Dolinskas, C., Uzzell, B. (1978*c*) 'Cranial computed tomography in diagnosis and management of acute head trauma.' *American Journal of Roentgenology*, **131**, 27–34.
—— —— Hackney, D.B., Goldberg, H.I., Grossman, R.I. (1986) 'Head injury: early results of comparing CT and high-field MR.' *American Journal of Neuroradiology*, **7**, 757–764.

115

6
INTRACRANIAL INFECTION

Robin E. Osborn

Intracranial abscess
An abscess is composed of a zone of central liquefaction necrosis surrounded by a collagenous and gliotic capsule. Intracranial abscesses may be parenchymal or within the epidural or subdural space. Abscesses are most commonly caused by pyogenic bacteria, but other bacteria such as *Myobacterium tuberculosis*, *Actinomyces* and *Nocardia* spp. are occasionally involved, as are fungi and parasites (Overturf 1986, Täuber *et al.* 1986, Sze and Zimmerman 1988, Haimes *et al.* 1989, Zimmerman and Haimes 1989, Jungreis and Grossman 1991, Zimmerman and Weingarten 1991).

Clinically, patients with intracranial abscess may present with fever, headache, seizure, focal neurologic findings or behavioral changes. Symptomatology depends on the location of the abscess and the amount of mass effect it elicits.

Pyogenic abscess
PARENCHYMAL ABSCESS
Cerebral abscess usually results from hematogenous spread of infection from another source in the body. The frontal and parietal lobes are most commonly involved. The cerebellum is not a common site. Posterior fossa abscess usually results from mastoid and middle ear infection. Cerebral abscess may result from sepsis, congenital calvarial or heart anomalies, paranasal or mastoid sinus disease, meningitis, trauma or surgery (Overturf 1986, Sze and Zimmerman 1988, Haimes *et al.* 1989, Zimmerman and Haimes 1989, Jungreis and Grossman 1991, Zimmerman and Weingarten 1991).

Cerebral abscess begins as a focal area of cerebritis. This first or early cerebritis stage produces significant degrees of inflammation and vasogenic edema. It is followed by the late cerebritis stage, which begins at about one week. During this second stage the central areas become necrotic and begin to form small cystic areas. The early abscess phase starts at the beginning of the third week. There is progressive encapsulation by a collagenous capsule and liquification of the central area. In the days and weeks that follow, the capsule becomes complete, isolating the infection. The adjacent inflammation outside the capsule then diminishes. This overall response of the brain is to limit the spread of infection and preserve the integrity of the uninfected tissues (Overturf 1986, Täuber *et al.* 1986, Sze and Zimmerman 1988, Haimes *et al.* 1989, Zimmerman and Haimes 1989, Jungreis and Grossman 1991, Zimmerman and Weingarten 1991). It has been noted by Volpe (1987) that abscesses occurring during the neonatal period tend to be relatively large and have a less developed capsule.

Most patients who present with brain abscess are usually first evaluated radio-

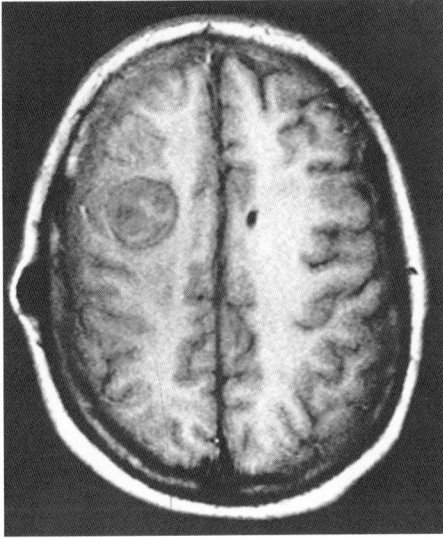

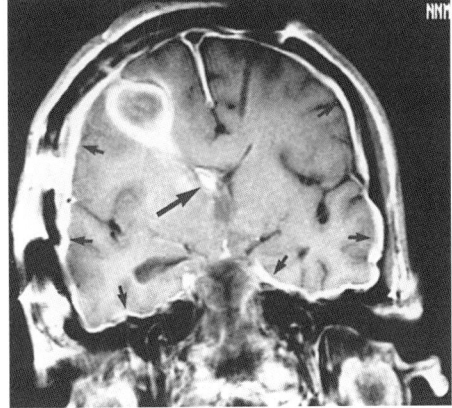

Fig. 6.1. Pyogenic parenchymal abscess. This patient developed a parenchymal abscess after presenting with meningitis, and subdural empyema which had previously been surgically treated. *(Left)* Short TR/TE axial image demonstrates a circular, well circumscribed area of diminished low intensity on the right side. *(Right)* Coronal, short TR/TE image after gadolinium enhancement demonstrates a ring enhancing lesion with smooth, even walls. Note also diffuse meningeal enhancement *(small arrows)* due to meningitis and ependymal enhancement *(large arrow)* in this patient whose cerebral abscess had ruptured into the right lateral ventricle.

logically with computed tomography and do not require magnetic resonance imaging. Patients are uncommonly evaluated with CT or MRI during the early stages of abscess formation. The MRI features of abscess include:

• corticomedullary mass with a central area of low intensity on T_1-weighted images and high intensity on long TR images, although the abscess fluid may have concentric layers of varying intensity

• well-formed, thin, regular, iso- or slightly hyperintense capsule on unenhanced T_1-weighted images which enhances brightly with gadolinium; the wall is thickest adjacent to the cortex and thinnest near the white matter; it is also hypointense relative to white matter on T_2-weighted and gradient echo images, which is thought to be due to the presence of free radicals

• perifocal vasogenic edema in varying amounts depending on the age and character of the abscess (Fig. 6.1). Daughter abscesses may be identified which actually represent adjacent smaller abscesses which formed concurrently with the larger area of involvement (Enzmann 1984, Sze and Zimmerman 1988, Haimes *et al.* 1989, Zimmerman and Haimes 1989).

The primary differential considerations when an abscess is encountered are primary and secondary neoplasm, infarction and contusion. Brain contusion may be excluded based on history alone in most cases. Infarction usually has typical findings including specific vascular distribution, cortical involvement, gyral enhancement, and appropriate history of sudden onset of symptoms. Although the initial CT or MRI findings may not exclude early cerebritis, later imaging will demonstrate encephalomalacic changes with infarction, whereas when infection is present there will be continued and increased mass effect and maturation of an abscess.

Cystic or necrotic glioma and metastases are the most difficult lesions to differentiate acutely from abscess. Abscess can nearly always be differentiated by the morphology of its capsule. Tumors tend to have irregular, thick walls which may enhance less homogeneously than those of abscesses. The amount of vasogenic edema present does not always assist in differentiation, although metastases usually have more associated edema. Tumors that are not cystic may be differentiated from early abscess by follow-up studies which do not demonstrate the typical progression of an abscess. Also, tumors are more likely to contain calcification and hemorrhage. Abscesses rarely contain either (Bach and Goldenberg 1983).

EPIDURAL AND SUBDURAL INFECTION

An abscess which forms outside the brain parenchyma usually results from contiguous spread from outside the cranial cavity. Epidural abscess is most commonly found in association with paranasal or mastoid sinus infection with extension through the outer table of the skull or secondary to postoperative changes or other trauma. Subdural abscess or empyema may also result from intracranial extension of infection or it may occur in association with meningitis. Complications which may arise due to these infections include dural sinus thrombosis with resultant brain infarction, superficial cortical venous thrombosis, meningitis, and brain abscess. Empyemas are surgical emergencies that are often difficult to diagnose due to the lack of specific symptoms (Enzmann 1984, Weingarten *et al.* 1989).

Epidural abscesses and subdural empyemas are composed of extra-axial fluid collections which commonly demonstrate mass effect. Epidural abscess may cross the midline, whereas subdural empyema does not. MRI has been shown to be more sensitive for detecting extra-axial fluid collections, delineating between subdural and epidural collections, better characterizing the location and extent of involvement, and demonstrating any associated brain involvement. The MRI appearance of these infections is variable, but they often demonstrate low signal, though higher than that of the cerebrospinal fluid (CSF), on T_1-weighted images. These collections show high signal on long TR sequences. Epidural abscess may demonstrate a hypointense rim, representing a displaced dura, between the abscess and brain. Enhancing membranes may be present with empyema, subdural effusion, or old subdural hematoma. The detection of such enhancement is therefore not a specific finding, and acute empyema may show no enhancement at all. Fortunately, MRI can assist in the delineation between infected and non-infected fluids based on the signal intensities. Non-infected fluid more typically is isointense to CSF, whereas higher signal is present when infection has occurred (Weingarten *et al.* 1989).

Nonpyogenic abscess
The most clinically important types of nonpyogenic abscesses are discussed in the sections that follow.

Encephalitis
Encephalitides are typically caused by a number of viruses and parasites. The congenital encephalitides and cerebral infections occurring in immunosuppressed patients will be discussed later. Encephalitis represents a diffuse infection of the brain causing edema, cell death and necrosis. Most viral encephalitides are acute, and sometimes they are fulminant infections. The radiologic appearance of encephalitis is usually nonspecific, and the exact etiology will not be determined with imaging alone.

Herpes simplex virus encephalitis
Herpes simplex virus (HSV) is found throughout nature. There are two serotypes. Type I HSV is the most commonly encountered and is well known for its perioral infections. Type II HSV is usually responsible for congenital and perinatally acquired encephalitis and will be discussed later (p. 135).

Patients with HSV type I encephalitis commonly present with low grade fever, seizure, memory loss and inability to form new memory, varying degrees of altered consciousness, and focal neurologic deficits. Early symptoms may include headache, lethargy, myalgia, anorexia, nausea, vomiting and sore throat. Focal neurologic findings may not develop, although neurologic decline may be rapid and irreversible and result in death (Enzmann 1984, Barkovich 1990, Smith and Kuharik 1990, Jordan and Enzmann 1991).

MRI usually demonstrates unilateral involvement, but bilateral, usually asymmetric, involvement may be seen. This infection originates within the medial aspect of the temporal lobes. Infection results from spread of HSV from the trigeminal ganglion to the temporal lobe. It then commonly spreads into the inferior frontal regions, laterally to involve the insula, superiorly through the white matter with sparing of the lentiform nuclei and curiously around the corpus callosum within the cingulate gyrus and adjacent white matter. All these areas of involvement are best delineated with long TR sequences where they are seen as high intensity. Hemorrhage within the uncal region may be identified. White matter or cortical infarction may occur, and parenchymal or meningeal enhancement may be seen after gadolinium is infused. Follow-up examinations will demonstrate prominent areas of encephalomalacia (Fig. 6.2). Calcification may occur within gray or white matter but may not be readily detected with MRI (Enzmann 1984, Barnes and Whitley 1986, Neils *et al.* 1986, Schroth *et al.* 1987*a,b*, Barkovich 1990, Smith and Kuharik 1990, Jordan and Enzmann 1991).

Subacute sclerosing panencephalitis
Subacute sclerosing panencephalitis (SSPE) is an inflammatory process that affects children and young adults. It results from a reactivation of measles infection. Laboratory investigation demonstrates increased titers of measles antibody in the serum and CSF.

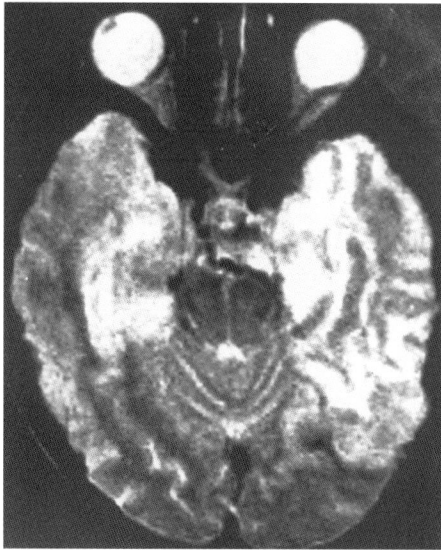

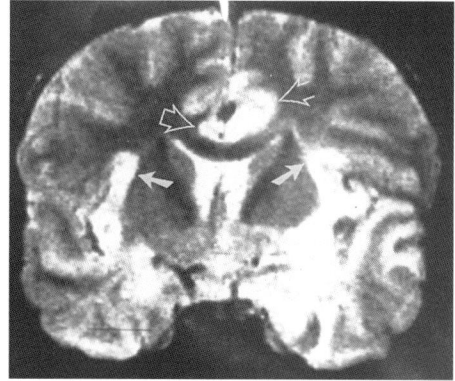

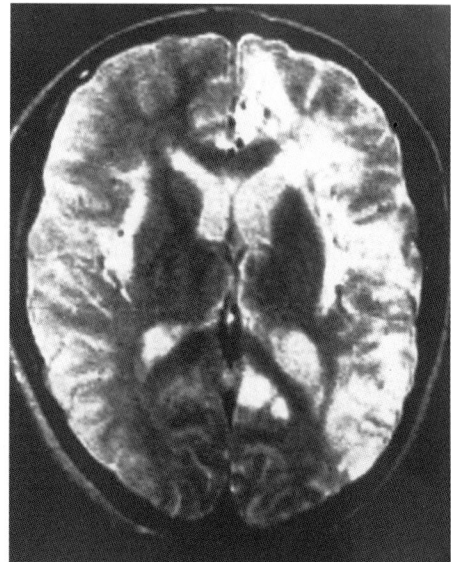

Fig. 6.2. HSV type 1 encephalitis. 13-year-old patient. Long TR/TE axial *(a)* and coronal *(b)* images during acute onset of symptoms. Bilateral temporal lobe white matter hyperintensity is identified with greater involvement on the left side. Note that the right-sided involvement is in the typical medial temporal distribution. The white matter edema/infection ascends into the external capsules *(white arrows)* and involves the insulae but spares the basal ganglia. Note also involvement of the cingulate gyrus bilaterally and adjacent white matter on the left *(open arrows)*. *(c)* Long TR/TE axial image three months after onset of the infection demonstrates high signal throughout the left cerebral hemisphere secondary to postinfectious demyelination and encephalomalacia. The left-sided abnormality remains more advanced than that on the right.

Pathologically there is panencephalitis or infection of gray and white matter including the brainstem. A mononuclear cellular infiltration, gliosis and diffuse cell death occurs (Gilden 1983, Barkovich 1990, Wolinsky 1990).

The MRI features of SSPE include patchy white matter areas of high intensity due to demyelination and basal ganglia infarction (Gilden 1983, Barkovich 1990, Wolinsky 1990, Jordan and Enzmann 1991) (Fig. 6.3). These findings are not specific for this infection.

120

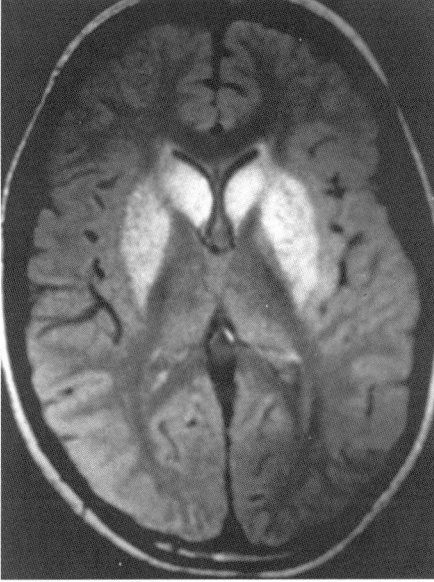

Fig. 6.3. Subacute sclerosing panencephalitis. Long TR/short TE image in 14-year-old boy demonstrates high white matter intensity in the periatrial regions and putaminal lacunar infarctions. This patient was acutely and severely emaciated. Extremely high titers of measles antibodies were present in the CSF.

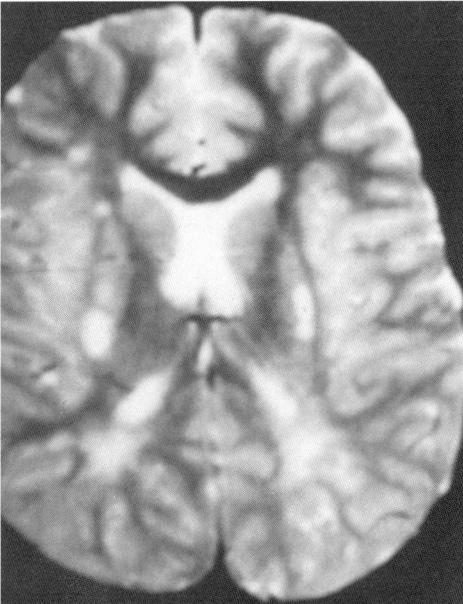

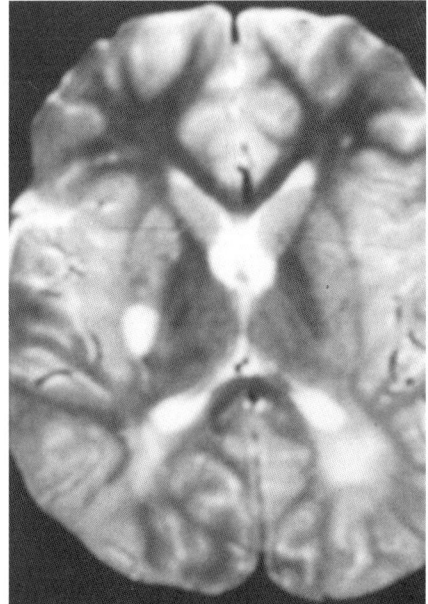

Fig. 6.4. Varicella encephalitis. Long TR *(left)* and long TE *(right)* images of 9-year-old male patient after resolution of the disorder demonstrating hyperintensity of the lentiform and caudate nuclei bilaterally, representing basal ganglia ischemic changes.

Other encephalitides

Other viral agents may cause encephalitis. These include the arboviruses which are carried and disseminated by arthropods, usually mosquitos and ticks; they are responsible for St. Louis, Japanese, California, Murray Valley, eastern and western equine, and tick-borne encephalitides. Enterovirus encephalitides include poliovirus, coxsackievirus and echovirus infections. Mumps, rubella, and varicella (Fig. 6.4) encephalitis may also occur. All these different types of viral encephalitis result in rather non-specific CT or MRI findings and cannot be differentiated reliably by this means (Gilden 1983, Wolinsky 1990).

Meningitis

Acute meningitis

Meningitis is an infection of the meninges or covering of the brain. This infection also involves the subarachnoid space which contains CSF. Meningitis may be caused by bacteria, viruses or fungi.

Bacterial meningitis after the neonatal period is commonly caused by three pathogens, *Haemophilus influenzae* type b, *Neisseria meningitidis* and *Streptococcus pneumoniae*. *H. influenzae* has been the most common form in young patients between the ages of 2 months and 10 years, although the recent introduction of the conjugated vaccine is considerably reducing its frequency. *N. meningitidis* is the most common cause of meningitis in older children and young adults and may occur in epidemics. *S. pneumoniae* is the most common cause of bacterial meningitis in adults (Syrogiannopoulos *et al.* 1986, Chang *et al.* 1990*b*, Harris and Edwards 1991).

Some viruses, notably enterovirus and mumps virus, may cause a self-limiting meningitis. The most favored routes for meningeal infection are via the neural pathways and olfactory tracts and hematogenously. The inflammatory reaction in viral meningitis is lymphocytic. Sequelae are rare (Harris and Edwards 1991).

Bacterial meningitis may result from direct extension from the paranasal or mastoid sinuses or the middle ear cavity. It may also result from trauma or previous surgery. The most common route, however, is hematogenous, with involvement of the choroid plexus followed by infection of the CSF and leptomeninges. Pathologically there is cellular infiltration accompanied by a fibrinous exudate. Infiltration of the walls of adjacent arteries and veins may occur and result in their thrombosis and occlusion, causing both arterial and venous infarction of brain substance. Further complications may include hydrocephalus, subdural empyema or effusion, ventriculitis, cerebritis and brain abscess (Syrogiannopoulos *et al.* 1986, Barkovich 1990, Chang *et al.* 1990*b*, Smith and Kuharik 1990, Harris and Edwards 1991).

The MRI appearance of early uncomplicated bacterial meningitis is commonly normal. There may be nominal meningeal enhancement with gadolinium. More advanced degrees may produce other transient or permanent sequelae. The most frequently detected abnormality is hydrocephalus. This is commonly extraventricular or 'communicating' and is caused by obstruction to CSF absorption over the convexity. Intraventricular or 'noncommunicating' hydrocephalus may occur, resulting from obstruction of the cerebral

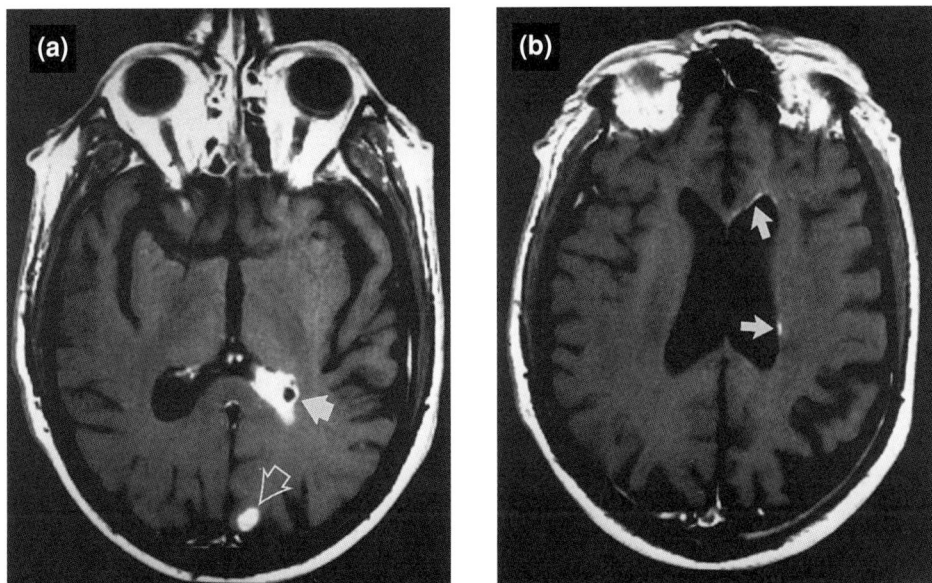

Fig. 6.5. Ventriculitis. Short TR/TE images with gadolinium enhancement demonstrate globular enhancement of the enlarged left choroid glomus *(a—white arrow)*. Note also small superficial parenchymal enhancement in the left parieto-occipital region *(a—open arrow)*. Ependymal enhancement was also identified *(b—arrows)*. This patient presented with symptoms of meningitis. No meningeal abnormality was identified and the symptoms resolved after antibiotic therapy. Therapy was instituted prior to the cultures that were obtained. These cultures were expectedly negative.

aqueduct of Sylvius by inflammatory exudate and/or gliosis or ependymal proliferation (Syrogiannopoulos *et al.* 1986, Chang *et al.* 1990*b*, Harris and Edwards 1991).

Meningeal enhancement and thickening due to infiltration of inflammatory exudate may be identified as well. This finding is usually not encountered during the early stages of the illness. Such enhancement may resolve after appropriate therapy or it may persist and contribute to other sequelae such as hydrocephalus. This is typically encountered in patients who have suffered tuberculous meningitis (Syrogiannopoulos *et al.* 1986, Chang *et al.* 1990*a*, Harris and Edwards 1991).

Ventriculitis occurs in approximately one third of patients with bacterial meningitis. It can be recognized with MRI as enhancement of the ependymal lining of the ventricular system (Fig. 6.5). Such infection may result in ventricular septa formation and hydrocephalus (Barkovich 1990).

Infarction and secondary infection of the brain are two of the most serious complications. They may be difficult to differentiate from one another initially and they may present simultaneously. Furthermore, cerebritis and eventual abscess may follow closely on the heels of infarction. Both arterial and venous infarctions are known to occur and are secondary to vasculitis and venous thrombosis. Small foci of hemorrhage may be detected as well as edema and mass effect. Cerebritis and abscess would follow the expected evolution, depending on the effectiveness of treatment (Syrogiannopoulos *et al.* 1986, Chang *et al.* 1990*b*, Harris and Edwards 1991).

Two types of subdural abnormalities may be encountered in patients with bacterial meningitis. These are effusions which represent uninfected collections of fluid and subdural empyema. Subdural effusion is regarded as reactive; the fluid may show a neutrophil leucocytosis and low glucose level, but is usually sterile (Syrogiannopoulos *et al.* 1986). The most common initiating organisms are *H. influenzae* and *S. pneumoniae*. The effusions are iso- or commonly hyperintense to CSF on T_1-weighted and intermediate images and isointense on T_2-weighted images.

Subdural empyema is composed of grossly purulent material within the subdural space. This is a serious complication of bacterial meningitis and requires timely surgical and medical therapy. With MRI, subdural empyema has a relatively low signal intensity on short TR/TE sequences, though it is hyperintense to CSF, and a high signal on long TR sequences (Syrogiannopoulos *et al.* 1986, Chang *et al.* 1990*b*, Harris and Edwards 1991).

Tuberculosis
Tuberculous meningitis
The most widely recognized type of chronic meningitis is that caused by *M. tuberculosis*, or tuberculous meningitis. It presents clinically in an already chronic state about half the time (Harris and Edwards 1991). It is believed to occur secondary to rupture of a cerebral or choroid plexus tuberculoma which may also be identified in these patients. Tuberculous meningitis produces a very thick, gelatinous exudate that has a predilection for the basal cisterns. Such involvement results in the well known cranial nerve deficits which may be present in up to 70 per cent of those affected (Clark *et al.* 1986, Wilhelm and Ellner 1986, Schoeman *et al.* 1988, Barkovich 1990, Chang *et al.* 1990*a*, Castro and Hesselink 1991, Harris and Edwards 1991).

The MRI appearance includes hydrocephalus which is present in virtually all cases. Meningeal enhancement represents another common and often striking finding in these patients. The basilar cisterns may appear completely filled with enhancing material (Fig. 6.6). Such inflammation may progress to calcification which has a fairly typical appearance on CT but may go undetected with MRI. Ventriculitis has been detected in these patients. Cerebral infarction may also result due to vasculitis similar to that found in acute pyogenic meningitis (Schoeman *et al.* 1988, Barkovich 1990, Chang *et al.* 1990*a*, Castro and Hesselink 1991).

Other causes of chronic meningitis include infections caused by *Brucella* spp., *Coccidioides* spp., *Treponema pallidum* and *Candida* spp. Noninfectious causes of chronic meningeal inflammation include sarcoid, subarachnoid hemorrhage, surgery and radiation (Ulmer and Elster 1991).

Tuberculoma
Tuberculoma represents the parenchymal form of intracranial tuberculous infection. It is found in isolation in 80 per cent of cases. It is spread hematogenously, and most often occurs at the gray–white matter junction. Clinically, a tuberculoma presents as a slowly

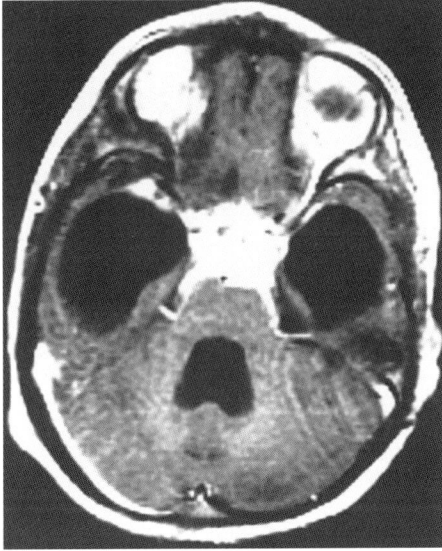

Fig. 6.6. Tuberculous meningitis. Short TR/TE, axial, gadolinium enhanced image demonstrates prominent enhancement of the basilar cisterns which have been replaced by thick exudate produced by tuberculous infection.

expanding intracranial mass. Specific symptoms may include headache, fever, seizures, and signs of increased intracranial pressure including papilledema, which is present in 90 per cent of cases. 50–70 per cent of patients have tuberculosis diagnosed at other sites, of which the lung is the most common. Pathologically mature tuberculomas are granulomatous with central caseation. Less advanced involvement demonstrates small tubercles, some with caseating or cystic centers surrounded by edema (Loizou and Anderson 1982, Sheller and Des Prez 1986, Draouat *et al.* 1987, Castro and Hesselink 1991).

MRI of a tuberculoma may demonstrate only edema on all imaging sequences, although a hypointense rim may separate its hyperintense center from the hyperintensity of the adjacent edema on T_2-weighted images. Gadolinium enhanced images demonstrate nodular or ring enhancing lesions (Barkovich 1990, Chang *et al.* 1990*a*, Castro and Hesselink 1991).

Tuberculous abscess and cerebritis
Tuberculous abscess represents a true abscess containing pus and viable organisms. Pathologically there is no evidence of the typical granulomatous reaction. This type of involvement is very rare. It is said to be difficult to differentiate from pyogenic abscess.

Tuberculous cerebritis is also rare and is composed of a segment of infected brain which exhibits microgranulomas, lymphocytic infiltrate, Langerhan's giant cells, epithelioid cells, and few organisms. MRI would be expected to demonstrate evidence of focal involvement with the appearance of cerebritis (Castro and Hesselink 1991).

Sarcoid
Neurosarcoid is a granulomatous process that is uncommon in childhood and most often

125

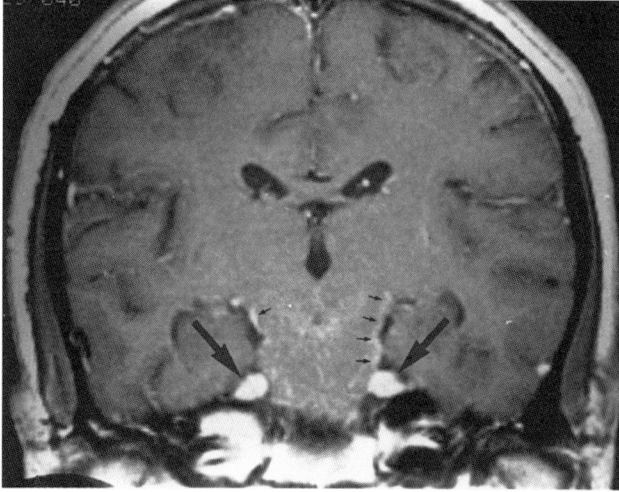

Fig. 6.7. Sarcoid meningitis. Short TR/TE, gadolinium enhanced coronal image demonstrates marked enhancement of the enlarged Vth cranial nerves *(large arrows)* and the basilar meninges *(small arrows)*. This patient presented clinically with intractable hiccups.

found in young adults. Neurosarcoid usually involves the region of the pituitary stalk and may present as a focal intracranial mass or diffuse meningeal involvement. Black persons are more commonly affected than other races.

Although most cases of neurosarcoid have other sites of involvement, isolated neurologic involvement does occur. Extraneural sites include the lung, lymph nodes, eyes and bone. Clinically, neurosarcoid may present as aseptic meningitis, cranial neuropathy, hydrocephalus or hypothalamic–pituitary axis anomalies. Sarcoid may produce intra-cranial vasculitis and present as an encephalopathy or with seizures.

The MRI appearance of sarcoid includes meningeal enhancement (Fig. 6.7), pituitary stalk enlargement, focal hypothalamic region mass, ependymitis, focal brain mass, and edema and mass effect secondary to cerebral vasculitis. The non-caseating granulomas of sarcoid are usually isointense to gray matter on short TR/TE sequences and iso- to hyper-intense to gray matter on long TR sequences, and prominently enhance with gadolinium (Barkovich 1990, Ulmer and Ester 1991).

Fungal infections
Fungal infections of the brain are usually an unexpected finding. They typically have a slow clinical course with no distinguishing characteristics. The rarity and lack of specific clinical or radiographic findings usually result in these lesions being initially diagnosed as abscess, tuberculoma, tumor, or other types of meningitis. Fungi are considered true pathogens when they are able to cause infection in an otherwise healthy host. Other fungi that are not true pathogens cause infection in debilitated or immunosupressed hosts. These fungi are opportunistic rather than true pathogens. The fungi which are considered

126

true pathogens include *Histoplasma, Blastomycoses, Coccidiomycoses, Paracoccidio-mycoses* and *Sporothrix* (Enzmann 1984, Lyons and Andriole 1986, Barkovich 1990, Bazan *et al*. 1991).

Fungi may present in three forms: yeast, hyphal and pseudohyphal. Since they enter the CNS via the arterial circulation their size causes them to affect the brain and meninges in different ways. The yeast form results in a chronic meningitis. Its small size allows it to pass to the small vessels of the subarachnoid space. The pseudohyphal forms are larger and obstruct arterioles, while the hyphal forms are larger still and obstruct large and intermediate sized arteries. The hyphal and pseudohyphal forms result in paren-chymal brain infection due to their size and resultant site of vascular obstruction (Lyons and Andriole 1986).

Histoplasmosis
Histoplasmosis is caused by the fungus *Histoplasma capsulatum*. It may result in diffuse brain and meningeal involvement in a miliary pattern, as a meningitis with vasculitis, or in focal brain involvement. Patients with such involvement usually have disseminated disease and commonly present with respiratory symptoms, the lungs being the site of initial infection (Bazan *et al*. 1991). The MRI appearance of intracranial histoplasmosis is not well documented. Dion *et al*. (1987) recorded a patient with a thalamic histo-plasmoma—a cystic mass with hypointense walls on T_1-weighted sequences which became hyperintense on T_2-weighted sequences. Gadolinium was not given in this case. Desai *et al*. (1991) reported a case of disseminated histoplasmosis with spinal involve-ment. The lesion was isointense to spinal cord on T_1-weighted images, hyperintense on T_2-weighted images and had prominent contrast enhancement with gadolinium. I have found no pediatric cases of intracranial histoplasmosis in the literature, and an insuf-ficient number of adult cases evaluated with MRI to be certain of its typical appearance.

Blastomycosis
Blastomycosis is caused by *Blastomyces dermatitidis*. Human infection is caused by the yeast form. It may cause meningitis, which is most common, or cerebral granulomas. It may occasionally coexist with other infections such as tuberculosis or histoplasmosis (Lyons and Andriole 1986, Roos *et al*. 1987, Bazan *et al*. 1991). It may also occur in patients with lymphoma or in those receiving steroid therapy (Loizou and Anderson 1982, Lyons and Andriole 1986, Sheller and Des Prez 1986, Wilhelm and Ellner 1986, Draouat *et al*. 1987, Castro and Hesselink 1991, Ulmer and Elster 1991). CNS involve-ment occurs in 3–10 per cent of patients with blastomycosis and in up to 33 per cent of patients with disseminated disease (Enzmann 1984, Lyons and Andriole 1986, Bazan *et al*. 1991). No MRI examples of this entity were found in the literature, and the CT findings are not distinguishable from other granulomatous infections (Enzmann 1984).

Coccidioidomycosis
Coccidioidomycosis is caused by *Coccidioides immitis* in its yeast form. It is found in the south-western USA, northern Mexico, and some parts of Central and South America.

CNS infection is usually in the form of a meningitis and is secondary to hematogenous spread from a pulmonary lesion. The CT appearance is of enhancing leptomeningeal thickening and hydrocephalus. These findings are very similar to those of tuberculous meningitis (Lyons and Andriole 1986, Bazan *et al.* 1991). No MRI demonstrations of this infection were found in the literature.

Aspergillosis
CNS aspergillosis is usually caused by hematogenous spread of hyphal elements of *Aspergillus* spp. from the lung. The disease may cause a low grade fever, it progresses slowly, and is accurately diagnosed only after biopsy. Intracranial involvement may include meningitis, meningoencephalitis, parenchymal granuloma, or abscess. There may also be associated cerebral infarction and hemorrhage due to vasculitis and vascular occlusion (Lyons and Andriole 1986, Bazan *et al.* 1991).

The MRI appearance of intracranial aspergillosis has been at least partially determined. Since CT of *Aspergillus* meningitis demonstrates thickened enhancing leptomeninges, MRI would be expected to demonstrate similar findings. Intraparenchymal lesions probably appear hypo- to isointense on long TR sequences and may have some surrounding high intensity edema (Grossman *et al.* 1981, Mikhael *et al.* 1985, Jinkins *et al.* 1987, Gupta *et al.* 1990). Enhancement of abscess walls and granulomas would be expected with enhanced MRI images.

Other fungal infections
Cryptococcosis is discussed later in the section on HIV-related infections. Fungal infections such as candidiasis, paracoccidioidomycosis and others have rarely or never been evaluated with MRI or appeared in the literature.

Parasitic infections
Parasitic infection of the brain is most common in underdeveloped countries. The radiographic diagnosis of these infections may be hindered due to the rarity with which they are encountered in more developed countries, although extensive travel and emigration mean that even some very rare parasitic infections will occasionally be imaged. The diagnosis of such infections must derive from pathologic analysis in order to ensure proper treatment. In the case of cysticercosis, its relative frequency, clinical history and radiographic findings allow treatment without the need for surgical intervention (Chang *et al.* 1991a,b).

Cysticercosis is the most common parasitic brain infection. Other parasites which may cause neural infection are *Paragonimus westerani*, which is a lung fluke, *Spirometra* tapeworms, *Echinococcus granulosus*, *Toxocara*, *Schistosoma*, *Trichinella spiralis* and *Entamoeba histolytica*.

Cysticercosis
PARENCHYMAL CYSTICERCOSIS
Neurocysticercosis is caused by *Taenia solium* which is the pork tapeworm. Only one

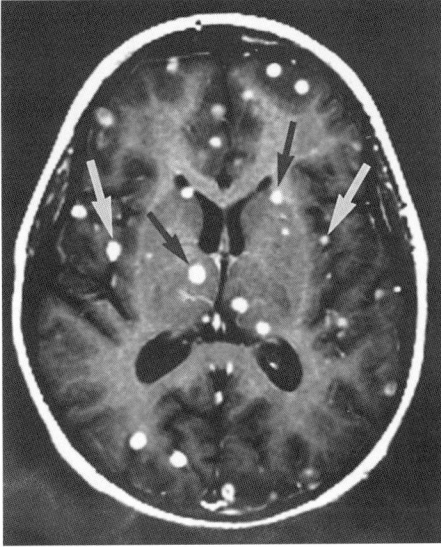

Fig. 6.8. Cysticercosis. Short TR/TE, gadolinium enhanced axial image demonstrates multiple, bilateral, enhancing intraparenchymal *(black arrows)* and subarachnoid *(white arrows)* nodular masses.

other rarely encountered tapeworm larva from the dog, *Multiceps*, may infect the human brain. This larva has multiple scolices, whereas the cysticercal larva has only one. Cysticercosis is endemic to Mexico, Chile, Spain, Africa, Poland and Asia. The cysticercus is the encysted form of the tapeworm. It typically lodges in the eye, muscle, and most often the brain. Pathologically, cysticercal infection causes local granulomatous inflammation and calcification. The most common clinical presentation is headache, nausea and vomiting, with seizures occurring in about 40 per cent of patients. Clinical signs include papilledema, mental status changes, cranial nerve and focal neurologic deficits. Diagnosis is dependent on history of appropriate exposure in an endemic area, CT and MRI findings, CSF lymphocytosis, immunoassays of blood and CSF, peripheral blood and/or CSF eosinophilia, and clinical evidence of other organ involvement (Loo and Braude 1982, Sotelo *et al.* 1985, Lotz *et al.* 1988, Kramer *et al.* 1989, Chang *et al.* 1991*a,b*).

Neurocysticercosis may be classified by location of intracranial infection. This may be ventriculocisternal, parenchymal or mixed. Parenchymal involvement is most common. It is usually bilateral and occurs at the gray–white matter junction. Initial infection causes no clinical or radiographic abnormality. Early changes include local inflammation and edema. By 3–12 months the lesions contain a cystic collection of clear fluid. A mural nodule which represents the scolex is also present. There is no adjacent inflammatory brain response at this time. This is what is termed the vesicular stage of the cysticercus. The next stage is called the colloidal–vesicular stage which corresponds to the time that the larva begins to degenerate and die. During this time inflammation reappears, the cyst wall thickens, and the cyst fluid becomes turbid. In the third or granular–nodular stage the larva retracts, calcifies, and develops a thick collagenous wall.

129

The final nodular–calcified stage demonstrates a focal calcified lesion with no edema or acute inflammation or mass effect. It may take from two to ten years to reach this final stage (Loo and Braude 1982, Salazar *et al.* 1983, Zee *et al.* 1984, Sotelo *et al.* 1985, Lotz *et al.* 1988, Kramer *et al.* 1989, Chang *et al.* 1991*a,b*).

The MRI appearance of the parenchymal form of cysticercosis depends on the stage of the infection. During the first or vesicular stage the larva presents as a thin walled, usually non-enhancing cyst with a mural nodule. The cystic fluid is isointense to CSF on both short and long TR sequences. In the study by Chang *et al.* (1991*a,b*), three of 54 cysticerci in this stage (6 per cent) had contrast enhancement. Cysticerci in the colloidal–vesicular stage are degenerating and may cause encephalitis. These lesions have surrounding edema and often show capsular enhancement. The cyst fluid is hyperintense to CSF on both short and long TR sequences. The granular–nodular stage lesions demonstrate a thick enhancing capsule. Some also have a central low intensity representing the scolex with surrounding capsular enhancement (Fig. 6.8). Unenhanced MRI shows isointensity of the lesions on T_1- and T_2-weighted images and possibly central high intensity on long TR sequences. In the final or calcified stage, MRI demonstrates low intensity on all sequences without contrast enhancement (Chang *et al.* 1991*a,b*).

VENTRICULAR–CISTERNAL CYSTICERCOSIS

Cysticercosis of the basilar cisterns may be composed of two different larval forms. The *Cysticercus cellulosae* has a bladder and a scolex while the racemose form lacks a scolex and comprises only the bladder or cyst component. The cysts usually present as a grape-like cluster up to several centimeters in size. The racemose form may be difficult to diagnose, since identification and adequate characterization of these lesions may be dependent on visualization of the scolex. The ventricular form of cysticercosis comprises around 15–20 per cent of cases of this disease. The ventricular form is caused by *C. cellulosae* (Salazar *et al.* 1983, Apuzzo *et al.* 1984, Zee *et al.* 1984, Chang *et al.* 1991*b*).

MRI is the best radiographic means of demonstrating these infections. The common MRI findings include identification of the scolex which is iso- or hyperintense relative to brain parenchyma on T_1-weighted images and iso- or hypointense on T_2-weighted images. The cyst fluid is usually isointense to CSF but may be mildly hyperintense on all imaging sequences. The cyst wall, subependymal reaction, focal ventricular enlargement and hydrocephalus may also be identified. The subependymal changes will be visualized only on long TR sequences. Subependymal reaction occurs at the attachment site of the cyst to the ventricle. Cisternal cysticercosis, when large enough, acts as a cystic mass which displaces adjacent brain tissue and widens fissures. The scolex and cyst wall are best delineated with T_1-weighted images, whereas tissue reaction caused by cyst attachment or larval degeneration are better delineated with long TR sequences. Gadolinium enhancement may occur in patients with ependymitis and meningitis (Chang *et al.* 1991*a,b*).

Congenital infections

Congenital CNS infections may be caused by many agents, more commonly *Toxoplasma gondii*, rubella virus, cytomegalovirus (CMV) and HSV. These congenital infections are usually acquired either via the maternal, hematogenous–transplacental route or ascending from the birth canal (Freij and Sever 1988, Klein and Remington 1990).

The type and degree of abnormality they cause depends to a large extent on the timing of the maternal infection (Desmonts 1982, Miller *et al.* 1982, Chowdhury 1986, Klein and Remington 1990). Initiation of the infection during the first or second trimester of pregnancy results in both destructive and developmental brain anomalies. Later onset during the third trimester and sometimes earlier may result in only a destructive process, or the fetus may escape infection (Miller *et al.* 1982). These agents are known for the typical brain abnormalities they cause including atrophy, infarction, cerebritis, hydrocephalus and calcification (Friede and Mikolasek 1978, Bale 1984, Bale *et al.* 1985, Diebler *et al.* 1985, Herman *et al.* 1985, Noorbehesht *et al.* 1987, Freij *et al.* 1988). It has also been known for some time, but more widely recognized recently, that these infections when occurring early in pregnancy may also result in neuronal migrational anomalies. Grossly, the brains in these patients have a diffuse asymmetric pachygyric appearance and a diffuse knobbly or bumpy appearance to the cortical surface. Pathologically, they are shown to have polymicrogyria (Crome and France 1959, Dennis and Alvord 1961, De Léon 1972, Manz 1977, Friede and Mikolasek 1978, Barth 1987, Galloway and Roessmann 1987, Osborn *et al.* 1988).

Toxoplasmosis
Toxoplasma gondii is a coccidian which is ubiquitous in nature. Up to one half of the entire world population has been infected with this agent (Chowdhury 1986). Approximately one in 10,000 infants born annually in the USA have congenital toxoplasmosis. Most do not demonstrate clinical evidence of the disease initially but may do so later in life (Remington and Desmonts 1990).

The infective agent is passed hematogenously through the placenta to the fetus. The parasite may thrive within the placenta some time after the maternal parasitemia has subsided, and then later gain access to the fetal circulation. Clinically, significant abnormalities are found when the fetus is infected prior to 26 weeks gestation. The earlier the fetus is infected, the more severe the fetal disease (Desmonts and Couvreur 1974, Diebler *et al.* 1985, Remington and Desmonts 1990). Previous studies have shown that the most severe fetal anomalies are produced when infection occurs between 10 and 24 weeks gestation (Desmonts 1982).

The typical triad of findings in an infant with congenital toxoplasmic encephalitis is hydrocephalus, choroidoretinitis and intracranial calcification. Choroidoretinitis is the most common single clinical finding in the infected newborn infant (Chowdhury 1986). The clinical presentation of these patients is diverse and may be very mild or quite severe. Clinically recognizable disease in the neonate is usually severe. Mild cases typically may go undetected; however, when mild disease is identified in the neonate, it is often suggested by choroidoretinal scars. These scars may be found only when they are specifically sought (Remington and Desmonts 1990). In very mild cases neurologic involvement may present late as seizures.

The neurologic anomalies associated with this infection include hydrocephalus, intracranial calcification, atrophy, microcephaly, infarction, hydranencephaly and neuronal

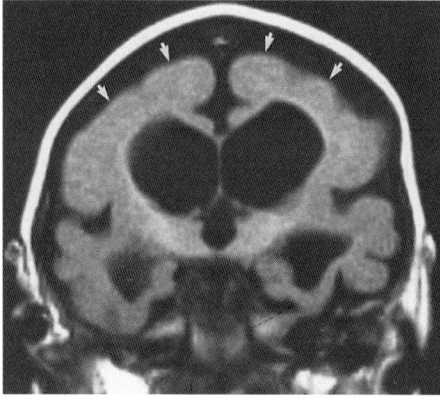

Fig. 6.9. Congenital toxoplasmic encephalitis with pachygyria. Short TR/TE coronal image demonstrates diffuse pachygyria *(arrows)*. No normal gyri are identified. The lateral ventricles are enlarged due to cerebral atrophy.

migrational anomalies (Diebler *et al.* 1985, Byrd *et al.* 1987, Remington and Desmonts 1990). Pathologically, there is infiltration of the pia–arachnoid with lymphocytes, plasma cells, macrophages and eosinophils. The underlying brain cortex is destroyed due to vascular involvement by the parasite. Calcification occurs due to deposition of calcium salts in the zones of brain necrosis (Remington and Desmonts 1990).

Hydrocephalus is common and may occur secondary to infection and gliosis in the region of the aqueduct of Sylvius. Generalized atrophy is also commonly present and is detected more often with early severe infection. Focal areas of brain infarction and even hydranencephaly may also be seen (Remington and Desmonts 1990). Neuronal migrational anomalies occur when there is interruption of migration of the subependymal neuroblast during the formation of the neocortex (Barkovich *et al.* 1987, Osborn *et al.* 1988).

The radiographic evaluation of the brain in patients congenitally infected with *T. gondii* is best effected with MRI (Fig. 6.9). Intracranial calcification is present in most cases and is better delineated with CT. Calcification has a predilection for the subependymal areas and basal ganglia, but may occur anywhere in the brain and tends to be somewhat more diffuse than that associated with CMV encephalitis. Hydrocephalus occurs secondary to aqueductal stenosis and presents as enlargement of the lateral and third ventricles with a normal sized fourth ventricle. Other findings include porencephaly at the site of previous infarction and hydranencephaly which is a manifestation of (near) total cerebral infarction (Diebler *et al.* 1985).

MRI is well suited for delineating demyelination secondary to the infective insult on long TR spin echo sequences. However, such changes can be recognized only in patients old enough to have a significant degree of myelination. Young patients with no significant myelination will normally exhibit high signal within the white matter.

MRI is the modality of choice for detecting and diagnosing the pachygyria associated with congenital brain infections. Pachygyria consists of large gyri which are too few in number. The cortex is thickened and the white matter is thin. The gray–white matter junction is more smooth than normal due to a decrease in the number and size of white matter digitations (Osborn *et al.* 1988).

132

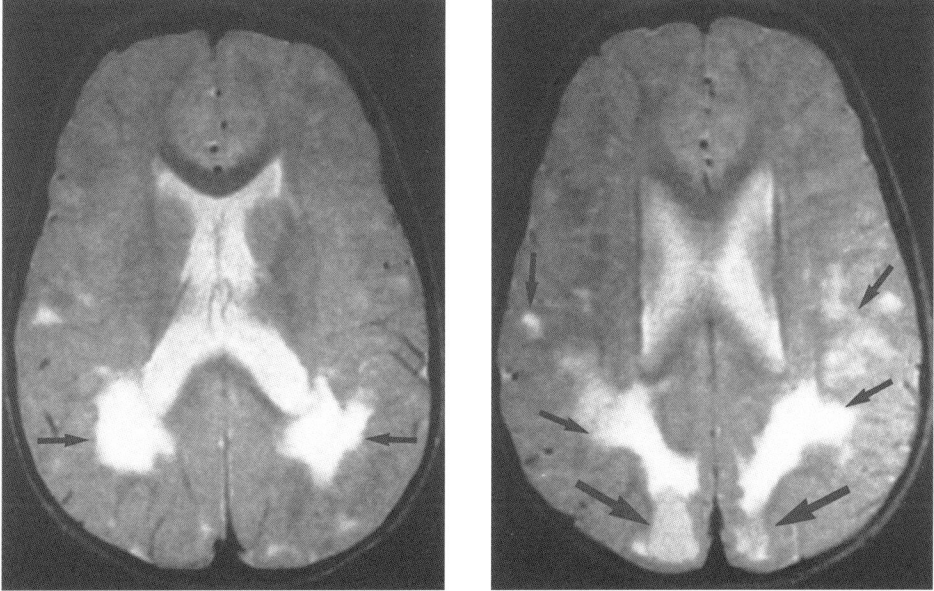

Fig. 6.10. Congenital cytomegalovirus encephalitis. 18-month-old patient. Long TR/TE axial images demonstrate hyperintensity within the periatrial and subcortical white matter representative of demyelination and gliosis *(small arrows)*. Some periventricular calcification, demonstrated on CT (not shown) was not detected with MRI. Parietal infarctions are delineated *(large arrows)*.

Cytomegalovirus

CMV, like *T. gondii*, is ubiquitous in nature and is similar to HSV. Human CMV is a DNA virus for which humans are the only reservoir. In the USA, anywhere from 50 to 85 per cent of women of childbearing age are seropositive.

It is believed that signs of infection recognizable at birth or soon after result from transplacental transmission. In the USA, between 0.2 and 2.2 per cent of all newborn infants have congenital CMV infection; this does not only occur during primary maternal infection in pregnancy, but can result from secondary infections as well (Bale 1984, Alford *et al.* 1990, Stagno 1990).

From a pathologic standpoint, CNS involvement is its most significant aspect (Bale 1984). The entire brain may be involved with an encephalitic process, with eventual gliosis and calcification. As in toxoplasmosis, calcification may occur anywhere in the brain, but is most frequently found in the periventricular zones.

Most babies infected with CMV, though, probably acquired it in their passage through the birth canal and have no outward signs. A low percentage of these patients will ultimately develop anomalies including choroidoretinitis, cerebral palsy, micro-cephaly and sensorineural hearing loss. Such clinical symptoms are usually apparent by 2 years of age (Bale 1984, Stagno 1990).

The MRI findings of CMV encephalitis, like those of toxoplasmosis, include

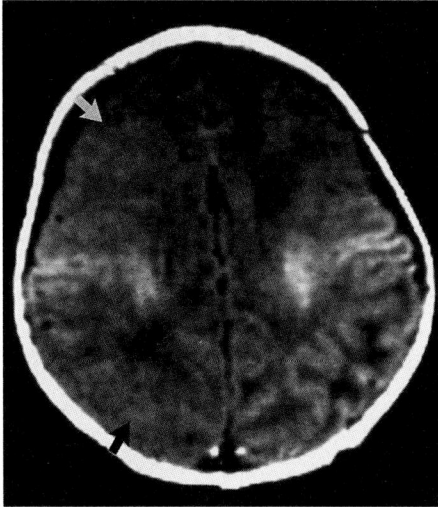

(a)

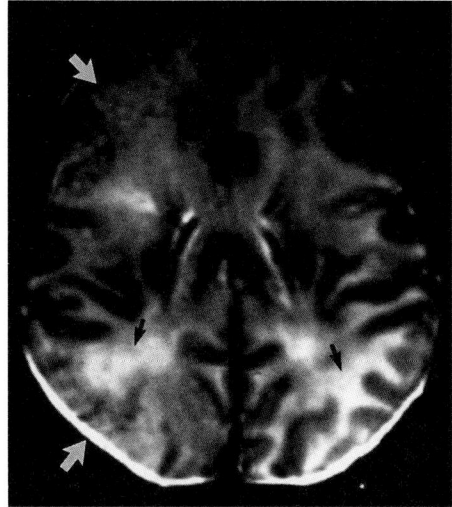

(b)

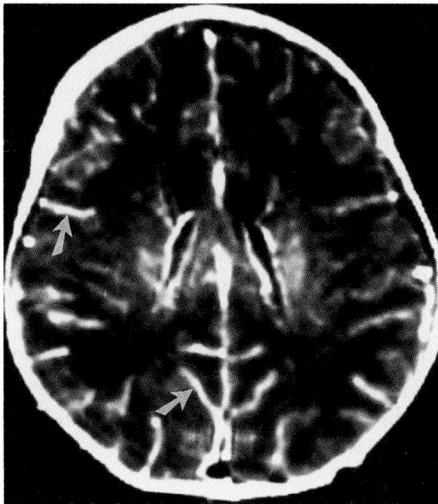

(c)

Fig. 6.11. Congenital HSV type II encephalitis. Acute findings. *(a)* Short TR/TE, and *(b)* long TR/TE axial images demonstrate loss of gray–white matter junction in right frontal and parietal areas *(arrows)*. Abnormal high intensity on the long TR/TE image is due to cerebral edema involving the white matter of the posterior parietal area bilaterally *(b—small black arrows)*. This can also be identified in the left posterior parietal white matter on the short TR/TE image as increased hypointensity. *(c)* Gadolinium enhanced image demonstrates diffuse meningeal enhancement *(arrows)*.

atrophy, hydrocephalus, infarction, calcification, gliosis, demyelination and neuronal migrational anomalies (Crome and France 1959, Navin and Angevine 1968, Friede and Mikolasek 1978, Anders *et al.* 1980, Bale *et al.* 1985, Barkovich 1990) (Fig. 6.10). Differentiation between toxoplasmosis and CMV infection based on the MRI findings cannot be done with any certainty.

MRI commonly does not or does not well delineate the intracranial calcification seen with CT. However, it will delineate diffuse white matter abnormalities, seen as high

134

signal on long TR spin echo sequences indicative of abnormal myelination and gliosis secondary to the infective process (Barkovich 1990). MRI also better demonstrates the neuronal migrational anomalies resulting from these infections (Osborn *et al.* 1988).

Herpes simplex virus
HSV is a DNA virus and its clinical manifestations in adults have been described for centuries. Neonatal HSV infection, however, was first described only 50 years ago. Most congenital infections are due to type II HSV. The virus may infect the fetus either hematogenously via the placenta or, more frequently, ascending from the birth canal before or during delivery (Freij and Sever 1988). HSV infection may have a devastating effect on the fetus and newborn infant.

Infection during the first trimester commonly results in microcephaly, cerebral atrophy, hydranencephaly, cerebral and cerebellar necrosis, intracranial calcification, choroidoretinitis and multiple other cutaneous and systemic anomalies (Whitley 1990).

Infection obtained via the birth canal during delivery may result in localized infection of the skin, eyes and oral cavity, or in a localized CNS involvement with or without cutaneous or eye lesions, or in disseminated multi-organ systemic disease involving the brain in around two-thirds of cases (Freij and Sever 1988, Whitley 1990). Infants with localized CNS involvement usually present clinically between 15 and 17 days of age, while those with disseminated infection usually present between 9 and 11 days of age. 20 per cent of patients with CNS involvement have no cutaneous lesions, making early diagnosis difficult (Freij and Sever 1988).

The MRI appearance of neonatal herpes encephalitis is sometimes difficult to appreciate because of the diffuse lack of myelination. On long TR spin echo images all the white matter is of high signal intensity. Because of this, white matter edema may be difficult to detect based on the signal characteristics. Long TR images, however, may show an increased signal (Figs. 6.11, 6.12), while short TR images may demonstrate subtle areas of low signal. Gadolinium enhanced images may demonstrate parenchymal or meningeal enhancement subacutely (Barkovich 1990). All imaging sequences may demonstrate cerebral infarction with loss of the gray–white matter interface. Hemorrhage and mass effect due to edema may also be seen. MRI is commonly not performed during the acute setting. Late findings include encephalomalacia, demyelination and calcification (Fig. 6.12).

Rubella
Because of immunization programs in the USA, UK and elsewhere, together with current screening methods, congenital rubella infection has become quite rare. Rubella virus may be transmitted to the fetus through the placenta during primary maternal infection. Maternal infection, however, usually does not result in fetal infection. The results of fetal infection are both teratogenic and destructive. Maternal infection may result in abortion, stillbirth, devastating or mild anomalies, or an apparently normal baby (Bakshi and Cooper 1989). As in the other congenital brain infections, a later onset of symptoms signifies milder abnormalities than in cases that present at birth (Dion *et al.* 1987).

135

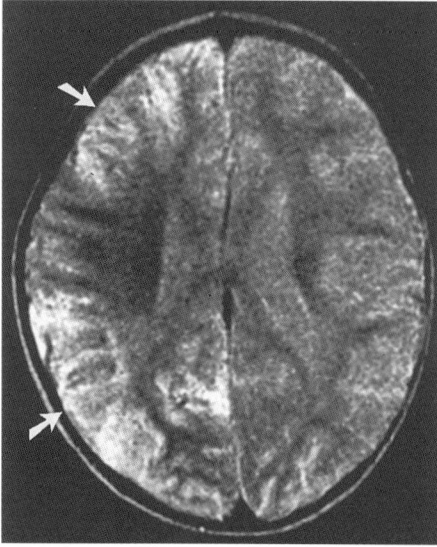

(a)

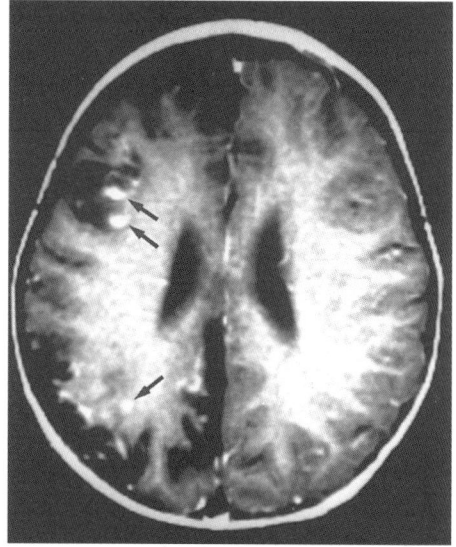

(b)

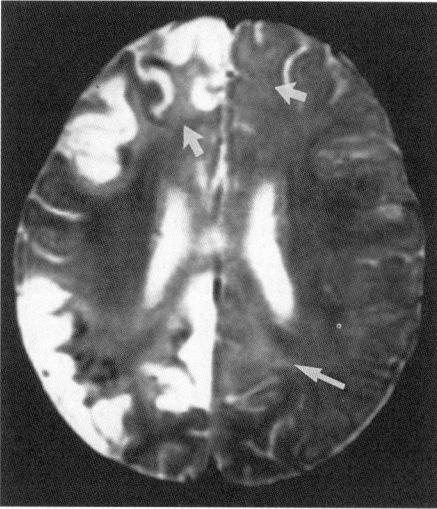

(c)

Fig. 6.12. Congenital HSV type II encephalitis. Acute and chronic findings. *(a)* Acute onset of disease delineated on long TR/TE image. High intensity edema involves parts of the entire right cerebral hemisphere *(arrows)*. *(b)* Gadolinium enhanced short TR/TE image at 13 months of age demonstrates encephalomalacia involving the right cerebral hemisphere and multiple small areas of parenchymal enhancement *(arrows)*. *(c)* Long TR/TE image at the same level as *(b)* demonstrates hyperintensity in the areas of right cerebral encephalomalacia and white matter hyperintensity bilaterally *(arrows)* denoting bilateral infection.

Fetal infection before 8–12 weeks gestation results in a greater percentage of infection and this tends to be more severe. Fetal infection occurring during the third trimester is relatively mild without significant lasting effects (Cooper *et al.* 1969, Miller *et al.* 1982, Freij *et al.* 1988, Bakshi and Cooper 1989, Preblud and Alford 1990).

Pathologically, the fetal organs tend to be hypoplastic and demonstrate a necrotizing angiopathy. There may also be cytolysis and tissue necrosis (Preblud and Alford 1990).

Clinically, infected neonates have multi-organ anomalies. Brain involvement results in a meningoencephalitis which may cause microcephaly secondary to diffuse brain atrophy, and rarely intracranial calcification, hydrocephalus, mental retardation and behavior disorders (Cooper *et al.* 1969, Freij *et al.* 1988, Preblud and Alford 1990).

Even the typical CT appearance of congenital CNS rubella infection is not known. Fitz (1985) illustrated a single case which demonstrated initially diffuse brain hypodensity due to edema and chronically diffuse lucency, probably encephalomalacic changes, and dense calcification in the basal ganglia, right temporal lobe and cortex adjacent to the interhemispheric fissure. I have found no MRI reports of congenital rubella encephalitis.

The sonographic appearance of congenital rubella syndrome has been reported in two cases by Beltinger and Saule (1988). Their findings consisted of bilateral cystic lesions in the subependymal germinal matrices. They noted that this finding had also been reported with congenital CMV infection.

Neuronal migrational disorders
Congenital infection of the brain occurring during the critical period of neuroblast migration may result in abnormal neuronal migration. Both CMV and *T. gondii* infections are known to cause such disordered neuronal migration (Crome and France 1959, Dennis and Alvord 1961, Navin and Angevine 1968, De Léon 1972, Friede and Mikolasek 1978, Marques Dias *et al.* 1984, Barth 1987, Byrd *et al.* 1987, Galloway and Roessmann 1987, Osborn *et al.* 1988, Hayward *et al.* 1991). Both CMV and *T. gondii* infect the entire brain but appear to have a predilection for the subependymal regions. Anomalous migration may result from injury at the subependymal region or anywhere in the brain parenchyma. The brains of patients thus affected grossly demonstrate pachygyria and microscopically demonstrate polymicrogyria. Polymicrogyria is very commonly present and is suspected in these patients when the cortical surface has a lumpy, bumpy or knobbly appearance. Occasionally the cortical surface is nearly smooth and has an agyric rather than a pachygyric appearance (Hayward *et al.* 1991).

Neuronal migrational disorders caused by congenital infection differ from those caused by other etiologies in that the infectious variety commonly also have intracranial calcification and more diffuse parenchymal high signal on long TR spin echo sequences. This high signal is secondary to demyelination and gliosis. Such white matter changes cannot be detected in neonates because their white matter is normally of high intensity on these sequences due to the lack of significant amounts of mature myelin. There may also be further intracranial abnormalities including infarction, atrophy and hydrocephalus.

CT and MRI findings in 14 patients with pachygyria induced by congenital brain infection were presented by Byrd *et al.* (1987). Two patients had congenital toxoplasmosis (Fig. 6.9) and the remainder had congenital CMV encephalitis (Fig. 6.10). This and other studies by the current and previous authors have found that MRI is the modality of choice for imaging all neuronal migrational disorders (Barkovich *et al.* 1987, Byrd *et al.* 1987, Osborn *et al.* 1988).

Pachygyria caused by infection tends to be less predictable or homogeneous in its appearance than that of an idiopathic etiology. The gyri tend not to be as regular and uniform as is often the case in idiopathic forms of pachygyria. The latter typically have larger gyri and deeper sulci. Infection-induced pachygyria typically exhibits gyri of varying size with scattered shallow sulci. Furthermore, idiopathic pachygyria usually has a smooth cortical surface, whereas infectious pachygyria usually has the knobbly cortical surface signifying the presence of polymicrogyria.

Human immunodeficiency virus (HIV) and related infections of the brain
Over 50 per cent of HIV infected individuals have neurologic symptoms. All patients with acquired immunodeficiency syndrome (AIDS) have brain involvement. HIV infection occurs early and results in a subacute encephalitis. Toxoplasmic encephalitis is the most common infection (with the exception of HIV itself) encountered in symptomatic patients. Other CNS infections found in HIV infected patients include cryptococcosis, pyogenic abscesses, tuberculosis, cysticercosis, progressive multifocal leukoencephalopathy, and those caused by CMV, HSV and *T. pallidum* (Price *et al.* 1986; Post *et al.* 1988, 1991; Chrysikopoulos *et al.* 1990; Flowers *et al.* 1990; Olsen 1991; Rovira *et al.* 1991).

The clinical picture ranges from nonfocal symptoms, including progressive dementia and AIDS encephalopathy, to focal effects caused by an intracranial mass of opportunistic infection or tumor.

HIV encephalitis
Patients with HIV encephalitis present with a progressive subcortical dementia (Price *et al.* 1986; Post *et al.* 1988, 1991; Chrysikopoulos *et al.* 1990; Flowers *et al.* 1990; Rovira *et al.* 1991). Children are affected as well as adults. Epstein *et al.* (1985) presented four pediatric cases of HIV encephalopathy. The symptoms included ataxia, loss of motor milestones and developmental delay. At autopsy these children's brains demonstrated cerebral atrophy, microglial nodules, and intranuclear inclusions.

The MRI appearance of HIV encephalitis includes cerebral atrophy and white matter lesions. Involvement of the deep white matter, which is best delineated with T_2-weighted imaging, appears as high intensity. The extent of white matter involvement correlates directly with the degree of cerebral atrophy and dementia (Tien *et al.* 1991). White matter lesions detected with MRI may be focal, diffuse, patchy or generalized. There is no mass effect or enhancement (Post *et al.* 1988, 1991; Chrysikopoulos *et al.* 1990; Flowers *et al.* 1990; Olsen 1991; Rovira *et al.* 1991).

Fig. 6.13. *(Opposite)* AIDS related toxoplasmosis. This 15-year-old male patient who had a factor VIII hematological deficiency acquired HIV infection through blood transfusions. *(a)* Short TR/TE axial image demonstrates a medial, bifrontal mass *(black arrows)* with associated hypointense white matter edema *(white arrows)*. *(b)* The centrally necrotic mass enhanced with gadolinium *(curved arrow)*; this lesion was proven to be toxoplasmosis. Enhancement of multiple, smaller lesions was also identified *(straight arrows)*. They responded to therapy appropriate for toxoplasmosis. *(c,d)* The frontal lesion was approximately isointense to gray matter on the long TR sequences *(black arrow)*. Prominent adjacent vasogenic edema is identified as well. Other small, etiologically nonspecific lesions appearing as high intensity foci were scattered throughout the brain *(white arrows)*.

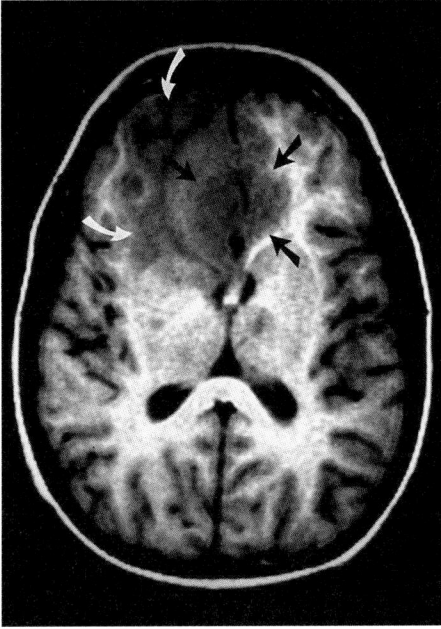

(a)

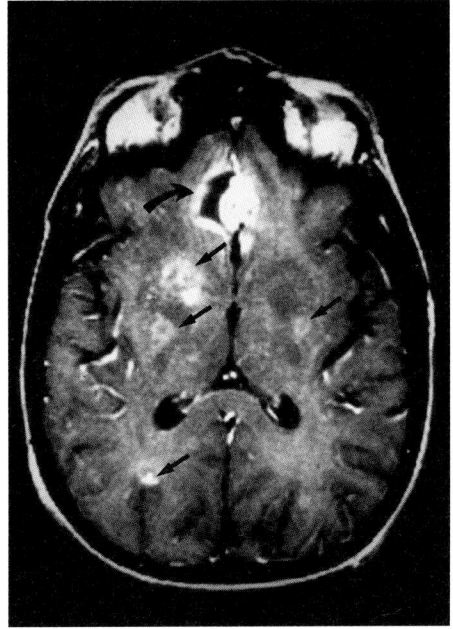

(b)

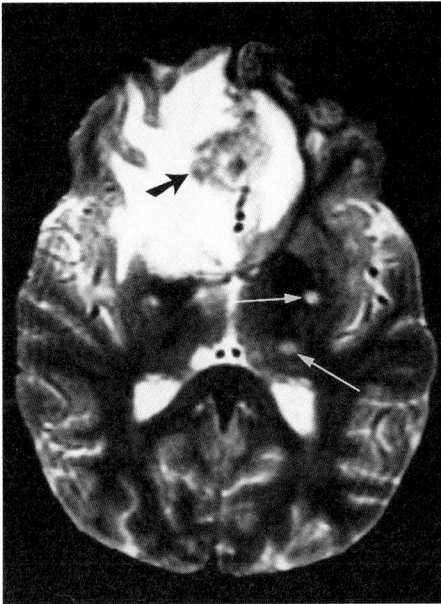

(c)

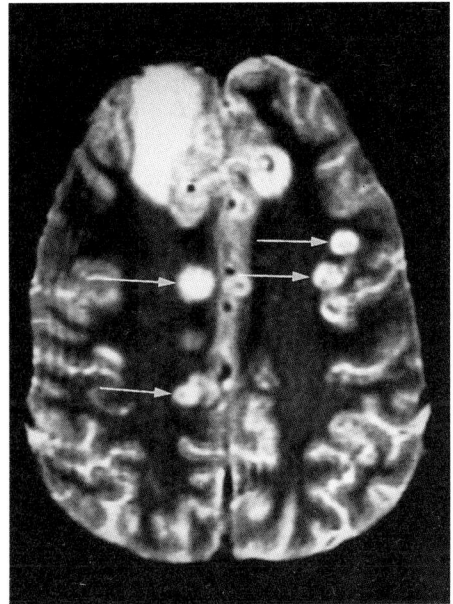

(d)

139

Toxoplasmosis

Toxoplasmosis in AIDS patients results in lesions that typically cause mass effect. They occur in approximately 10 per cent of HIV infected patients and are usually multiple and bilateral (Rovira *et al.* 1991). MRI demonstrates both well- and ill-defined lesions, which may be solid and cystic or centrally necrotic. The most common presentation is multiple thin-walled abscesses. These lesions enhance with gadolinium. T_1-weighted images demonstrate isointense lesions with surrounding hypointense edema. Long TR images demonstrate an iso- to hyperintense lesion with prominent high intensity surrounding edema. The thin-walled cystic lesions demonstrate a hypo- or isointense wall on T_2-weighted images (Olsen 1991, Rovira *et al.* 1991) (Fig. 6.13). Cerebral atrophy is commonly identified secondary to the existing HIV encephalitis. The primary differential consideration when toxoplasmosis is considered is lymphoma (Olsen 1991, Rovira *et al.* 1991). Lymphoma is more common than toxoplasmosis in children with AIDS (Smith and Kuharik 1990).

Fungal infections

Cryptococcosis is the most common fungal infection encountered in HIV infected individuals. It is the third most common infection after HIV and toxoplasmosis. *Cryptococcus* usually causes a meningitis rather than brain abscess. Although crytococcomas occur, an apparently pathognomonic finding in these patients is dilated Virchow–Robin spaces in the basal ganglia. The diagnosis of cryptococcosis is made by elevated cryptococcal antigen titers in the CSF and serum (Rovira *et al.* 1991, Tien *et al.* 1991).

The MRI appearance of cryptococcosis usually shows no abnormality if only meningitis is present. The low degree of inflammatory response that this infection incites in the meninges does not produce contrast enhancement when gadolinium is given, nor is there enhancement in the regions of the dilated Virchow–Robin spaces in the basal ganglia. Contrast enhancement is identified when a crytococcoma is present. Parenchymal lesions cannot be delineated from other infections such as toxoplasmosis.

Other fungal infections, including *Candida albicans*, *Aspergillus fumigatus* and *Coccidioides immitis*, are rare (Rovira *et al.* 1991, Tien *et al.* 1991).

Progressive multifocal leukoencephalopathy

Progressive multifocal leukoencephalopathy (PML) is a viral disease involving the white matter of immunosuppressed patients. The infection is caused by human papovavirus which affects myelin-producing oligodendrocytes. Fewer than 5 per cent of AIDS patients present with symptoms due to PML. Any neurologic symptom may be dominant, and they are not specific for this disease (Gilden 1983, Aksamit *et al.* 1986, Wolinsky 1990).

The earliest MRI finding with PML is focal areas of subcortical infection which appear as relative hypointensity on short TR sequences and hyperintensity on long TR sequences. The posterior centrum semiovale region is commonly involved. The lesions tend to increase in size over time and coalesce to form larger ones. Infection may cross from one hemisphere to the other via the corpus callosum (Fig. 6.14). PML does not enhance with gadolinium. Differential considerations when the diagnosis of AIDS has been made include other viral or non-enhancing infection or tumor. The diagnosis of

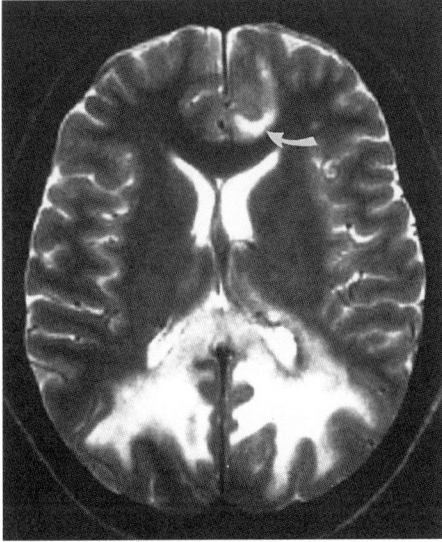

Fig. 6.14. Progressive multifocal leukoencephalopathy in a patient with AIDS. Long TR/TE axial image demonstrates high intensity white matter edema in both posterior parietal regions which communicates across the midline via the splenium of the corpus callosum. Multiple other white matter high intensity foci were present. One of these is identified in the left frontal region *(arrow)*.

PML can be suggested based on the MRI findings, predominately due to the pattern of involvement and lack of enhancement (Olsen 1991, Rovira *et al.* 1991).

Cytomegalovirus
CMV is a herpes virus which commonly infects the brains of AIDS patients. This infection is usually a subclinical one and therefore of less significance than other symptom-producing opportunistic infections. It is possible that CMV encephalitis might contribute to white matter changes including demyelination, with resultant high intensity on long TR images. It has been stated that CMV occasionally produces periventricular enhancement on gadolinium enhanced MR sequences (Olsen 1991).

Other infections
Some other infections found in immunosuppressed patients include pyogenic abscess, cysticercosis and tuberculosis. They do not differ in appearance from those found in non-immunosuppressed patients.

Other rare viral infections include those caused by HSV and the varicella–zoster virus. Few data are available for characterizing them. Neurosyphilis has been described and represents a vaso-occlusive process which produces cerebral infarction. Any meningoencephalitis may produce vasculitis and resultant infarction, therefore a pattern of infarction and vaso-occlusive disease is not pathognomonic for syphilis. The diagnosis of neurosyphilis requires clinical and pathologic methods (Pachner 1986).

REFERENCES

Aksamit, A.J., Sever, J.L., Major, E.O. (1986) 'Progressive multifocal leukoencephalopathy: JC virus detection *in situ* hybridization compared with immunohistochemistry.' *Neurology*, **36**, 499–504.

Alford, C.A., Stagno, S., Pass, R.F., Britt, W.J. (1990) 'Congenital and perinatal cytomegalovirus infections.' *Reviews of Infectious Diseases*, **12**, S745–S753.

Anders, B.J., Lauer, B.A., Foley, L.C. (1980) 'Computerized tomography to define CNS involvement in congenital cytomegalovirus infection.' *American Journal of Diseases of Children*, **134**, 795–797.

Apuzzo, M.L.J., Dobkin, W.R., Zee, C-S., Chan, J.C., Giannotta, S.L., Weiss, M.H. (1984) 'Surgical considerations in treatment of intraventricular cysticercosis. An analysis of 45 cases.' *Journal of Neurosurgery*, **60**, 400–407.

Bach, D., Goldenberg, M.H. (1983) 'Hemorrhage into a brain abscess.' *Journal of Computer Assisted Tomography*, **7**, 1067–1069.

Bakshi, S.S., Cooper, L.Z. (1989) 'Rubella.' *Clinical Dermatology*, **7**, 8–18.

Bale, J.F. (1984) 'Human cytomegalovirus infection and disorders of the nervous system.' *Archives of Neurology*, **41**, 310–320.

—— Bray, P.F., Bell, W.E. (1985) 'Neuroradiographic abnormalities in congenital cytomegalovirus infection.' *Pediatric Neurology*, **1**, 42–47.

Barkovich, A.J. (1990) 'Infections of the nervous system.' *In: Pediatric Neuroimaging.* New York: Raven Press, pp. 293–325.

—— Chuang, S.H., Norman, D. (1987) 'MR of neuronal migration anomalies.' *American Journal of Neuroradiology*, **8**, 1009–1017.

Barnes, D.W., Whitley, R.J. (1986) 'CNS diseases associated with varicella zoster virus and herpes simplex virus infection. Pathogenesis and current therapy.' *Neurologic Clinics*, **4**, 265–283.

Barth, P.G. (1987) 'Disorders of neuronal migration.' *Canadian Journal of Neurological Sciences*, **14**, 1–16.

Bazan, C., Rinaldi, M.G., Rauch, R.R., Jinkins, J.R. (1991) 'Fungal infections of the brain.' *Neuroimaging Clinics of North America*, **1**, 57–88.

Beltinger, C., Saule, H. 'Sonography of subependymal cysts in congenital rubella syndrome.' *European Journal of Pediatrics*, **148**, 206–207.

Byrd, S.E., Osborn, R.E., Naidich, T.P., Bohan, T.P. (1987) 'CT and MR imaging evaluation of the inherited and prenatally acquired migrational disorders of the brain.' *Radiology*, **165** (Suppl.), 99. *(Abstract.)*

Castro, C.C., Hesselink, J.R. (1991) 'Tuberculosis.' *Neuroimaging Clinics of North America*, **1**, 119–139.

Chang, K.H., Han, M.H., Roh, J.K., Kim, I.O., Han, M.C., Choi, K.S., Kim, C-W. (1990*a*) 'Gd-DTPA enhanced MR imaging of intracranial tuberculosis.' *Neuroradiology*, **32**, 19–25.

—— —— —— —— —— Kim, C-W. (1990*b*) 'Gd-DPTA-enhanced MR imaging of the brain in patients with meningitis: comparison with CT.' American Journal of Roentgenology, 154, 809–816.

—— Cho, S.Y., Hesselink, J.R., Han, M.H., Han, M.C. (1991*a*) 'Parasitic diseases of the central nervous system.' *Neuroimaging Clinics of North America*, **1**, 159–178.

—— Lee, J.H., Han, M.H., Han, M.C. (1991*b*) 'The role of contrast-enhanced MR imaging in the diagnosis of neurocysticercosis.' *American Journal of Neuroradiology*, **12**, 509–512.

Chowdhury, M.N.H. (1986) 'Toxoplasmosis: a review.' *Journal of Medicine; Clinical, Experimental and Theoretical*, **17**, 373–396.

Chrysikopoulos, H.S., Press, G.A., Grafe, M.R., Hesselink, J.R., Wiley, C.A. (1990) 'Encephalitis caused by human immunodeficiency virus: CT and MR imaging manifestations with clinical and pathologic correlation.' *Radiology*, **175**, 185–191.

Clark, W.C., Metcalf, J.C., Muhlbauer, M.S., Dohan, F.C., Robertson, J.H. (1986) '*Mycobacterium tuberculosis* meningitis: a report of twelve cases and a literature review.' *Neurosurgery*, **18**, 604–610.

Cooper, L.Z., Ziring, P.R., Ockerse, A.B., Fedun, B.A., Kiely, B., Krugman, S. (1969) 'Rubella: clinical manifestations and management.' *American Journal of Diseases of Children*, **118**, 18–29.

Crome, L., France, N.E. (1959) 'Microgyria and cytomegalic inclusion disease in infancy.' *Journal of Clinical Pathology*, **12**, 427–434.

De Léon, G.A. (1972) 'Observations on cerebral and cerebellar microgyria.' *Acta Neuropathologica*, **20**, 278–287.

Dennis, J.P., Alvord, E.C. (1961) 'Microcephaly with intracerebral calcification and subependymal ossification: radiologic and clinico-pathologic correlation.' *Journal of Neuropathology and Experimental Neurology*, **20**, 412–426.

Desai, S.P., Bazan, C., Hummell, W., Jinkins, J.R. (1991) 'Disseminated CNS histoplasmosis.' *American Journal of Neuroradiology*, **12**, 290–292.

Desmonts, G. (1982) 'Toxoplasmose acquise de la femme enceinte. Estimation du risque de transmission du parasite et de toxoplasmose congénitale.' *Lyon Medical*, **248**, 115–123.

142

—— Couvreur, J. (1974) 'Congenital toxoplasmosis. A prospective study of 378 pregnancies' *New England Journal of Medicine*, **290**, 1110–1116.

Diebler, C., Dusser, A., Dulac, O. (1985) 'Congenital toxoplasmosis: clinical and neuroradiological evaluation of the cerebral lesions.' *Neuroradiology*, **27**, 125–130.

Dion, F.M., Venger, B.H., Landon, G. (1987) 'Thalamic histoplasmoma: CT and MR imaging.' *Journal of Computer Assisted Tomography*, **11**, 193–195.

Draouat, S., Abdenabi, B., Ghanem, M., Bourjat, P. (1987) 'Computed tomography of cerebral tuberculoma.' *Journal of Computer Assisted Tomography*, **11**, 594–597.

Enzmann, D.R. (1984a) 'Focal parenchymal infection.' *In: Imaging of Infections and Inflammation of the Central Nervous System: Computed Tomography, Ultrasound and Nuclear Magnetic Resonance.* New York: Raven Press, pp. 27–102.

—— (1984b) 'Extracerebral infection.' *In: Imaging of Infections and Inflammation of the Central Nervous System: Computed Tomography, Ultrasound and Nuclear Magnetic Resonance.* New York: Raven Press, pp. 234–249.

—— (1984c) 'Diffuse parenchymal infections.' *In: Imaging of Infections and Inflammation of the Central Nervous System: Computed Tomography, Ultrasound and Nuclear Magnetic Resonance.* New York: Raven Press, pp. 128–175.

Epstein, L.G., Sharer, L.R., Joshi, V.V., Fojas, M.M., Koenigsberger, M.R., Oleske, J.M. (1985) 'Progressive encephalopathy in children with acquired immune deficiency syndrome.' *Annals of Neurology*, **17**, 488–496.

Fitz, C.R. (1985) 'Inflammatory diseases.' *In:* Gonzalez, C.F., Grossman, C.B., Masdeu, J.C. (Eds.) *Head and Spine Imaging.* New York: Wiley, pp. 537–554.

Flowers, C.H., Mafee, M.F., Crowell, R., Raofi, B., Arnold, P., Dobben, G., Wycliffe, N. 'Encephalopathy in AIDS patients: evaluation with MR imaging.' *American Journal of Neuroradiology*, 11, 1235–1245.

Freij, B.J., Sever, J.L. (1988) 'Herpesvirus infections in pregnancy: risks to embryo, fetus, and neonate.' *Clinics in Perinatology*, **15**, 203–231.

—— South, M.A., Sever, J.L. (1988) 'Maternal rubella and the congenital rubella syndrome.' *Clinics in Perinatology*, **15**, 247–257.

Friede, R.L., Mikolasek, J. (1978) 'Postencephalitic porencephaly, hydranencephaly or polymicrogyria: a review.' *Acta Neurologica Pathologica*, **43**, 161–168.

Galloway, P.G., Roessmann, U. (1987) 'Diffuse dysplasia of cerebral hemispheres in a fetus. Possible viral cause?' *Archives of Pathology and Laboratory Medicine*, **111**, 143–145.

Gilden, D.H. (1983) 'Slow virus diseases of the CNS. 1. Subacute sclerosing panencephalitis, progressive rubella panencephalitis, and progressive multifocal leukoencephalopathy.' *Postgraduate Medicine*, **73** (1), 99–108.

Grossman, R.I., Davis, K.R., Taveras, J.M., Beal, M.F., O'Carroll, C.P. (1981) 'Computed tomography of intracranial aspergillosis.' *Journal of Computer Assisted Tomography*, **5**, 646–650.

Gupta, R., Singh, A.K., Bishnu, P., Malhotra, V. (1990) 'Intracranial *Aspergillus* granuloma simulating meningioma on MR imaging.' *Journal of Computer Assisted Tomography*, **14**, 467–469.

Haimes, A.B., Zimmerman, R.D., Morgello, S., Weingarten, K., Becker, R.D., Jennis, R., Deck, M.D.F. (1989) 'MR imaging of brain abscesses.' *American Journal of Roentgenology*, **152**, 1073–1085.

Harris, T.M., Edwards, M.K. (1991) 'Meningitis.' *Neuroimaging Clinics of North America*, **1**, 39–56.

Hayward, J.C., Titelbaum, D.S., Clancy, R.R., Zimmerman, R.A. (1991) 'Lissencephaly–pachygyria associated with congenital cytomegalovirus infection.' *Journal of Child Neurology*, **6**, 109–114.

Herman, T.E., Cleveland, R.H., Kushner, D.C., Taveras, J.M. (1985) 'CT of neonatal herpes encephalitis.' *American Journal of Neuroradiology*, **6**, 733–775.

Jinkins, J.R., Siqueira, E., Al-Kawi, M.Z. (1987) 'Cranial manifestations of aspergillosis.' *Neuroradiology*, **29**, 181–185.

Jordan, J., Enzmann, D.R. (1991) 'Encephalitis.' *Neuroimaging Clinics of North America*, **1**, 17–38.

Jungreis, C.A., Grossman, R.I. (1991) 'Intracranial infections and inflammatory diseases.' *In:* Latchaw, R.E. (Ed.) *MR and CT Imaging of the Head, Neck and Spine, 2nd Edn.* St. Louis, MI: Mosby Year Book, pp. 303–346.

Klein, J.O., Remington, J.S. (1990) 'Current concepts of infections of the fetus and newborn infant.' *In:* Remington, J.S., Klein, J.O. (Eds.) *Infectious Diseases of the Fetus and Newborn Infant, 3rd Edn.* Philadelphia: W.B. Saunders, pp. 1–16.

Kramer, L.D., Locke, G.E., Byrd, S.E., Daryabagi, J. (1989) 'Cerebral cysticercosis: documentation of natural history with CT.' *Radiology*, **171**, 459–462.

143

Loizou, L.A., Anderson, M. (1982) 'Intracranial tuberculomas: correlation of computerized tomography with clinico-pathological findings.' *Quarterly Journal of Medicine*, **51**, 104–114.

Loo, L., Braude, A. (1982) 'Cerebral cysticercosis in San Diego. A report of 23 cases and a review of the literature.' *Medicine*, **61**, 341–359.

Lotz, J., Hewlett, R., Alheit, B., Bowen, R. (1988) 'Neurocysticercosis: correlative pathomorphology and MR imaging.' *Neuroradiology*, **30**, 35–41.

Lyons, R.W., Andriole, V.T. (1986) 'Fungal infections of the CNS.' *Neurologic Clinics*, **4**, 159–170.

Manz, H.J. (1977) 'Pathology and pathogenesis of viral infections of the central nervous system.' *Human Pathology*, **8**, 3–26.

Marques Dias, M.J., Harmant-van Rijckevorsel, G., Landrieu, P., Lyon, G. (1984) 'Prenatal cytomegalovirus disease and cerebral microgyria: evidence for perfusion failure, not disturbance of histogenesis, as the major cause of fetal cytomegalovirus encephalopathy.' *Neuropediatrics*, **15**, 18–24.

Mikhael, M.A., Rushovich, A.M., Ciric, I. (1985) 'Magnetic resonance imaging of cerebral aspergillosis.' *Computerized Radiology*, **9**, 85–89.

Miller, E., Cradock-Watson, J.E., Pollock, T.M. (1982) 'Consequences of confirmed maternal rubella at successive stages of pregnancy.' *Lancet*, **2**, 781–784.

Navin, J.J., Angevine, J.M. (1968) 'Congenital cytomegalic inclusion disease with porencephaly.' *Neurology*, **18**, 470–472.

Neils, E.W., Lukin, R., Tomsick, T.A., Tew, J.M. (1987) 'Magnetic resonance imaging and computed tomography scanning of herpes simplex encephalitis. Report of two cases.' *Journal of Neurosurgery*, **67**, 592–594.

Noorbehesht, B., Enzmann, D.R., Sullinder, W., Bradley, J.S., Arvin, A.M. (1987) 'Neonatal herpes simplex encephalitis: correlation of clinical and CT findings.' *Radiology*, **162**, 813–819.

Olsen, W.L. (1991) 'MRI of the brain in patients with AIDS.' *MRI Decisions*, **5**, 19–28.

Osborn, R.E., Byrd, S.E., Naidich, T.P., Bohan, T.P., Friedman, H. (1988) 'MR imaging of neuronal migrational disorders.' *American Journal of Neuroradiology*, **9**, 1101–1106.

Overturf, G.D. (1986) 'Pyogenic bacterial infections of the CNS.' *Neurologic Clinics*, **4**, 69–90.

Pachner, A.R. (1986) 'Spirochetal diseases of the CNS.' *Neurologic Clinics*, **4**, 207–222.

Post, M.J.D., Tate, L.G., Quencer, R.M., Hensley, G.T., Berger, J.R., Sheremata, W.A., Maul, G. (1988) 'CT, MR, and pathology in HIV encephalitis and meningitis.' *American Journal of Roentgenology*, **151**, 373–380.

—— Berger, J.R., Quencer, R.M. (1991) 'Asymptomatic and neurologically symptomatic HIV-seropositive individuals: prospective evaluation with cranial MR imaging.' *Radiology*, **178**, 131–139.

Preblud, S.R., Alford, C.A. (1990) 'Rubella.' *In:* Remington, J.S., Klein, J.O. (Eds.) *Infectious Diseases of the Fetus and Newborn Infant, 3rd Edn.* Philadelphia: W.B. Saunders, pp. 196–240.

Price, R.W., Navia, B.A., Cho, E.S. (1986) 'AIDS encephalopathy.' *Neurologic Clinics*, **4**, 285–301.

Remington, J.S., Desmonts, G. (1990) 'Toxoplasmosis.' *In:* Remington, J.S., Klein, J.O. (Eds.) *Infectious Diseases of the Fetus and Newborn Infant, 3rd Edn.* Philadelphia: W.B. Saunders, pp. 89–195.

Roos, K.L., Bryan, J.P., Maggio, W.W., Jane, J.A., Scheld, W.M. (1987) 'Intracranial blastomycoma.' *Medicine*, **66**, 224–235.

Rovira, M.J., Post, M.J.D., Bowen, B.C. (1991) 'Central nervous system infections in HIV-positive persons.' *Neuroimaging Clinics of North America*, **1**, 179–200.

Salazar, A., Sotelo, J., Martinez, H., Escobedo, F. (1983) 'Differential diagnosis between ventriculitis and fourth ventricle cyst in neurocysticercosis.' *Journal of Neurosurgery*, **59**, 660–663.

Schoeman, J., Hewlett, R., Donald, P. (1988) 'MR of childhood tuberculous meningitis.' *Neuroradiology*, **30**, 473–477.

Schroth, G., Gawehn, J., Thron, A., Vallbracht, A., Voigt, K. (1987*a*) 'Early diagnosis of herpes simplex encephalitis by MRI.' *Neurology*, **37**, 179–183.

—— Kretzschmar, K., Gawehn, J., Voigt, K. (1987*b*) 'Advantage of magnetic resonance imaging in the diagnosis of cerebral infections.' *Neuroradiology*, **29**, 120–126.

Sheller, J.R., Des Prez, R.M. (1986) 'CNS tuberculosis.' *Neurological Clinics*, **4**, 143–158.

Smith, R.R., Kuharik, M.A. (1990) 'Inflammation and infection of the brain.' *In:* Cohen, M.D., Edwards, M.K. (Eds.) *Magnetic Resonance Imaging of Children.* Philadelphia: B.C. Decker, pp. 221–275.

Sotelo, J., Guerrero, V., Rubio, F. (1985) 'Neurocysticercosis: a new classification based on active and inactive forms.' *Archives of Internal Medicine*, **145**, 442–445.

Stagno, S. (1990) 'Cytomegalovirus.' *In:* Remington, J.S., Klein, J.O. (Eds.) *Infectious Diseases of the Fetus and Newborn Infant, 3rd Edn.* Philadelphia: W.B. Saunders, pp. 241–281.

Syrogiannopoulos, G.A., Nelson, J.D., McCracken, G.H. (1986) 'Subdural collections of fluid in acute bacterial meningitis: a review of 136 cases.' *Pediatric Infectious Disease*, **5**, 343–352.

Sze, G., Zimmerman, R.D. (1988) 'The magnetic resonance imaging of infections and inflammatory diseases.' *Radiologic Clinics of North America*, **26**, 839–859.

Täuber, M.G., Brooks-Fournier, R.A., Sande, M.A. (1986) 'Experimental models of CNS infections. Contributions to concepts of disease and treatment.' *Neurologic Clinics*, **4**, 249–264.

Tien, R.D., Chu, P.K., Hesselink, J.R., Duberg, A., Wiley, C. (1991) 'Intracranial cryptococcosis in immunocompromised patients: CT and MR findings in 29 cases.' *American Journal of Neuroradiology*, **12**, 283–289.

Ulmer, J.L., Elster, A.D. (1991) 'Sarcoidosis of the central nervous system.' *Neuroimaging Clinics of North America*, **1**, 141–158.

Weingarten, K., Zimmerman, R.D., Becker, R.D., Heier, L.A., Haimes, A.B., Deck, M.D.F. (1989) 'Subdural and epidural empyemas: MR imaging.' *American Journal of Roentgenology*, **152**, 615–621.

Whitley, R.J. (1990) 'Herpes simplex virus infections.' *In:* Remington, J.S., Klein, J.O. (Eds.) *Infectious Diseases of the Fetus and Newborn Infant, 3rd Edn.* Philadelphia: W.B. Saunders, pp. 282–305.

Wilhelm, C., Ellner, J.J. (1986) 'Chronic meningitis.' *Neurologic Clinics*, **4**, 115–141.

Wolinsky, J.S. (1990) 'Subacute sclerosing panencephalitis, progressive rubella panencephalitis, and multifocal leukoencephalopathy.' *In:* Waksman, B.H. (Ed.) *Immunologic Mechanisms in Neurologic and Psychiatric Disease.* New York: Raven Press, pp. 259–268.

Zee, C-S., Segall, H.D., Apuzzo, M.L.J., Ahmadi, J., Dobkin, W.R. (1984) 'Intraventricular cysticercal cysts: further neuroradiologic observations and neurosurgical implications.' *American Journal of Neuroradiology*, **5**, 727–730.

Zimmerman, R.D., Haimes, A.B. (1989) 'The role of MR imaging in the diagnosis of infections of the central nervous system.' *Current Clinical Topics in Infectious Diseases*, **10**, 82–108.

—— Weingarten, K. (1991) 'Neuroimaging of cerebral abscesses.' *Neuroimaging Clinics of North America*, **1**, 1–16.

7
CEREBROVASCULAR MRI

Michele H. Johnson

Computed tomography (CT) was the first non-invasive modality to provide cross-sectional imaging of cerebrovascular pathologic processes. Magnetic resonance imaging (MRI), with its multiplanar, cross-sectional imaging capacity, together with magnetic resonance angiography (MRA) provide information about cerebrovascular structures previously only available with conventional angiography. Improvements in MRA technology may significantly reduce the need for conventional angiography in children with the exception of those cases requiring endovascular therapeutic procedures.

Vascular disorders in children have been classified into a variety of different categories (Chaung 1989). Many lesions present with stroke syndromes as a result of either occlusive disease or intracerebral hemorrhage. Others are discovered incidentally during the evaluation of headache or seizure disorders. MRI and MRA are uniquely suited for the evaluation of cerebrovascular disorders in children.

Stroke

Stroke can be defined as a loss of neurologic function due to ischemic injury, resulting in parenchymal destruction. Stroke syndromes are often apoplectic, although significant clinical syndromes may result as sequelae of chronic ischemia. Although stroke is less commonly seen in children than in adults, in one study children with stroke represented 2.52 per 100,000 patients (Schoenberg *et al.* 1978). Smith and Baumann (1991) reviewed the clinical and MRI findings of stroke in 53 children, which in the majority (69 per cent) occurred during the neonatal period. Stroke in childhood occurs at a rate equivalent to one half the incidence of pediatric brain tumors (Schoenberg *et al.* 1978).

Strokes in children can be characterized in the same manner as those in adults. They may be hemorrhagic or non-hemorrhagic, focal, multifocal or global, and may result from either direct or indirect vascular compromise. Clinically, stroke syndromes in young patients are often referred to as 'acute hemiplegia of childhood'. This term may refer to infarcts of any etiology, but commonly refers to those caused by vascular occlusion. Infarcts of idiopathic origin are often placed in this category. Vascular occlusion may be the result of intracranial vasculitis or vasculopathy (*i.e.* systemic lupus erythematosus and sickle cell disease), metabolic diseases (*i.e.* homocystinuria), or embolic occlusion secondary to cardiac disease or extracranial vascular disorders (*i.e.* fibromuscular dysplasia or dissection).

The MRI characteristics of stroke have been thoroughly described in the adult patient (Yuh *et al.* 1991). Wiznitzer and Masaryk (1991) reviewed the MRI and MRA findings in 24 pediatric stroke patients, 18 of whom had arterial stenosis or occlusion. Alterations in vascular flow may be detected prior to detection of parenchymal ischemia (Bradley and

Waluch 1985). The finding of increased signal intensity within major vessels or their branches suggests flow reduction or vascular occlusion (Fig. 7.1). T_2-weighted images have been found to be most sensitive in this regard. Arterial enhancement following gadolinium administration may be identified in the setting of slow arterial flow due to stenosis or distal occlusion (Yuh 1991). Tissue response to ischemia (edema, infarction) is typically identified following detection of flow alterations. Both cytotoxic edema, occurring within the first six hours after infarction, and vasogenic edema, occurring at approximately six hours, manifest as increased signal intensity on T_2-weighted images (Fig. 7.2) (Inagaki *et al.* 1992). With cortical infarction, sulcal effacement may be present. Other manifestations of mass effect from edema, such as ventricular effacement and subfalcine or transtentorial herniation, may also be identified. Contrast enhancement is classically seen at the five to seven day period (as with CT) due to breakdown of the blood–brain barrier (Fig. 7.3). Sometimes, however, irregular enhancement may be seen within several hours of infarction (Fig. 7.4). This may be related to localized loss of autoregulation, which allows the enhancement to occur, despite an 'intact' blood–brain barrier (Yuh *et al.* 1991).

Occlusive vascular disease
Major vessel occlusion
Internal carotid artery occlusion may occur as a primary lesion, usually located just above the level of the ophthalmic artery origin. Intimal webs and clefts, as well as abrupt occlusions, have been demonstrated angiographically, although the exact etiology of the occlusion may never be determined. MRI demonstrates a lack of blood flow (absence of flow void) in the occluded internal carotid artery and the presence of ischemic changes in the involved hemisphere.

Occlusive disease involving the *middle cerebral artery* may occur as an isolated lesion, resulting in infarction of the corresponding vascular territory. A range of lesions are demonstrable on MRI, depending on the point of occlusion and the adequacy of collateral vascular supply to the ischemic territory (Figs. 7.1–7.4). Lack of flow void in the middle cerebral artery or its branches may be observed on the cross-sectional images. MRA may allow direct demonstration of the lesion in the middle cerebral artery (Fig. 7.3). MRI is particularly useful for the evaluation of vertebrobasilar occlusive disease (Fig. 7.5).

Moyamoya syndrome refers to a specific constellation of collateral channels identified in the setting of proximal vascular occlusive disease (Fig. 7.6). First reported in the 1960s (Kudo 1965, Takeuchi *et al.* 1982), moyamoya (which translates as 'puff of smoke' in Japanese), refers to a pattern of basal collaterals occurring secondary to proximal vascular occlusions of multiple cerebral vessels. CT scans on patients with moyamoya circulation are notable for cerebral infarctions, most commonly in watershed vascular territories (Bruno *et al.* 1988). These are evident in 60–80 per cent of patients (Takeuchi *et al.* 1982, Chaung 1989). MRI not only reveals areas of infarction, but also allows direct visualization of these collateral vessels as multiple small flow voids at the base of the brain and basal ganglia (Welch *et al.* 1988, Storm and Uhlenbrock 1989, Wilms *et al.* 1989, Suto *et al.* 1990).

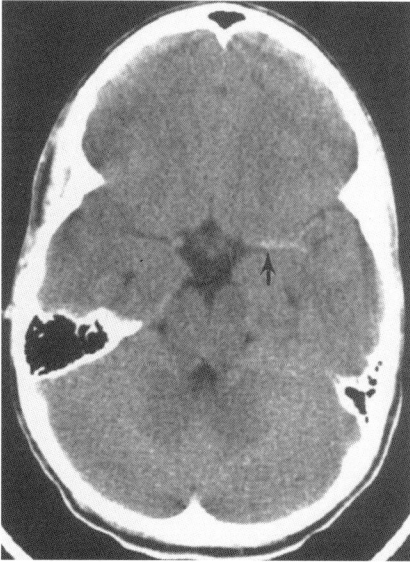

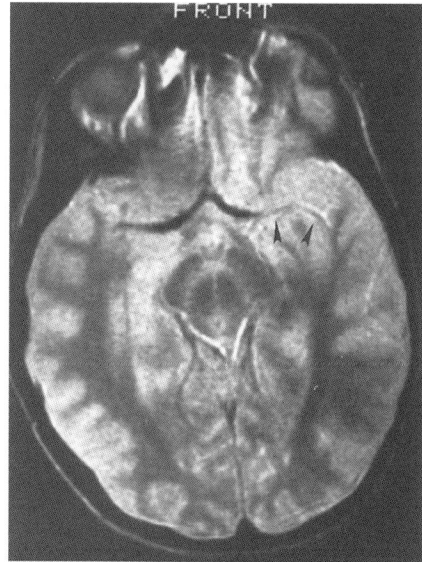

Fig. 7.1. Homocystinuria. *(Left)* Axial CT in this 12-year-old female demonstrates hyperdensity in the left middle cerebral artery (MCA), consistent with MCA thrombosis *(arrow)*. *(Right)* The MRI (TE 45/TR 3000) demonstrates absence of the flow void normally seen in the MCA and its branches *(arrowheads)*, along with hyperintense signal in the lentiform nucleus, indicative of infarction.

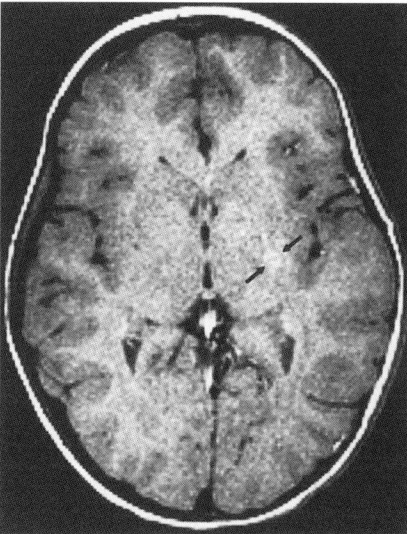

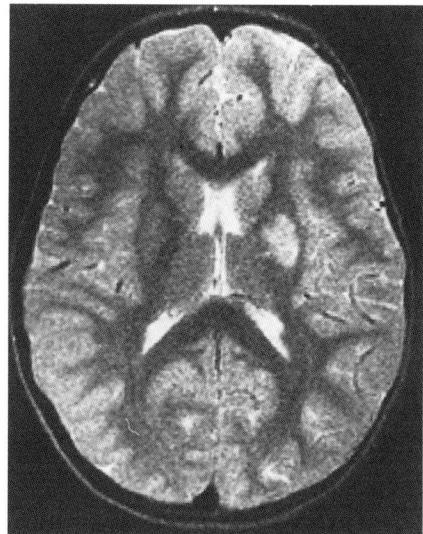

Fig. 7.2. Middle cerebral artery infarction. *(Left)* Axial T_1-weighted image (TE 20/TR 700) after contrast administration demonstrates heterogenous increased signal in the left basal ganglia with a small area of contrast enhancement *(arrows)*. *(Right)* On T_2-weighted image (TE 90/TR 3000) there is increased signal intensity in the basal ganglia. This extended upward to involve the corona radiata, consistent with cerebral infarction in this 11-year-old child.

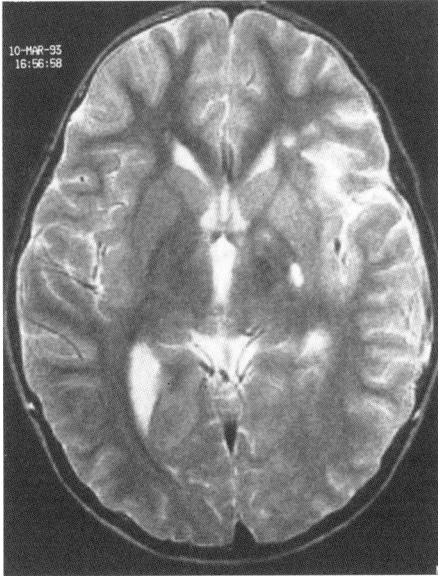

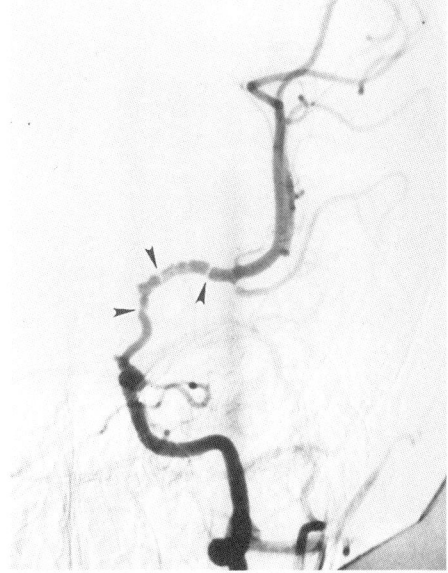

Fig. 7.3. Middle cerebral artery (MCA) occlusive disease with infarction. *(Left)* On the T_2-weighted image there is an area of increased signal intensity in the MCA territory on the left, involving both the cortical and basal ganglia regions. *(Right)* Anteroposterior view of the left internal cerebral artery (ICA) demonstrates a small ICA which terminates in a beaded, irregular proximal (M-1) segment of the MCA *(arrowheads)*. Note that only the proximal branches of the MCA are filled.

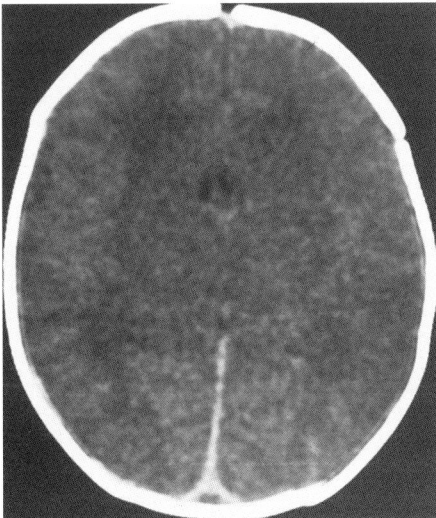

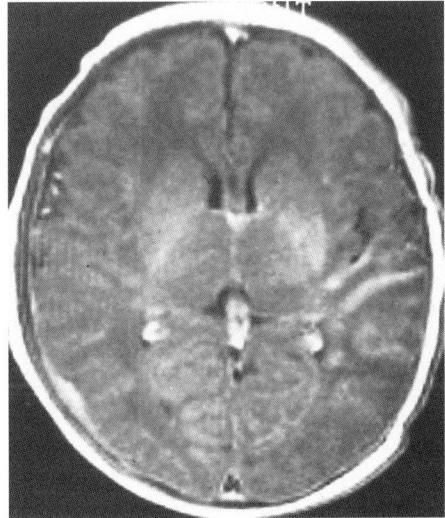

Fig. 7.4. Acute middle cerebral artery (MCA) infarction with early contrast enhancement. *(Left)* Non-contrast CT in a newborn infant demonstrates loss of gray–white matter differentiation in the left MCA distribution. *(Right)* T_1-weighted axial MRI scan following contrast administration demonstrates irregular enhancement in the MCA distribution.

149

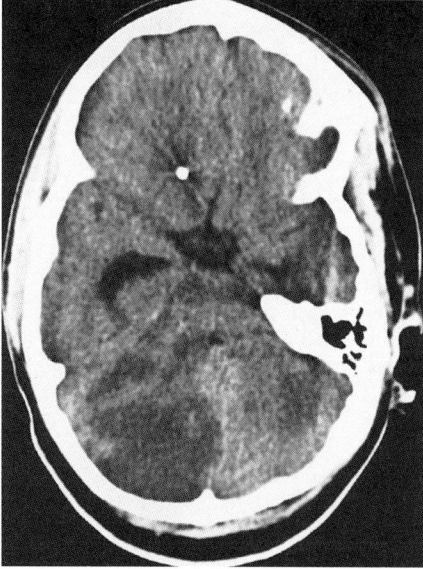

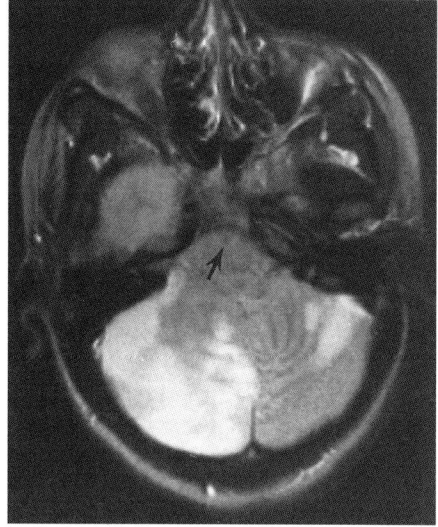

Fig. 7.5. Vertebrobasilar occlusive disease with infarction. *(Left)* Non-contrast CT demonstrates infarction of both cerebellar hemispheres with edema causing compression of the fourth ventricle and hydrocephalus (see large temporal horns and ventriculostomy catheter). *(Right)* On the proton density (TE 45/TR 3000) MR image the areas of infarction are hyperintense with respect to normal brain. The fourth ventricle is not visible. Note the absence of flow void in the region of the basilar artery *(arrow)*. Vertebral arteriography demonstrated marked irregularity of the basilar artery without normal filling of posterior cerebral branches.

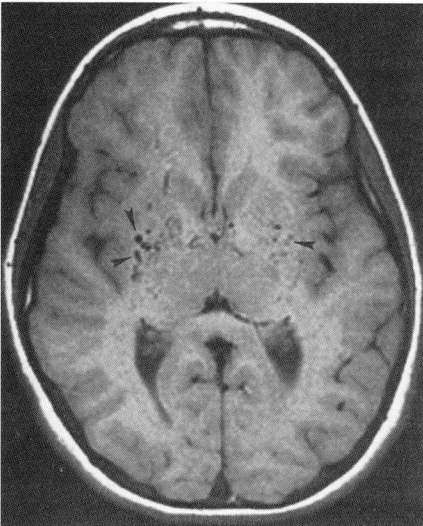

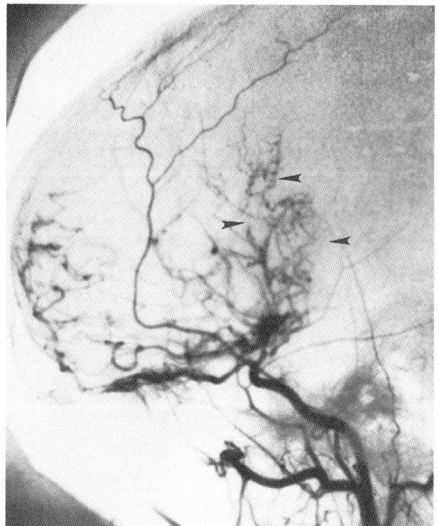

Fig. 7.6. Moyamoya circulation. *(Left)* T_1-weighted axial image demonstrates multiple flow voids in the basal ganglia *(arrowheads)*. *(Right)* Note the correlation between the sagittal MRI and the lateral carotid arteriogram *(arrowheads)*. (Courtesy of W.R.K. Smoker, Richmond, VA.)

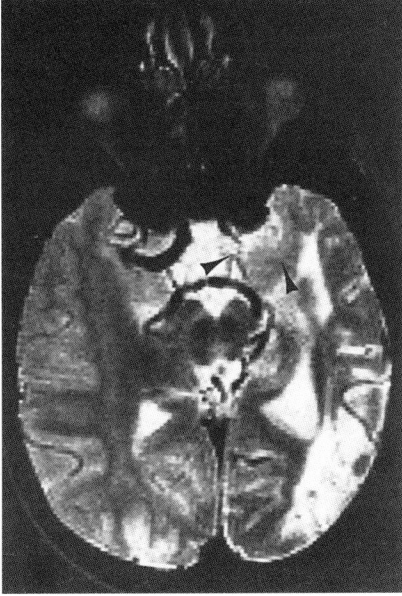
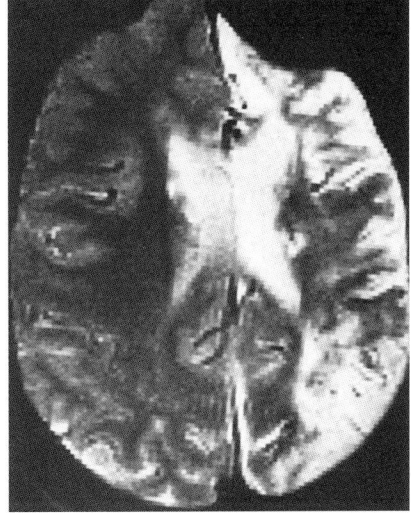

Fig. 7.7. Sickle cell hemoglobinopathy with infarction. T_1-weighted MRI in this 13-year-old demonstrated marked atrophy of the left cerebral hemisphere, involving principally the middle (MCA) and anterior cerebral artery (ACA) territories. The ipsilateral ventricle was normal in size. *(a)* T_2-weighted image (TE 90/TR 3000) demonstrates absence of the flow void in the region of the left ICA and left MCA *(arrowheads) (b)* Areas of encephalomalacia are present resulting from proximal vascular occlusion.

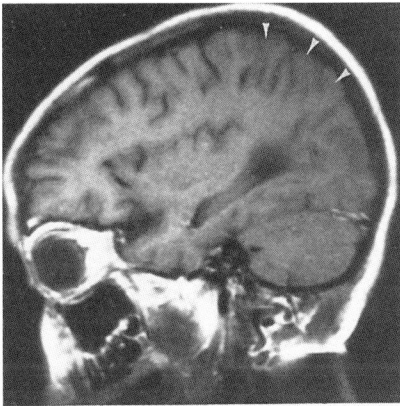
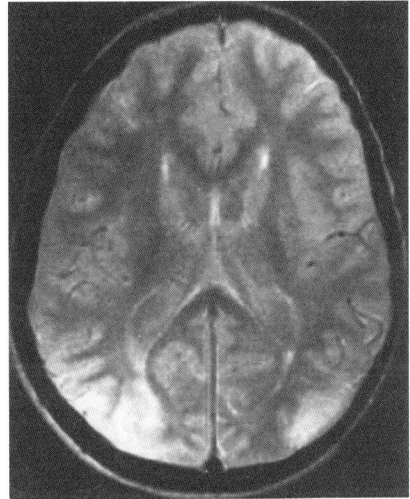

Fig. 7.8. Lupus vasculitis. *(Left)* T_1-weighted MRI (TE 20/TR 700) demonstrates decreased signal intensity in the parieto-occipital region *(arrowheads)*. *(Right)* T_2-weighted image (TE 45/TR 3000) demonstrates hyperintensity in the watershed vascular territories secondary to infarction. Right carotid anteriography in the arterial phase demonstrated a branch occlusion and multiple branches with irregular widening and narrowing typical of vasculitis.

151

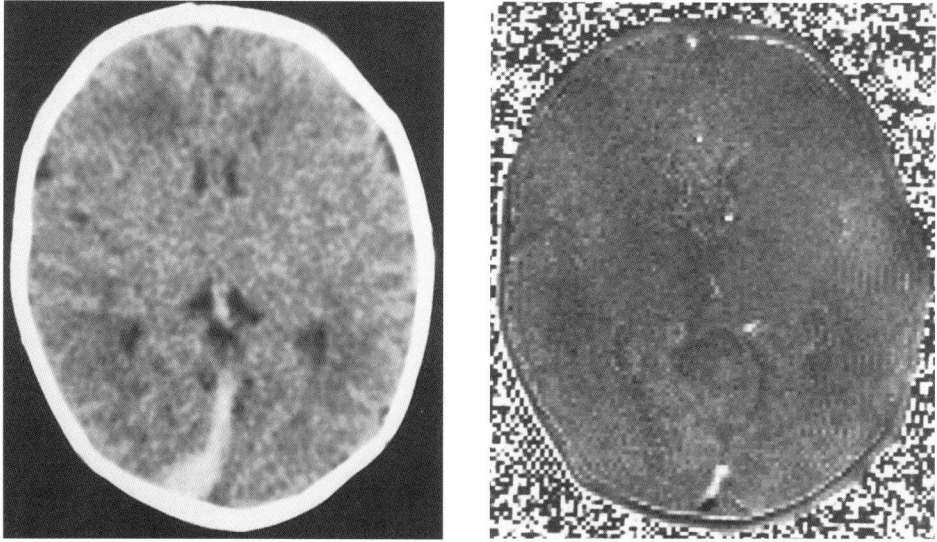

Fig. 7.9. Dehydrated 3-day-old infant with apparent sinus thrombosis on CT. *(Left)* Axial CT examination without contrast demonstrates increased density in the straight sinus and transverse sinus. *(Right)* The phase contrast MRI (TE 20/TR 700) demonstrates normal flow within the dural venous sinuses.

Sickle cell vasculopathy is one of the identifiable causes of cerebrovascular occlusive disease and infarction. Cerebrovascular complications of sickle cell anemia occur in 6–17 per cent of patients, often running in families (Powars *et al.* 1978, Wood 1978, Zimmerman *et al.* 1987). MRI and MRA may demonstrate both the vaso-occlusive disease and the resultant infarction in patients with sickle cell disease (Zimmerman *et al.* 1987, Adams *et al.* 1988, Pavlakis *et al.* 1988) (Fig. 7.7). The proximal vascular occlusive disease most commonly involves the proximal middle cerebral or internal carotid arteries, resulting in cortical infarction, typically in the watershed (border zone) regions of the brain (Pavlakis *et al.* 1988). Pathologic evidence of occlusive disease in the penetrating arterioles may account for the patchy deep white matter lesions seen in many patients with sickle cell anemia (El Gammel *et al.* 1986, Zimmerman *et al.* 1987).

Vasculitis in the CNS may be either idiopathic or caused by a connective tissue disease such as systemic lupus erythematosus. Arteriography demonstrates irregularity of medium or small vessels, ranging from areas of widening and narrowing to areas of frank 'beading'. MRI may demonstrate multiple areas of increased signal intensity on T_2-weighted images, corresponding to areas of ischemia and/or infarction usually in watershed vascular territories (Fig. 7.8).

Dural sinus and cerebral venous thrombosis
Dehydration from any cause (prolonged vomiting, starvation, diabetic ketoacidosis) may lead to dural sinus and/or cerebral venous thrombosis. The resulting increased intracranial

152

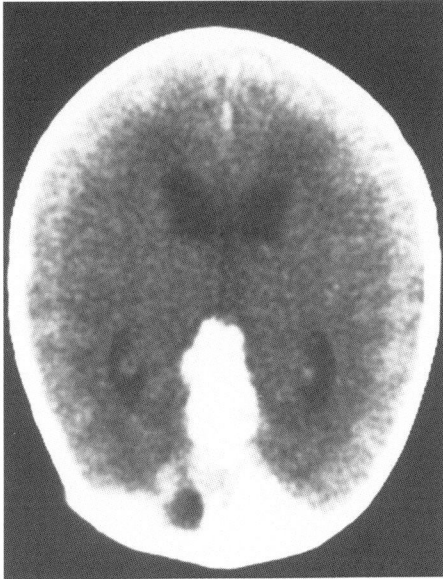
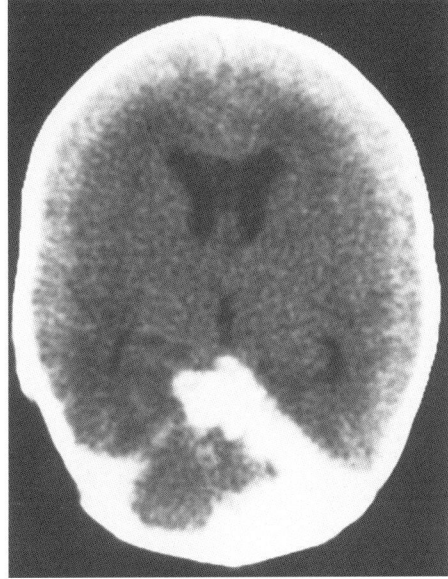

(a)   (b)

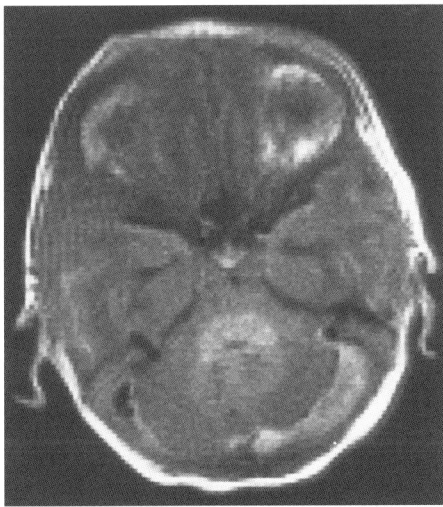
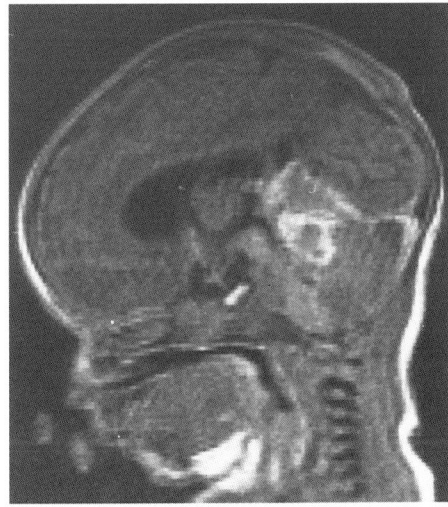

(c)   (d)

Fig. 7.10. Dural sinus thrombosis. *(a,b)* CT examination demonstrates increased density in the transverse and straight sinus as well as the sigmoid sinus. Mild increase in ventricular size is apparent. *(c)* Axial T_1-weighted image (TE 17/TR 700) demonstrates hyperintensity in the transverse sinus on the left. *(d)* The sagittal T_1-weighted image (TE 17/TR 700) demonstrates increased signal intensity in the region of the vein of Galen, straight sinus and torcular.

153

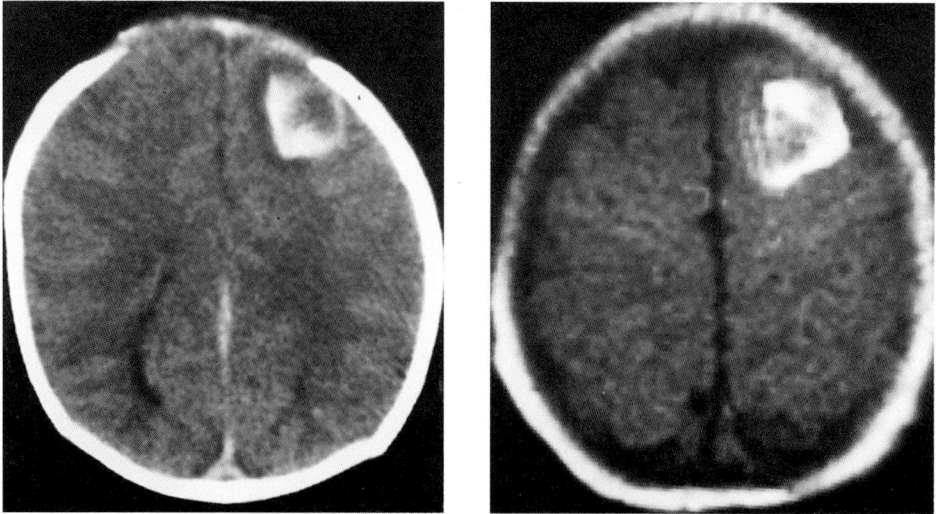

Fig. 7.11. Hemorrhagic cerebral infarction. *(Left)* CT shows an area of hemorrhage with peripheral edema in the watershed region of the left frontal lobe. *(Right)* Axial T_1-weighted image (TE 20/TR 700) demonstrates a matching area of increased signal intensity with central areas of hypointensity consistent with hemorrhagic infarction.

pressure manifests initially as obtundation, and later, venous infarctions may lead to focal neurologic deficits, seizures or both. CT signs of sinus thrombosis, such as the 'empty delta sign', are not always reliable (Fig. 7.9). Prior to MRI, definitive diagnosis of cerebral dural sinus or venous thrombosis required conventional arteriography. The ability to non-invasively evaluate these structures with MRI has made it the procedure of choice for the diagnosis of cerebral dural sinus or venous thrombosis (Macchi *et al.* 1986, Baram *et al.* 1988). Early thrombosis manifests as signal within the sinus which is isointense with brain on T_1-weighted images and hypointense on T_2-weighted images (Figs. 7.9, 7.10). Hyperintensity develops within the thrombosed sinus as the deoxyhemoglobin changes to methemoglobin, progressing peripherally to centrally. Thrombosed medullary veins may be detected in severe cases. Later, recanalization of the clot may occur creating a laminar appearance of blood and clot within the sinus. Serial MRI and MRA can be utilized to assess treatment efficacy (Medlock *et al.* 1992).

Intracranial hemorrhage
The most common cause of intracranial hemorrhage in childhood is trauma. Subdural and other extra-axial hematomas may occur in addition to parenchymal and intraventricular hematomas. Child abuse, particularly shaking injury, may result in intracranial hemorrhages or global anoxia with diffuse cerebral edema.

Hemorrhagic stroke syndromes may be caused by vascular malformations of all types, blood dyscrasias, aneurysms, tumors and infectious processes (Hecht-Leavitt *et al.* 1986) (Fig. 7.11). Imaging assessment of stroke syndromes generally begins with CT

154

TABLE 7.1
Intracranial hemorrhage

MRI appearance of hemorrhage*	T₁-weighted	T₂-weighted
Hyperacute: <24 hours, oxyhemoglobin begins changing to deoxyhemoglobin in 3 hours	Isointense	Initially hyperintense, becoming hypointense within 1–2 days
Acute: 1–3 days, deoxyhemoglobin	Iso- to hypointense	Hypointense
Subacute: intracellular methemoglobin (early 1–2 weeks) to extracellular methemoglobin (late 2–4 weeks)	Hyperintensity begins peripherally, solid hyperintensity at 2–3 weeks	Hypointense until 2 weeks, then peripheral hypointensity progresses to solid hyperintensity at 2–3 weeks
Chronic: ≥1 month	Isointense to mildly hypointense periphery becoming more hypointense with time	Hypointense periphery progresses to complete hypointensity

*These are general patterns which may vary with location and source of hemorrhage as well as pulse sequence and field strength.

scanning, which is useful in defining the extent of the hemorrhage, although the etiology may not be apparent. MRI is less useful in the acute setting due to its relative insensitivity to small amounts of acute hemorrhage. However, once the hemorrhage has been demonstrated, MRI is more sensitive in the detection of the causative lesion (Jenkins *et al.* 1988, Imakita *et al.* 1989). Many otherwise occult vascular malformations may be identified on MRI, adjacent to or within areas of hematoma (Gomori *et al.* 1986, Ebeling *et al.* 1988, Turjman *et al.* 1992). Multiple lesions, as seen with embolic strokes of cardiac origin, may also be demonstrated. Extracranial or intracranial arterial dissection may also result in embolic strokes. In such cases, the dissection itself, the vascular occlusion, and parenchymal infarction may all be demonstrated on MRI (Goldberg *et al.* 1986, Kobayashi *et al.* 1989). Although no MRI characteristics are specific for lesions resulting from blood dyscrasias such as hemophilia, hematomas in multiple compartments or in varying stages of hemoglobin degradation may be indicative of an underlying hematologic condition. (Lesions resulting from child abuse may also fit this description.) The MRI characteristics of hemorrhage and the stages of hemoglobin degradation are described in detail elsewhere (Gomori 1985, Bydder *et al.* 1988) and are summarized in Table 7.1.

Aneurysms
Aneurysms are rare in the pediatric age group, representing only 0.6 per cent of the symptomatic aneurysms in the Cooperative Study (Locksley 1966). Approximately one third are post-traumatic, mycotic or idiopathic, while the remainder are congenital (Thompson *et al.* 1973, Kaplan and Hahn 1984). Slightly more common in females, aneurysms may be

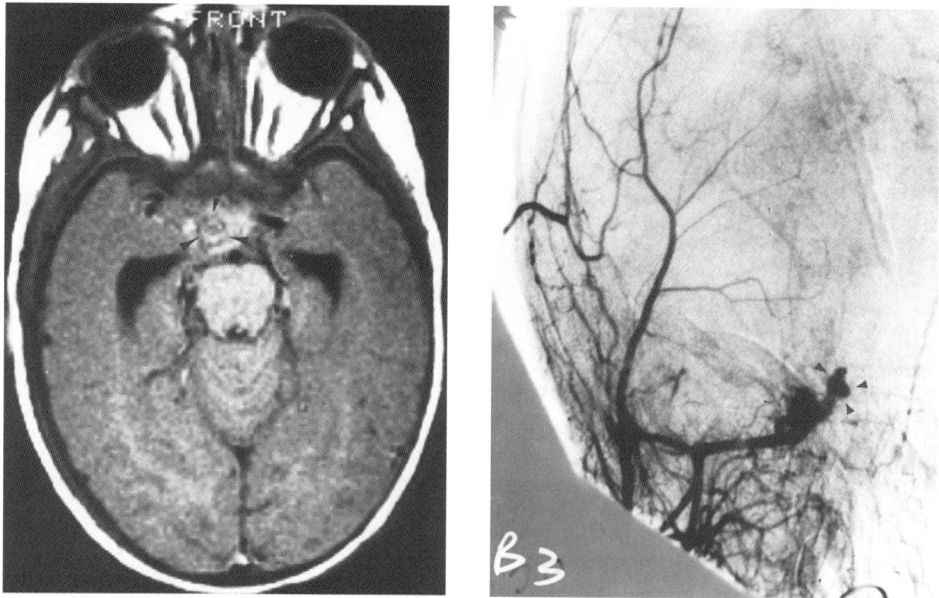

Fig. 7.12. Aneurysm and subarachnoid hemorrhage. *(Left)* Axial T$_1$-weighted image demonstrates the lack of a flow void in the region of the supraclinoid internal carotid artery in this 6-month-old infant. An area of increased signal is identified in the supraclinoid region, consistent with thrombosis in an aneurysm *(arrowheads)*. *(Right)* Anteroposterior arteriogram demonstrates a hypoplastic right internal carotid artery terminating in an irregularly shaped aneurysm *(arrowheads)*.

associated with other congenital lesions, such as polycystic kidneys (16 per cent), co-arctation of the aorta (16 per cent), multiple angiomas (9 per cent), neurofibromatosis (9 per cent), and arteriovenous malformations (9 per cent). Pathologically, congenital aneurysms in adults and children differ (Heiskanen and Vilkki 1981). A congenital medial defect is usually present in children, with tapering of the internal elastic lamina as it enters the aneurysm. In adults, the internal elastic lamina and media end at the mouth of the aneurysm. Fusiform aneurysms are more commonly observed in children, in which case the entire vessel wall is usually aneurysmal (Kaplan and Hahn 1984). Congenital aneurysms in childhood have a predilection for the internal carotid artery bifurcation, a distinctly uncommon location in the adult population (Fig. 7.12) (Patel and Richardson 1973, Thompson *et al.* 1973, Putty *et al.* 1990–91). Basilar artery aneurysms are also common, as are aneurysms involving primitive anastomotic vessels (*i.e.* trigeminal, otic and hypoglossal arteries). Congenital aneurysms in children also tend to be large (>5 mm in diameter). Embolism from thrombus within an unruptured aneurysm has been reported in childhood with both intraluminal clot and cortical infarction demonstrated on MRI (Kobayashi *et al.* 1989). MRA may facilitate the non-invasive diagnosis of aneurysms. Conventional angiography is generally required for delineation of the aneurysm neck prior to surgery.

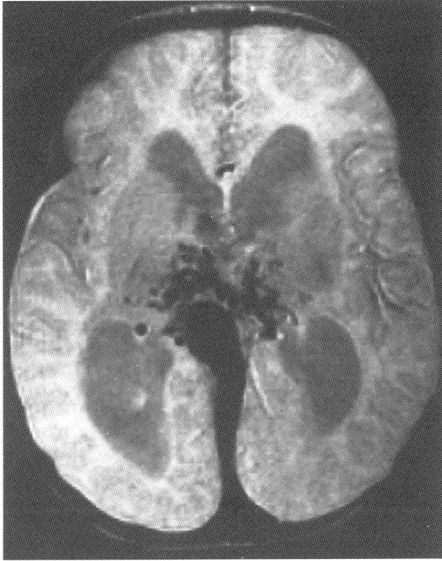

Fig. 7.13. Vein of Galen arteriovenous malformation (AVM): racemose type. Axial proton density image demonstrates the multiple serpentine flow voids of this bilateral thalamic AVM. Note the dilated vein of Galen.

Vascular malformations

Arteriovenous malformations (AVMs) are three times as common as aneurysms in the pediatric population. Children usually present with seizures or intracranial hemorrhage (Gerosa *et al.* 1980, Celli *et al.* 1984, Trussart *et al.* 1989). AVMs are supratentorial in 90 per cent of cases and infratentorial in the remainder (Harwood-Nash and Fitz 1976). Deep seated AVMs (basal ganglia, corpus callosum, thalamus and brainstem) occur in only 10 per cent of cases. AVMs occur most frequently in the areas of greatest vascular supply. Thus, lesions occur more commonly in the middle cerebral artery territory (Russell and Rubinstein 1989).

Pial AVMs are visualized on MRI as a tangled network of tubular structures with absent luminal signal, which are visible on both T_1- and T_2-weighted images (Lee *et al.* 1985, Imakita *et al.* 1989) (Fig. 7.13). Dural AVMs are the exception to these generalizations because they may not be visualized except by arteriography. Large draining veins form the largest volume of the true AVM, with a lesser contribution from the smaller caliber arterial feeders. Large cortical AVMs tend to be conical or pyramidal in shape with the apex pointing toward the midline, often adjacent to the ventricular system. The multiplanar capabilities of MRI are invaluable in treatment planning for stereotactic radiosurgery (Phillips *et al.* 1991).

Increased or decreased signal due to hemorrhage may be detected surrounding any vascular malformations. The actual signal characteristics are dependent upon the timing of the previous hemorrhage and the type of hemoglobin present. Increased signal on T_2-weighted images within cerebral tissue adjacent to the malformation may be identified, with or without adjacent hemorrhage. Anoxia, ischemia and/or gliosis may be the explanation for this finding in the absence of hemorrhage (Crain *et al.* 1991).

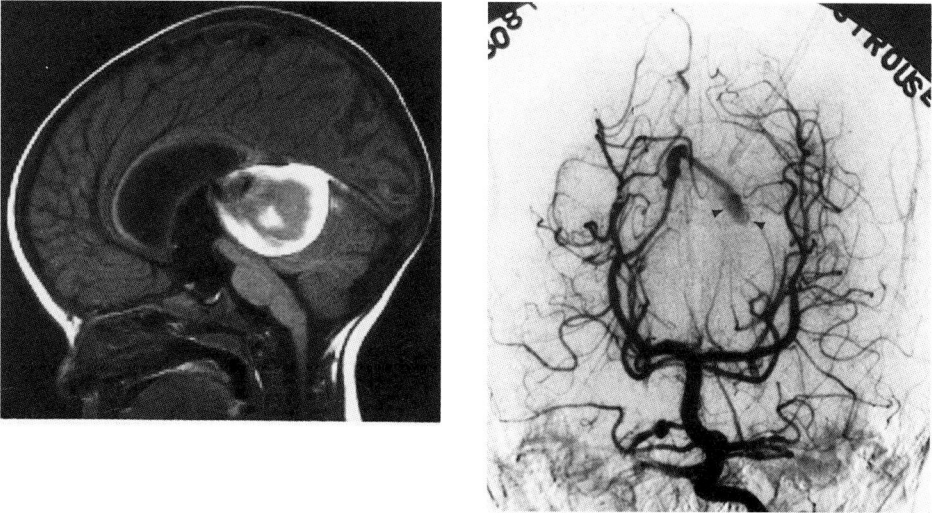

Fig. 7.14. Vein of Galen arteriovenous malformation: partially thrombosed. *(Left)* Sagittal T₁-weighted image (TE 20/TR 500) demonstrates a posterior third ventricular mass in continuity with the straight sinus. Evidence of peripheral high signal and central isointensity confirms the presence of thrombus. *(Right)* Anteroposterior arteriogram in early arterial phase demonstrates rapid shunting, via the posterior cerebral artery, into the small residual lumen of a thrombosed vein of Galen *(arrowheads)*.

Aberrant communications between primitive choroidal arteries, veins and venous sinuses result in the development of midline vascular malformations, such as vein of Galen AVM. Vein of Galen AVM or vein of Galen aneurysm (a descriptive misnomer) is a vascular malformation involving the galenic system of veins whereby the vein of Galen is markedly dilated, forming a varix (Figs. 7.13, 7.14). Vascular supply is principally derived from the posterior cerebral, anterior pericallosal, superior cerebellar and thalamic perforating arteries. Occasionally, middle cerebral artery supply is also present. Thrombosis, with closure of the fistula, may occur rarely in these lesions (Fig. 7.14). There are two patterns of vein of Galen AVM. One consists of a large varix with a single or multi-hole fistula (Fig. 7.15). The other has a racemose appearance typical of a small vessel AVM (Fig. 7.13). If these lesions present at birth, they are generally associated with severe cardiac failure and an intracranial bruit. Late in infancy, lesions may present with mild heart failure and cranial enlargement with cranial bruits developing within six months. Older children and adolescents may present with headache, syncope, hydrocephalus, exercise intolerance and/or congestive heart failure. MRA may be useful to follow patients with vein of Galen malformations and other deep AVMs and fistulae, both prior to and following treatment, although, at present, this technique does not obviate the need for conventional arteriography for complete evaluation of the lesion (Fig. 7.15).

Crawford and Russell (1956) coined the term *'cryptic angiomas'* in the setting of idiopathic intraparenchymal hemorrhage in young patients. These are angiographically occult vascular malformations which include cavernous angiomas and telangiectasia (capillary

158

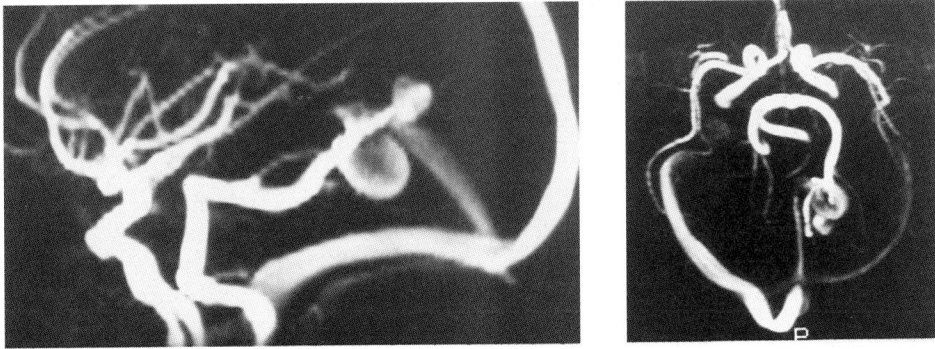

Fig. 7.15. Central arteriovenous fistula. *(Left)* Sagittal MRA image clearly demonstrates enlargement of the vertebral, basilar and posterior cerebral arteries with filling of a venous structure with two pouches. The smaller pouch lies superior to the straight sinus and the larger pouch inferior to the straight sinus. *(Right)* Axial MRA image demonstrates filling of the posterior cerebral artery, with the location of the venous pouches just lateral to the location of the vein of Galen and straight sinus.

malformations). They are commonly located in the brainstem, where hemorrhage may be devastating. Cavernous angiomas are one of the least common varieties of angiomas, ranging from 1 mm to 3 cm in size. Patients frequently will present with seizures or hemorrhage. The cavernous angioma is composed of a sinusoidal network of stagnant and sequestered blood with no intervening parenchymal tissue. This leads to hyalinization of vessel walls, calcification, thrombosis and even ossification in some cases. The MRI appearance of cavernous angiomas is characterized by a heterogeneous pattern of increased and decreased signal, due to a combination of flow-related enhancement, calcification, and hemoglobin in varying stages of degradation (Figs. 7.16, 7.17). *Telangiectasias* are capillary angiomas measuring from 3 mm to 1 cm, separated by intervening neural tissue, unlike cavernous angiomas. Lesions predominate in the pons and in the roof of the fourth ventricle. They may be multiple and familial (Osler–Weber–Rendu syndrome). On MRI, these lesions may be identifiable only by the localized region of hemorrhage.

Venous angiomas consist of one or more central veins draining a series of veins in a spoke-wheel or radial pattern. The central vein drains peripherally towards either a dural venous sinus or a cortical vein. Venous angiomas are typically located in the frontal or parietal lobes and are less common in the cerebellar white matter. Supratentorial venous angiomas are usually of little clinical significance, although those in the posterior fossa more commonly cause hemorrhage, particularly in adolescent athletes (Rothfus *et al.* 1984). Venous malformations or venous angiomas present as curvilinear flow voids on T_1-weighted images, without the tangled network of vessels seen with AVMs. The T_2 appearance is more variable, ranging from the flow voids seen on T_1-weighted images, to serpentine regions of increased signal, reflecting slow flow within the angioma (Lee *et al.* 1985) (Fig. 7.18).

Scalp AVMs present as pulsatile masses, with or without discoloration, and prominent vessels. These are usually supplied by branches of the external carotid artery without an

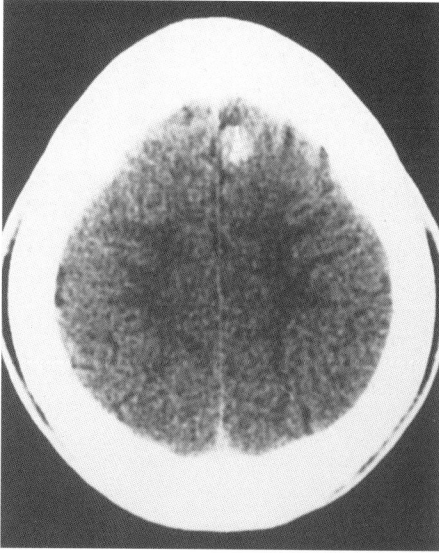

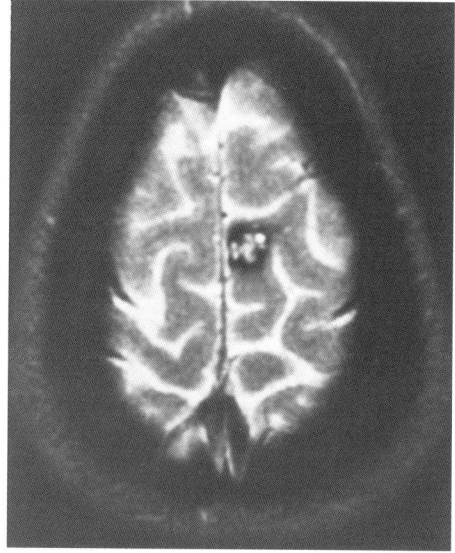

Fig. 7.16. Cavernous angioma. *(Left)* CT examination of the brain demonstrates a calcific mass in the medial frontal cortex on the left. No mass effect or hemorrhage is associated. *(Right)* Axial T$_2$-weighted image (TE 60/TR 2600) demonstrates heterogenous lesion in the medial frontal cortex which is hypointense peripherally and hyperintense centrally in an irregular pattern typical of cavernous hemangioma.

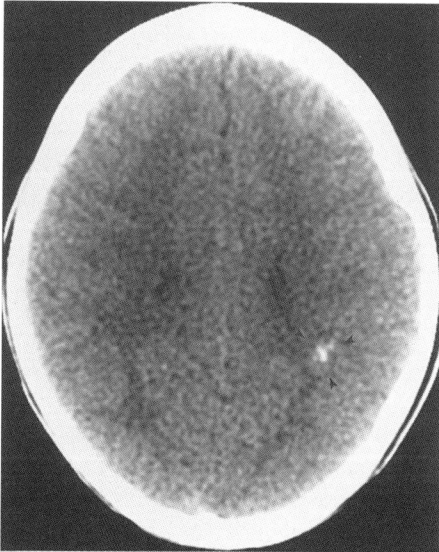

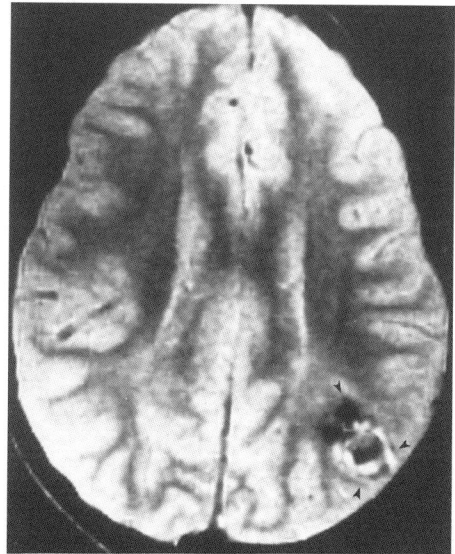

Fig. 7.17. Cavernous angioma with hemorrhage. *(Left)* CT examination obtained without contrast demonstrates an area of increased density in the periventricular region on the left. *(Right)* T$_2$-weighted proton density image (TE 45/TR 3000) demonstrates heterogenous signal intensity in the white matter, extending out towards the cortical surface, consistent with cavernous angioma with hemorrhage *(arrowheads)*.

160

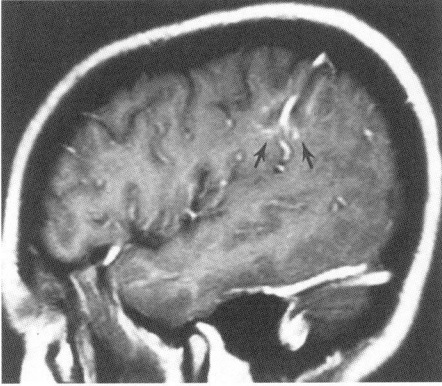

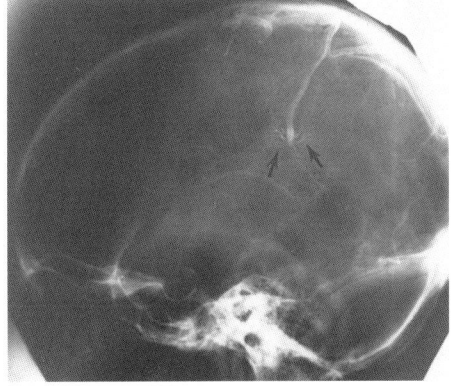

Fig. 7.18. Venous angioma. *(Left)* T$_1$-weighted image (TE 22/TR 700) obtained following contrast administration demonstrates a prominent cortical vain with an area of enhancement centrally *(arrows)*. *(Right)* Atypical venous angioma is seen on the lateral arteriogram *(arrows)*.

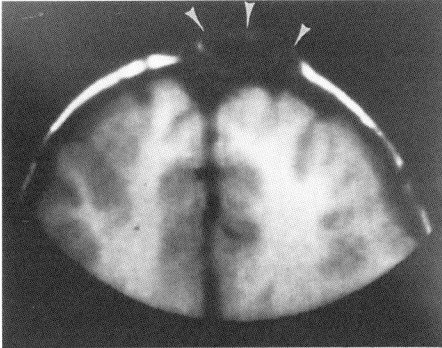

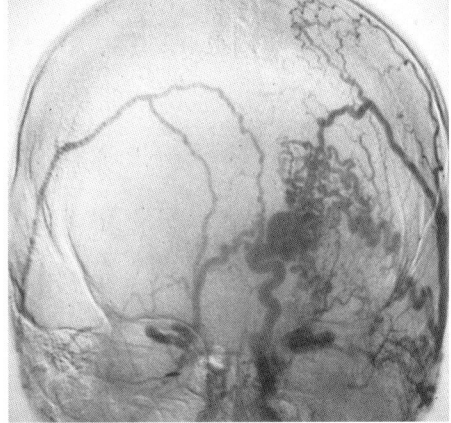

Fig. 7.19. Scalp arteriovenous malformation (AVM). *(Left)* On this axial T$_1$-weighted image (TE 20/TR 700) a mass composed of multiple flow voids is identified in the subcutaneous tissues, without brain involvement. *(Right)* Anteroposterior arteriogram demonstrates a large scalp AVM with a central venous pouch accounting for the mass seen on MRI.

associated intracranial component. MRI demonstrates the flow voids in the subcutaneous region of the scalp and may allow detection of associated calvarial extension (Fig. 7.19).

MRI is particularly well-suited for evaluation of cerebrovascular disease in the pediatric population, despite the need for sedation in younger patients. The detection of flow abnormalities on routine T$_1$- and T$_2$-weighted images permits early diagnosis of vascular stenoses and occlusive disease. MRA is a non-invasive method for delineating normal and abnormal vasculature, allowing conventional arteriography to be reserved for the more complicated diagnostic or therapeutic uses.

REFERENCES

Adams, R.J., Nichols, F.T., McKie, V., McKie, K., Milner, P., Gammal, T.E. (1988) 'Cerebral infarction in sickle cell anemia: mechanism based on CT and MRI.' *Neurology*, **38**, 1012–1017.

Baram, T.Z., Butler, I.J., Nelson, M.D., McArdle, C.B. (1988) 'Transverse sinus thrombosis in newborns: clinical and magnetic resonance imaging findings.' *Annals of Neurology*, **24**, 792–794.

Bradley, W.G., Waluch, V. (1985) 'Blood flow: magnetic resonance imaging.' *Radiology*, **154**, 443–450.

Bruno, A., Yuh, W.T.C., Biller, J., Adams, H.P., Cornell, S.H. (1988) 'Magnetic resonance imaging in young adults with cerebral infarction due to moyamoya.' *Archives of Neurology*, **45**, 303–306.

Bydder, G.M., Pennock, J.M., Porteous, R., Dubowitz, L.M.S., Gadian, D.G., Young, I.R. (1988) 'MRI of intracerebral haematoma at low field (0.15 T) using T_2-dependent partial saturation sequences.' *Neuroradiology*, **30**, 367–371.

Celli, P., Ferrante, L., Palma, L., Cavedon, G. (1984) 'Cerebral arteriovenous malformations in children. Clinical features and outcome of treatment in children and in adults.' *Surgical Neurology*, **22**, 43–49.

Chaung, S. (1989) 'Vascular diseases of the brain in children.' *In:* Edward, M.S.B., Hoffman, H.J. (Eds.) *Cerebral Vascular Disease in Children and Adolescents.* Baltimore: Williams & Wilkins, pp. 69–94.

Crain, M.R., Yuh, W.T.C., Greene, G.M., Loes, D.J., Ryals, T.J., Sato, Y., Hart, M.N. (1991) 'Cerebral ischaemia: evaluation with contrast-enhanced MR imaging.' *American Journal of Neuroradiology*, **12**, 631–639.

Crawford, J.V., Russell, D.S.. (1956) 'Cryptic arteriovenous and venous hamartomas of the brain.' *Journal of Neurology, Neurosurgery and Psychiatry*, **19**, 1-11.

Ebeling, J.D., Tranmer, B.I., Davis, K.A., Kindt, G.W., DeMasters, B.K. (1988) 'Thrombosed arteriovenous malformations: a type of occult vascular malformation. Magnetic resonance imaging and histopathological correlations.' *Neurosurgery*, **23**, 605–610.

El Gammal, T., Adams, R.J., Nichols, F.T., McKie, V., Milner, P., McKie, K., Brooks, B.S. (1986) 'MR and CT investigation of cerebrovascular disease in sickle cell patients.' *American Journal of Neuroradiology*, **7**, 1043–1049.

Gerosa, M., Licata, C., Fiore, D.L., Iraci, G. (1980) 'Intracranial aneurysms of childhood.' *Child's Brain*, **6**, 295–302.

Goldberg, H.I., Grossman, R.I., Gomori, J.M., Asbury, A.K., Bilaniuk, L.T., Zimmerman, R.A. (1986) 'Cervical internal carotid artery dissecting hemorrhage: diagnosis using MR.' *Radiology*, **158**, 157–161.

Gomori, J.M., Grossman, R.I., Goldberg, H.I., Zimmerman, R.A., Bilaniuk, L.T. (1985) 'Intracranial hematomas: imaging by high-field MR.' *Radiology*, **157**, 87–93.

—— —— —— Hackney, D.B., Zimmerman, R.A., Bilaniuk, L.T. (1986) 'Occult cerebral vascular malformations: high-field MR imaging.' *Radiology*, **158**, 707–713.

Harwood-Nash, D.C., Fitz, C.R. (1976) *Neuroradiology in Infants and Children. Vol 3.* St. Louis: C.V. Mosby.

Hecht-Leavitt, C., Gomori, J.M., Grossman, R.I., Goldberg, H.I., Hackney, D.B., Zimmerman, R.A., Bilaniuk,. L.T. (1986) 'High-field MRI of hemorrhagic cortical infarction.' *American Journal of Neuroradiology*, **7**, 581–585.

Heiskanen, O., Vilkki, J. (1981) 'Intracranial arterial aneurysms in children and adolescents.' *Acta Neurochirurgica*, **59**, 55–63.

Imakita, S., Nichimura, T., Yamada, N., Naito, H., Takamiya, M., Yamada, Y., Kikuchi, H., Yonekawa, Y., Sawada, T., Yamaguchi, T. (1989) 'Cerebral vascular malformations: applications of magnetic resonance imaging to differential diagnosis.' *Neuroradiology*, **31**, 320–325.

Inagaki, M., Koada, T., Takeshita, K. (1992) 'Prognosis and MRI after ischemic stroke of the basal ganglia.' *Pediatric Neurology*, **8**, 104–108.

Jenkins, A., Hadley, D.M., Teasdale, G.M., Condon, B., Macpherson, P., Patterson, J. (1988) 'Magnetic resonance imaging of acute subarachnoid hemorrhage.' *Journal of Neurosurgery*, **68**, 731–736.

Kaplan, P.A., Hahn, F.J. (1984) 'Aneurysms of the posterior cerebral artery in children.' *American Journal of Neuroradiology*, **5**, 771–774.

Kobayashi, H., Hayashi, M., Kawano, H., Handa, Y., Kabuto, M., Ishii, Y. (1989) 'Magnetic resonance imaging of embolism from intracranial aneurysms.'. *Surgical Neurology*, **32**, 225–230.

Kudo, T. (1965) 'Juvenile occlusion of the circle of Willis.' *In: Proceedings of the 8th International Congress of Neurology, Vienna. Vol. IV. Free Communications.* pp. 503–504.

Lee, B.C.P., Herzberg, L., Zimmerman, R.A., Deck, M.D.F. (1985) 'MR imaging of cerebral vascular malformations.' *American Journal of Neuroradiology*, **6**, 863–870.

162

Locksley, H.B. (1966) 'Natural history of subarachnoid hemorrhage, intracranial aneurysms and arteriovenous malformations. Based on 6368 cases in the Cooperative Study.' *Journal of Neurosurgery*, **25**, 219–239.

Macchi, P.J., Grossman, R.I., Gomori, J.M., Goldberg, H.I., Zimmerman, R.A., Bilaniuk, L.T. (1986) 'High-field MR imaging of cerebral venous thrombosis.' *Journal of Computer Assisted Tomography*, **10**, 10–15.

Medlock, M.D., Olivero, W. C., Hanigan, W.C., Wright, R.M., Winek, S.J. (1992) 'Children with cerebral venous thrombosis diagnosed with magnetic resonance imaging and magnetic resonance angiography.' *Neurosurgery*, **31**, 870–876.

Patel, A.N., Richardson, A.E. (1971) 'Ruptured intracranial aneurysms in the first two decades of life. A study of 58 patients.' *Journal of Neurosurgery*, **35**, 571–576.

Pavlakis, S.G., Bello, J., Prohovnik, I., Sutton, M., Ince, C., Mohr, J.P., Piomelli, S., Hilal, S., DeVivo, D.C. (1988) 'Brain infarction in sickle cell anemia: magnetic resonance imaging correlates.' *Annals of Neurology*, **23**, 125–130.

Phillips, M.H., Kessler, M., Chuang, F.Y., Frankel, K.A., Lyman, J.T., Fabrikant, J.I., Levy, R.P. (1991) 'Imaging correlation of MRI and CT in treatment planning for radiosurgery of intracranial vascular malformations.' *International Journal of Radiation Oncology, Biology, Physics*, **20**, 881–889.

Powars, D., Wilson, B., Imbus, C., Pegelow, C., Allen, J. (1978) 'The natural history of stroke in sickle cell disease.' *American Journal of Medicine*, **65**, 461–471.

Putty, T.K., Luerssen, T.G., Campbell, R.L., Boaz, J.C., Edwards, M.K. (1990–91) 'Magnetic resonance imaging diagnosis of a cerebral aneurysm in an infant. Case report and review of the literature.' *Pediatric Neurosurgery*, **16**, 48–51.

Rothfus, W.E., Albright, A.L., Casey, K.F., Latchaw, R.E., Roppolo, H.M.N. (1984) 'Cerebellar venous angioma: "benign" entity?' *American Journal of Neuroradiology*, **5**, 61–66.

Russell, D.S., Rubinstein, L.J. (1989) *Pathology of Tumours of the Nervous System. 5th Edn, Revised.* London: Edward Arnold.

Schoenberg, B.S., Mellinger, J.F., Schoenberg, D.G. (1978) 'Cerebrovascular disease in infants and children: a study of incidence, clinical features, and survival.' *Neurology*, **28**, 763–768.

Smith, C.D., Baumann, R.J. (1991) 'Clinical features and magnetic resonance imaging in congenital and childhood stroke.' *Journal of Child Neurology*, **6**, 263–272.

Storm, W., Uhlenbrock, D. (1989) 'Magnetic resonance imaging of moyamoya disease in a child with Down's syndrome.' *Journal of Mental Deficiency Research*, **33**, 507–510.

Suto, Y., Caner, B.E., Nakatsugawa, S., Katsube, Y., Ishii, Y., Torizuka, K. (1990) 'Evaluation of MRI in moyamoya disease.' *Radiation Medicine*, **8**, 92–95.

Takeuchi, S., Kobayashi, K., Tsuchida, T., Imamura, H., Tanaka, R., Ito, J. (1982) 'Computed tomography in moyamoya disease.' *Journal of Computer Assisted Tomography*, **6**, 24-32.

Thompson, J.R., Harwood-Nash, D.C., Fitz, C.R. (1973) 'Cerebral aneurysms in children.' *American Journal of Roentgenology, Radium Therapy and Nuclear Medicine*, **118**, 163–175.

Trussart, V., Berry, I., Manelfe, C., Arrue, P., Castan, P. (1989) 'Epileptogenic cerebral vascular malformations and MRI.' *Journal of Neuroradiology*, **16**, 273–284.

Turjman, F., Arteaga, C., Tavernier, T., Bossard, D., Bochu, M., Jouvet, A., Froment, J.C. (1992) 'Haemorrhagic complications of intracerebral cavernomas: value of MRI.' *Journal of Neuroradiology*, **19**, 107–117.

Welch, W.C., McBride, M., Kido, D.K., Nelson, C.N. (1988) 'Moyamoya disease in an infant with autonomic dysfunction: angiographic and MRI findings.' *Journal of Child Neurology*, **3**, 110–113.

Wilms, G., Marchal, G., Van Fraeyenhoven, L., Demaerel, P., Casaer, P., Van Elderen, S., Baert, A.L. (1989) 'Unilateral moya-moya disease: MRI findings.' *Neuroradiology*, **31**, 442.

Wiznitzer, M., Masaryk, T.J. (1991) 'Cerebrovascular abnormalities in pediatric stroke: assessment using parenchymal and angiographic magnetic resonance imaging.' *Annals of Neurology*, **29**, 585–589.

Wood, D.H. (1978) 'Cerebrovascular complications of sickle cell anemia.' *Stroke*, **9**, 73–75.

Yuh, W.T.C., Crain, M.R., Loes, D.J., Greene, G.M., Ryals, T.J., Sato, Y. (1991) 'MR imaging of cerebral ischemia: findings in the first 24 hours.' *American Journal of Neuroradiology*, **12**, 621–629.

Zimmerman, R.A., Gill, F., Goldberg, H.I., Bilaniuk, L.T., Hackney, D.B., Johnson, M., Grossman, R.I., Hecht-Leavitt, C. (1987) 'MRI of sickle cell cerebral infarction.' *Neuroradiology*, **29**, 232–237.

8
INTRACRANIAL TUMORS

Eric N. Faerber

Primary neoplasms of the CNS are the most common solid tumors in children (Heideman *et al.* 1989). They account for one fifth of all pediatric malignancies and are exceeded only by leukemia and lymphoma as a cause of malignant disease in this age group.

Although the tumors may occur at any age, the peak incidence is between 5 and 10 years, with a slight male preponderance (Van Eys 1984).

During the first year of life, the majority of intracranial tumors are supratentorial in origin (Tomita and McLone 1985, Asai *et al.* 1989). In infants and children a preponderantly infratentorial location (two thirds of cases) was reported by Naidich and Zimmerman (1984), although in more recent studies using CT and MRI, supratentorial tumors have been more prevalent, accounting for almost two thirds of the cases of Zimmerman (1990*b*) and 52 per cent of those of Harwood-Nash (1991).

The great majority (approximately 75 per cent) of childhood brain tumors are glial in origin (Duffner *et al.* 1985). The most common tumors, classified by specific histologic type, are astrocytomas (20–49 per cent), medulloblastomas (16–29 per cent), ependymomas (6–17 per cent) and glioblastomas (4–20 per cent) (Mueller and Gurney 1992). This distribution appears to be similar for histologically confirmed cases in most countries (Dohrmann and Farwell 1976).

Neuroimaging approach

The advent of MRI has had a major impact in the diagnosis and subsequent management of intracranial tumors in infants and children. Prior to this, ultrasound and CT scanning were the most frequently used technologies. Although MRI is generally more sensitive, it is also more costly and less widely available. CT thus remains valuable for neuroimaging, with reports attesting to the complementary roles of CT and MRI (Brody 1991, Barkovich 1992).

CT is more sensitive than MRI for the detection of calcification. Larger areas of calcification are detected on MRI as foci of signal void or decreased signal intensity. Cortical bone involvement, especially for the orbits, paranasal sinuses, otomastoid region, petrous temporal bone, skull base and cranial calvarial lesions, is better demonstrated by CT (Barnes 1990).

The superior contrast sensitivity of MRI enables detection of tumors that are often not demonstrated by CT or ultrasound (Barnes 1990). These include mesial or basal temporal lobe tumors, periaqueductal tumors, cervicomedullary junction tumors and leptomeningeal neoplastic dissemination.

MRI is extremely sensitive to free tissue water (edema). Minor alterations in the

164

blood–brain barrier may be detected earlier by MRI than by CT, as water transgresses the blood–brain barrier before the larger contrast molecules (Brant-Zawadzki 1988, Lizak and Woodruff 1992).

The use of gadolinium contrast enhancement has been shown to be of great value in the diagnosis and subsequent management of intracranial tumors in children (Bird *et al.* 1988).

Brain tumors in neonates and infants

Neonatal brain tumors are rare, comprising 0.5–1.9 per cent of all pediatric brain tumors (Jellinger and Sunder-Plassmann 1973, Sato *et al.* 1975, Honda *et al.* 1984). The location is mostly supratentorial (Buetow *et al.* 1990).

An enlarged head is the most frequent initial sign (Jellinger and Sunder-Plassmann 1973). The paucity of signs and symptoms with lack of specificity may result in delayed diagnosis. Papilledema and vomiting are infrequent late signs of tumor due to expansion of the infant calvaria to accommodate the intracranial mass (Radkowski *et al.* 1988). Nonspecific signs such as seizures, lethargy, fever and gastroenteritis are more common.

There is usually displacement of the brain rather than infiltration by neonatal tumors which may account for the absence of focal deficits in many cases (Jellinger and Sunder-Plassmann 1973).

Teratoma is the single most common tumor in the neonatal period, representing one third to one half of all cases reported (Jellinger and Sunder-Plassmann 1973, Takaku *et al.* 1978, Jooma and Kendall 1982, Buetow *et al.* 1990).

Neuroepithelial tumors as a group constituted the majority of neonatal tumors in the series of Buetow *et al.* (1990). These were mainly glial tumors, especially astrocytomas, supratentorial primitive neuroectodermal tumors (PNETs) and medulloblastomas. Less commonly encountered were single cases of ependymoma, medulloepithelioma germinoma, angioblastic meningioma and ganglioglioma. Supratentorial choroid plexus papilloma was the most common neonatal tumor in the series of Radkowski *et al.* (1988).

Tumors in very young children are often large and highly malignant with a poor overall prognosis (Buetow *et al.* 1990). Common brain tumors in children under 2 years of age include PNETs, astrocytomas, teratomas and choroid plexus papillomas.

Posterior fossa tumors

MRI is especially useful for investigating the posterior fossa due to its multiplanar imaging capability, the lack of bone artifact encountered with CT, and greater contrast resolution.

The four common tumors occurring in the posterior fossa are medulloblastoma, cerebellar astrocytoma, brainstem glioma and ependymoma. Medulloblastoma occurred most frequently in the series of Gusnard (1990) and Zee *et al.* (1993), whereas cerebellar astrocytoma predominated in the series of Maroldo and Barkovich (1992). Less common tumors include hemangioblastoma, choroid plexus papilloma, ganglioglioma, acoustic neuroma, meningioma and chordoma.

The common symptoms of posterior fossa tumors, other than brainstem gliomas, are

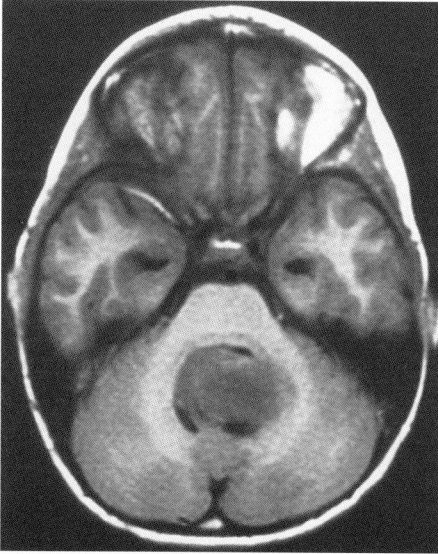

(a)

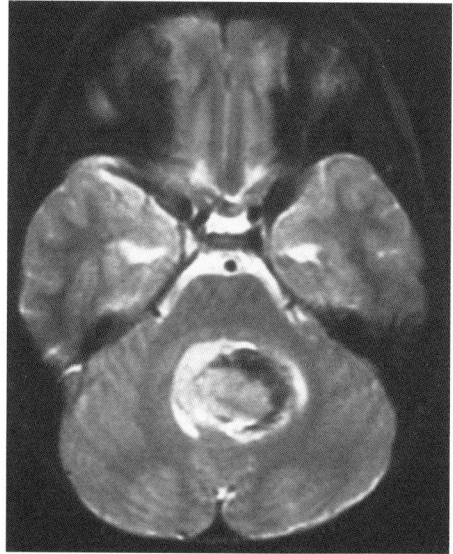

(b)

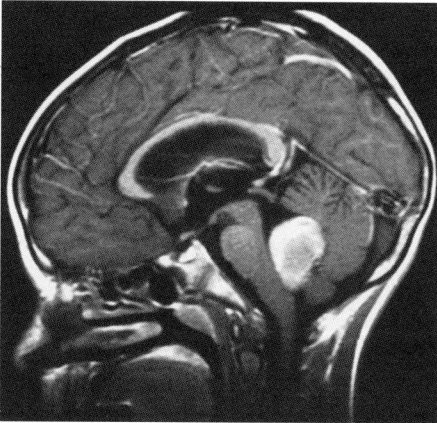

(c)

Fig. 8.1. Medulloblastoma. *(a)* T$_1$-weighted spin echo non-contrast axial scan demonstrates a low signal intensity mass posterior to the fourth ventricle. *(b)* T$_2$-weighted spin echo axial scan demonstrates predominantly high signal within the mass. Areas of low signal intensity are due to calcification and necrosis. *(c)* T$_1$-weighted spin echo contrast enhanced sagittal scan demonstrates marked contrast enhancement within the tumor.

due to hydrocephalus resulting from the tumor (Albright 1992). Hydrocephalus is present in virtually all children with cerebellar astrocytoma and in the vast majority of children with medulloblastoma (Albright *et al.* 1989). Brainstem gliomas manifest insidiously leading to long tract signs, ataxia and cranial neuropathies (Panitch and Berg 1970).

Medulloblastoma
Medulloblastomas are PNETs arising from cells which may originate either in the fetal granular layer of the cerebellum or the posterior medullary velum (Raaf and Kernohan

166

1944). The tumors may occur at any site along the path of migration of the poorly differentiated cells between these two locations.

They occur mainly in childhood, with a second peak in young adulthood. The usual site of origin in childhood is in the cerebellar vermis in the midline with growth into the fourth ventricle. In later life the site of origin is more lateral within the cerebellar hemisphere (Zimmerman et al. 1978).

Medulloblastoma may be associated with hereditary and familial diseases. The most frequent of these is the basal cell nevus syndrome (Gorlin syndrome). Other associations include Turcot syndrome, ataxia–telangiectasia, xeroderma pigmentosum, and the blue-rubber-bleb nevus syndrome (Russell and Rubinstein 1989).

Medulloblastoma has a variable, nonspecific appearance on MRI (Barkovich 1992). The most common appearance is of a midline mass located in the cerebellar vermis inferiorly. It is hypointense compared to normal brain on T_1-weighted images and hypo-, iso- or hyperintense on T_2-weighted images (Fig. 8.1). A hypointense appearance on T_2-weighted images should suggest the diagnosis of medulloblastoma as it is unusual in astrocytomas (Barkovich and Edwards 1990).

Signal heterogeneity may result from cystic or necrotic foci or intramural calcification (Meyers et al. 1992). Clump-like calcification has been reported in 21 per cent of medulloblastomas (Nelson et al. 1991).

There is usually marked enhancement following gadolinium administration. The pattern of enhancement is similar to that after injection of iodinated contrast with CT (Gusnard 1990).

Medulloblastomas may readily disseminate through the subarachnoid space. On the precontrast scan this manifests as blurring of the folia and gyral surfaces, with subsequent areas of dense linear or nodular extra–axial enhancement after gadolinium administration (Gusnard 1990).

Drop metastases appear as brightly enhanced foci in the intradural and extramedullary spaces and occasionally in the intramedullary spaces (Barkovich 1992). If MRI is unavailable, CT myelography is the best imaging approach.

A review of medulloblastomas in the postoperative period showed that not all recurrent tumor enhanced and that the absence of gadolinium enhancement did not necessarily exclude residual or recurrent tumor. T_2-weighted images should thus be obtained in all patients (Rollins et al. 1990).

Cerebellar astrocytoma

Cerebellar astrocytomas in infants and children account for around 38 per cent of cerebellar tumors (Farwell et al. 1977). Astrocytomas of the cerebellum differ from those in the cerebral hemispheres in several ways. They are mainly tumors of early age, circumscribed with a tendency to be grossly cystic, and are less likely to undergo anaplastic change (Russell and Rubinstein 1989).

The peak incidence is from birth to 9 years of age (Gjerris and Klinken 1978). Most of these tumors arise in the midline with extension into the cerebellar hemispheres in about one third of cases (Ringertz and Nordenstam 1951). The tumors may be cystic or

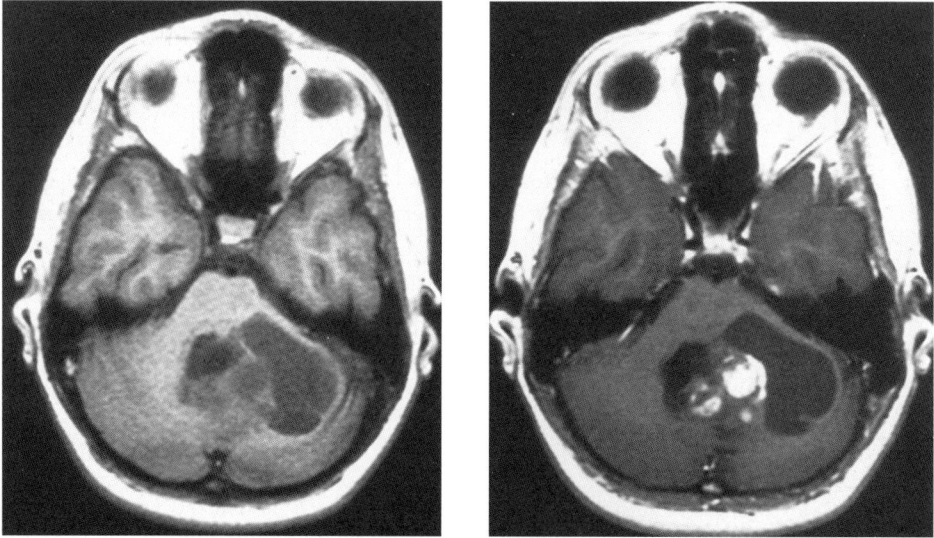

Fig. 8.2. Cerebellar astrocytoma. T₁-weighted spin echo axial non-contrast *(left)* and contrast enhanced *(right)* scans demonstrate a contrast enhancing mass compressing and displacing the fourth ventricle. There are both cystic and solid components within the tumor mass.

solid. The solid tumor may have a necrotic center (Gol and McKissock 1959). Nearly half of the tumors may be grossly cystic with a tumor module in the cyst wall. Compressed non–neoplastic cerebellar tissue is found in the cyst wall (Gol and McKissock 1959). Calcification is found in 20 per cent of these tumors (Gusnard 1990). Hemorrhage is rare.

Cerebellar astrocytomas may be classified into two main types. The benign juvenile pilocystic astrocytoma which constitutes 75–85 per cent of cases occurs in the first decade of life and has a 94 per cent 25 year survival rate (Zee *et al.* 1993). The diffuse fibrillary type is more frequently associated with anaplastic change (Steinberg *et al.* 1985, Lee *et al.* 1989, Russell and Rubinstein 1989); it has a peak incidence in adolescents and young adults, with a 40 per cent 25 year survival rate (Gjerris and Klinken 1978).

The MRI appearances of these tumors are as variable as the gross morphology (Lizak and Woodruff 1992). The solid portion of the tumor is hypo- to isointense to cerebral parenchyma on T₁-weighted images and iso- to hyperintense on T₂-weighted images (Fig 8.2).

The solid portion will enhance after gadolinium administration, in the same way as after iodinated contrast media administration for CT. The cystic portion of the tumor is isointense to CSF on T₁-weighted images and hyperintense on T₂-weighted images.

Brainstem glioma
Brainstem tumors are relatively common in children although uncommon in adults. The majority are gliomas (Bilaniuk *et al.* 1980). They constitute 10–20 per cent of all child-

168

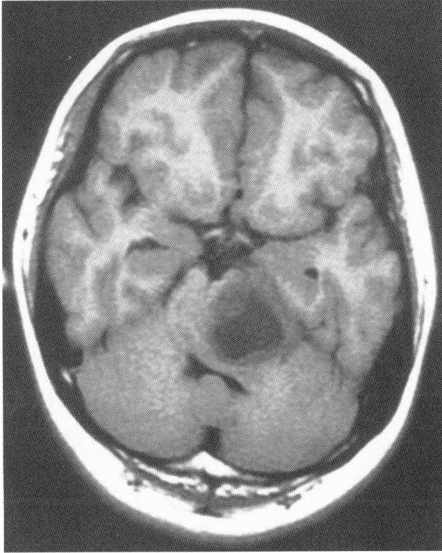

(a)

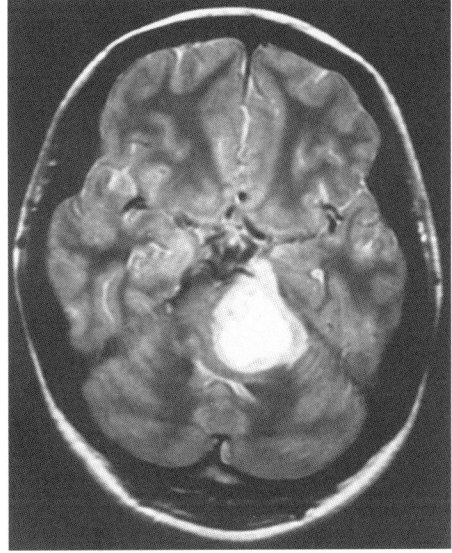

(b)

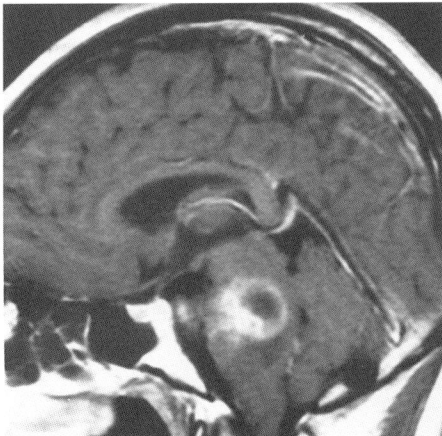

(c)

Fig. 8.3. Pontine glioma. T_1-weighted spin echo non-contrast *(a)* and T_2-weighted *(b)* axial scans demonstrate a pontine mass displacing and compressing the fourth ventricle posteriorly. *(c)* T_1-weighted spin echo contrast enhanced sagittal scan demonstrates ring enhancement within the tumor. There is anterior extension into the prepontine cistern.

hood CNS tumors (Panitch and Berg 1970). Males and females are equally affected. They may occur at any time of life, but the peak incidence is in the latter half of the first decade (Packer *et al.* 1992). Cranial nerve palsies are the presenting sign in up to 90 per cent of cases, and symptoms relating to hydrocephalus will be present in almost 30 per cent of patients at the time of presentation (Albright *et al.* 1983).

The pons is the most common site of origin of brainstem gliomas, followed in frequency by the midbrain and medulla (Barkovich and Edwards 1990). Exophytic growth of the pons occurs in approximately 60 per cent of cases. There are three major directions of extension (Barkovich and Edwards 1990): (i) anteriorly into the prepontine cistern; (ii) posteroinferiorly into the vallecula and cisterna magna; and (iii) posterolaterally into the cerebellopontine angle cistern.

There are two types of brainstem gliomas. Fibrillary astrocytoma is the most common, accounting for up to 80 per cent of cases, with a significant incidence of anaplastic change (Albright et al. 1983). Pilocytic astrocytoma accounts for the minority, with infrequent anaplastic change.

The advent of magnetic resonance imaging has greatly improved the diagnosis of brainstem tumors (Smith 1990) because bone artifact associated with CT is eliminated and there is increased sensitivity to intratumoral water. The tumor mass is characterized on MRI by low signal intensity on T_1-weighted images and high signal intensity on T_2-weighted images (Fig. 8.3). Contrast enhancement in focal tumors may be homo- or heterogeneous (Barkovich 1992).

Diffuse tumors are poorly marginated, involving more than half of the brainstem in the axial plane at the level of maximal involvement (Barkovich 1992). There is minimal or no contrast enhancement. The basilar artery is often engulfed by anterior extension of the tumor.

The associated findings seen with brainstem tumors such as hemorrhage, cyst formation or exophytic components are best demonstrated by MRI (Smith et al. 1987).

Ependymoma

Ependymomas account for around 9 per cent of intracranial tumors of childhood, and are the third most common posterior fossa tumors of childhood (Farwell et al. 1977). The majority of ependymomas (60–70 per cent) are infratentorial in location (Kun et al. 1988, Russell and Rubinstein 1989). There are two age peaks for this tumor. The first is in childhood under 5 years of age; the second occurs in adulthood, between 30 and 40 years (Zee et al. 1983, Kun et al. 1988). There is a male predominance of 2.5:1 (Farwell et al. 1977).

The tumors arise from ependymal cells, most commonly from the floor of the fourth ventricle, but also from any part of the ventricular system or the central canal of the spinal cord. Some ependymomas may arise directly from ependymal rests within the cerebellopontine angle (Amador 1983).

Ependymomas may frequently extend out of the fourth ventricle into adjacent cisterns and foramina. Approximately 15 per cent of these tumors extend through the foramina of Luschka to the cerebellopontine angles, and 60 per cent may extend through the foramina of Magendie into the cisterna magna, through the foramen magnum, and also into the cervical spinal cord (Barkovich and Edwards 1990). The cerebellar parenchyma is invaded in 30–40 per cent of cases.

On T_1-weighted images the MRI appearance of an ependymoma is that of a hypo- to isointense mass (Spoto et al. 1990) (Fig. 8.4). Foci of hyperintensity due to necrotic areas or cysts, and foci of hypointensity due to calcification or hemorrhage are seen on T_2-weighted images (Barkovich 1992). Signal heterogeneity is characteristic of ependymomas (Spoto et al. 1990, Barkovich 1992). Tumor vascularity and encasement or dis-

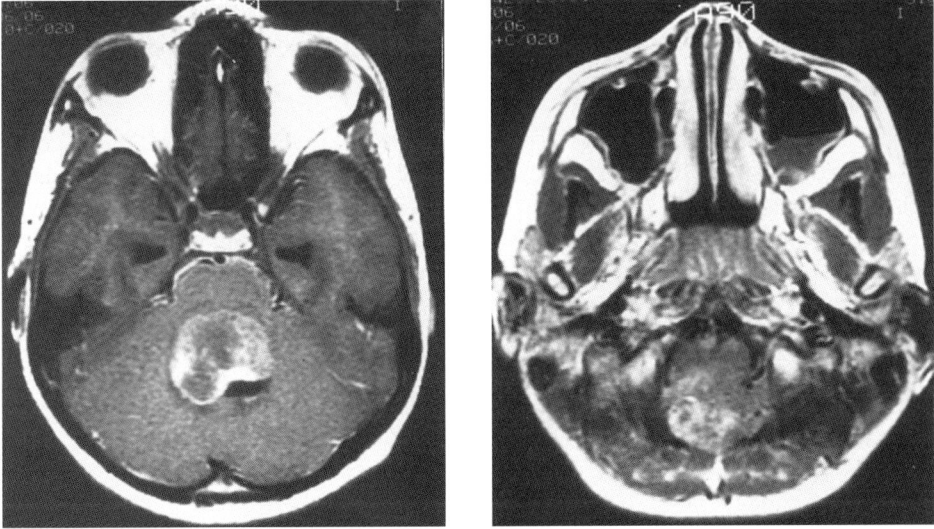

Fig. 8.4. Ependymoma. T_1-weighted spin echo contrast enhanced axial scans demonstrate a contrast enhancing mass within the posterior fossa with inferior extension through the foramen magnum. (By courtesy of James Elder, MD, Philadelphia, PA.)

placement of normal vessels are well demonstrated by MRI (Spoto *et al.* 1990). Calcification occurs in 25–50 per cent of posterior fossa ependymomas (Armington *et al.* 1985), although this may be missed on MRI (Spoto *et al.* 1990).

The cystic portions of the tumor are uniformly hyperintense to CSF on T_1-weighted images and isointense to hyperintense to CSF on T_2-weighted images (Lizak and Woodruff 1992). This dissimilarity to CSF is attributed to a higher protein content and also to lack of flow in the cystic component (Spoto *et al.* 1990).

The MRI appearances of ependymoma are generally not specific enough to allow differentiation from other gliomas; however, the 'melted wax' appearance of an ependymoma extending along the margins of the fourth ventricle and into the adjacent cisterns and enveloping the brainstem is characteristic (Gusnard 1990).

Schwannoma
Schwannomas are relatively rare tumors arising from Schwann cells that form the myelin sheaths of the axons of nerve roots. They account for 2 per cent of posterior fossa tumors in children (Amador 1983). The VIIIth cranial nerve is most frequently involved, followed by the Vth cranial nerve, and infrequently by other cranial nerves (Pinto and Kricheff 1984). Solitary schwannomas are usually incidental. Multiple schwannomas are characteristic of neurofibromatosis. The MRI appearances are discussed in Chapter 4.

Choroid plexus papilloma
Choroid plexus papilloma occurs less commonly in the fourth ventricle in infants and

171

children than in adults. The MRI appearances of this tumor are described in the section on supratentorial tumors, below.

Hemangioblastoma

Hemangioblastoma is a rare benign vascular tumor which may present at any age, though it is less common in children than in adults (Russell and Rubinstein 1989). There is a male predominance.

The most common site is the cerebellum, most frequently involving the paramedian region and also commonly the lateral lobes and vermis. Hemangioblastomas of the vermis deform and may infiltrate the cavity of the fourth ventricle (Russell and Rubinstein 1989). Other locations in decreasing order of frequency are the medulla, in the area postrema, spinal cord and cerebrum.

A multiplicity of tumors suggests von Hippel–Lindau disease. There are associations with multiple endocrine neoplasia syndrome and pheochromocytoma (Russell and Rubinstein 1989), and also with secondary polycythemia (Cramer and Kimsey 1952).

The MRI appearance is of a cystic mass with a vascular mural nodule (Lee et al. 1989). The cyst is usually hypointense on T_1-weighted images, and hyperintense on T_2-weighted images (Elster and Arthur 1988, Lee et al. 1989). If the mural nodule is small it may not be possible to differentiate hemangioblastoma from an arachnoid cyst without the use of contrast medium (Barkovich 1992). Contrast enhanced MRI is now a suitable replacement for angiography in the detection of the small tumor nodules.

Embryonic tumors

Dermoid tumors

Dermoid tumors occur more commonly in the spinal canal than within the cranium. When they occur intracranially they are more often located in the posterior fossa, especially in the vermis or in the fourth ventricle (Barkovich and Edwards 1990).

The MRI appearance of a dermoid tumor is usually identical to that of a lipoma with shortened T_1 and T_2 relaxation times (Barkovich and Edwards 1990). Fat saturation techniques may be useful to differentiate fat from blood or proteinaceous cysts (Simon et al. 1988).

Epidermoid tumors

Epidermoids are the most common embryonic tumors. They can occur in numerous sites, most frequently the cerebellopontine angle, followed by the parapituitary region and the middle cranial fossa (Barkovich and Edwards 1990).

The MRI appearance is of an extra-axial mass which typically exhibits prolonged T_1 and T_2 values (Vion-Drury et al. 1987), with signal characteristics similar to CSF (Figs. 8.5, 8.6).

Supratentorial tumors

Neuroepithelial tumors

Neuroepithelial tumors include glial cell tumors (gliomas), neuronal (ganglion) cell

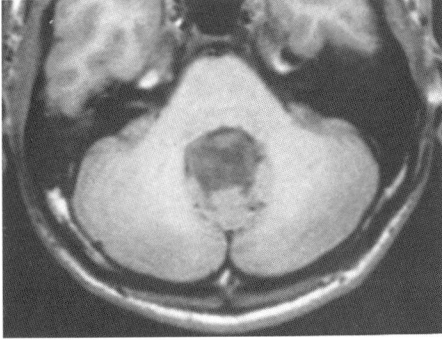

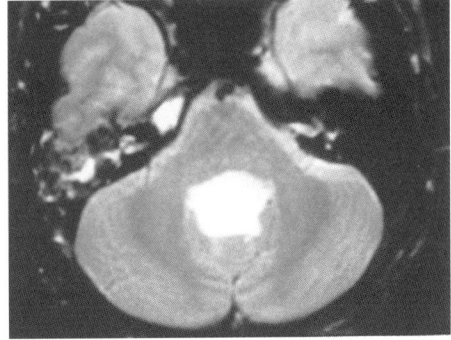

Fig. 8.5. Epidermoid. T_1-weighted *(left)* and T_2-weighted *(right)* spin echo non-contrast axial scans demonstrate a mass posterior to the fourth ventricle. The signal characteristics of the mass follow that of CSF. (By courtesy of Howard Rosenberg, Allentown, PA.)

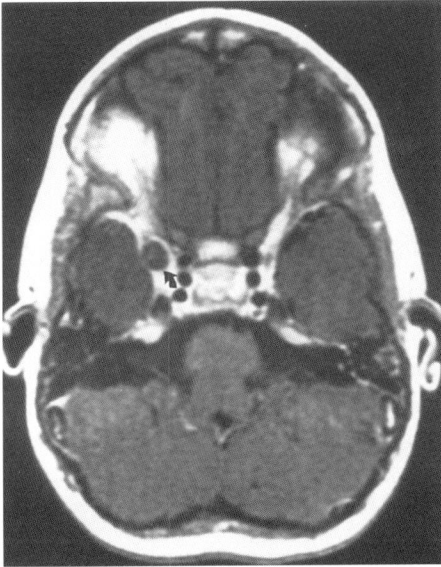

Fig. 8.6. Epidermoid. T_1-weighted spin echo contrast enhanced axial scan demonstrates a well-defined mass of low signal intensity *(arrow)* lateral to the right cavernous sinus. There was no contrast enhancement within the mass.

tumors, mixed neuronal–glial tumors, PNETs and pineal tumors (Zulch 1979). Collectively they constitute the largest group of tumors of the CNS in all ages (Cohen and Duffner 1989, Heideman *et al.* 1989).

Astrocytoma

Astrocytic tumors account for around one third to one half of childhood CNS tumors (Rorke *et al.* 1985, Cohen and Duffner 1989, Heideman *et al.* 1989). There is a male to female ratio approaching 2:1 (Farwell *et al.* 1977, Gjerris 1978). There are two age peaks, occurring at ages 2–4 years and in early adolescence.

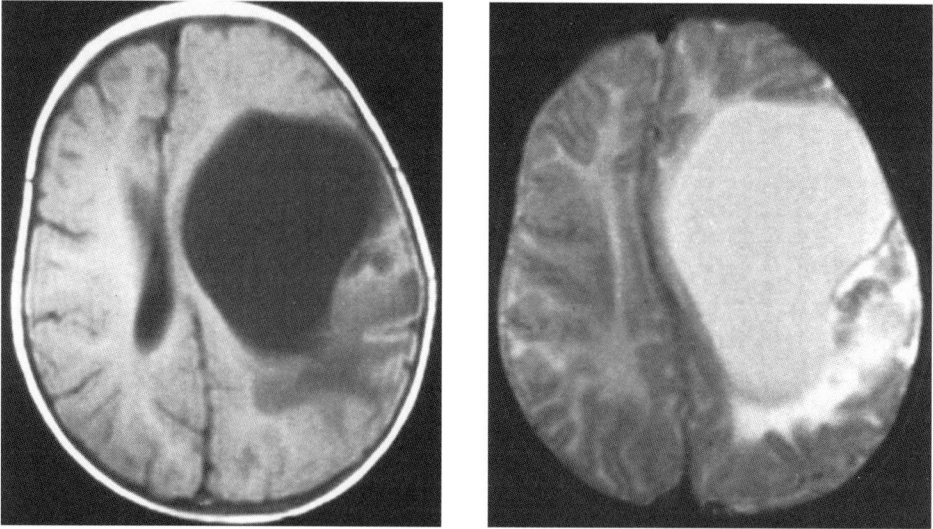

Fig. 8.7. Desmoplastic astrocytoma. T_1-weighted *(left)* and T_2-weighted *(right)* spin echo axial scans demonstrate a mass of mixed signal intensity representing both solid and cystic components.

The majority of lesions are located in the cerebral hemispheres, the remainder in the ventricles, thalami, hypothalamus and basal ganglia (Heideman *et al.* 1989).

The large and heterogeneous group of astrocytomas has been classified by Russell and Rubinstein (1989) into eight groups: protoplasmic, fibrillary, pilocystic, gemistocytic, subependymal giant cell, pleomorphic xantho-astrocytoma, desmoplastic cerebral astrocytoma of infancy, and anaplastic.

Certain astrocytomas may be associated with dysgenetic or malformative conditions (Russell and Rubinstein 1989). These include pilocystic astrocytomas of the third ventricle and of the anterior optic structures with neurofibromatosis, giant cell astrocytomas with tuberous sclerosis, and spinal cord astrocytomas with syringomyelia.

Differentiation between astrocytic tumors and other glial tumors, and also between low grade benign tumors and high grade (malignant) tumors, may often not be possible by neuroimaging (Barnes *et al.* 1992).

The MRI appearance of astrocytomas varies from low signal intensity or isointensity to surrounding brain on T_1-weighted images to high signal intensity on T_2-weighted images (Barkovich 1990, Davis 1990) (Fig. 8.7). Gadolinium enhancement is variable. The enhancement of pattern is similar to that seen on CT after intravenous administration of iodinated contrast medium (Barkovich 1992).

Giant cell astrocytoma
These tumors are characteristically associated with tuberous sclerosis but may frequently occur independently (Bonnin *et al.* 1984). They are usually found in the first and second

decades of life, with an earlier presentation in patients with tuberous sclerosis than in those in whom the tumors occur alone (Russell and Rubinstein 1989).

On MRI, giant cell astrocytomas show as hypo- or isointense signal masses on T_1-weighted images, becoming hyperintense on T_2-weighted images. Uniform enhancement occurs after intravenous administration of gadolinium (Barkovich and Edwards 1990). The MRI appearance of tuberous sclerosis is described in Chapter 4.

Oligodendroglioma
Oligodendrogliomas are composed of cells resembling oligodendrocytes. Although found mostly in adults, they are not uncommon in childhood and adolescence (Favier *et al.* 1985). They account for around 5 per cent of intracranial gliomas (McKeran and Thomas 1980). The majority are found in the cerebral hemispheres, most often in the fronto-temporal region. The cerebellum and spinal cord are less common sites (Fortuna *et al.* 1980).

Neuroimaging studies often show the tumor as a circumscribed mass of uniform density that is more solid than cystic, commonly containing calcification (Barnes *et al.* 1992). The MRI appearance is of a hypo- or isointense signal on T_1-weighted images and an iso- or hyperintense signal on T_2-weighted images. Cerebral edema and enhancement have been more frequently appreciated with MRI than with CT in the pediatric and adolescent population (Tice *et al.* 1993). Calcification, contrast enhancement and edema are seen less frequently in the pure oligodendrogliomas (without mixed elements) of childhood as compared to those found in adults (Tice *et al.* 1993).

Ganglioglioma
Gangliogliomas comprise well differentiated atypical neuronal elements and glial cells (Benitez *et al.* 1990). They have been reported in patients up to 80 years of age but are most common in children and young adults (Russell and Rubinstein 1989). They account for around 4–5 per cent of CNS tumors in children (Sutton *et al.* 1983).

Ganglioglioma is most commonly located within the cerebrum, involving especially the temporal lobes (Garrido *et al.* 1978). Other common sites are the frontal and parietal lobes, third ventricle and hypothalamus. The cerebellum, brainstem and spinal cord may also be involved (Barkovich and Edwards 1990). The tumor is usually solitary, although multiple lesion have been reported (Courville 1930).

Floccular and/or linear calcification may occur in 10 per cent of gangliomas: this is the most common manifestation of these tumors on plain radiographs (Sutton *et al.* 1983, Dorne *et al.* 1986).

The peripheral location within the hemispheres combined with erosion of the adjacent calvarium helps to establish the diagnosis of ganglioglioma (Demierre *et al.* 1986).

The MRI appearance of a ganglioglioma is an iso- or hypointense signal mass on T_1-weighted images with iso- to hyperintense signal on T_2-weighted pulse sequences (Benitez *et al.* 1990, Barnes *et al.* 1992). The lesions may be solid or partly cystic (Fig. 8.8). The signal intensity of the cystic component varies with the fluid content and may thus have the appearance of CSF, proteinaceous fluid or blood (Barnes *et al.* 1992).

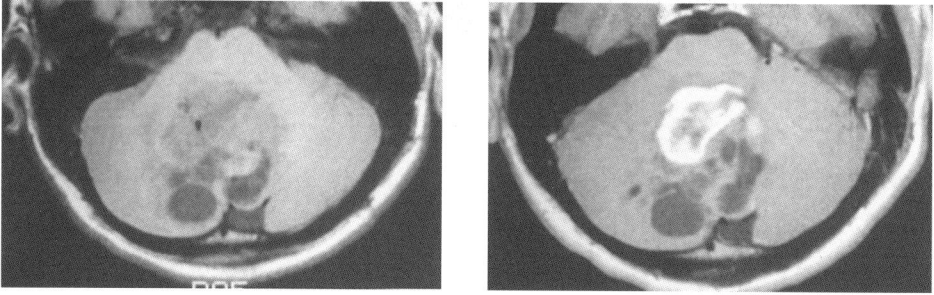

Fig. 8.8. Ganglioglioma. T$_1$-weighted spin echo axial non-contrast *(left)* and contrast enhanced *(right)* axial scans demonstrate a mass with both solid and cystic components. Inhomogeneous enhancement within the tumor mass is demonstrated in the contrast enhanced image. (By courtesy of Howard Rosenberg, MD, Allentown, PA.)

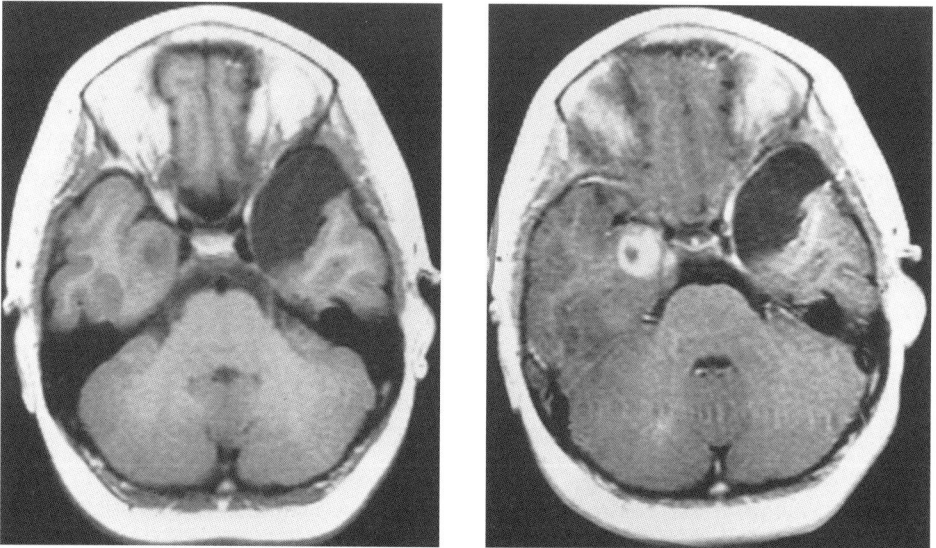

Fig. 8.9. Ganglioglioma. T$_1$-weighted spin echo axial non-contrast *(left)* and contrast enhanced *(right)* axial scans demonstrate a contrast enhancing mass within the right temporal lobe. The arachnoid cyst in the left middle cranial fossa was an incidental finding.

Contrast enhancement within the mass is highly variable (Barkovich and Edwards 1990, Castillo *et al*. 1990) (Fig. 8.9).

Most gangliogliomas grow slowly and produce symptoms from tumor expansion. Dissemination into the subarachnoid space is rare. Tumor spread within the basal cisterns and caudal end of the thecal sac has been demonstrated by contrast enhanced MRI (Wacker *et al*. 1992).

176

Glioblastoma multiforme

Glioblastoma multiforme occurs less commonly in children than in adults (Zulch 1965). It accounts for approximately 7 per cent of all intracranial tumors of childhood (Dohrmann *et al.* 1976). The frontal and parietal lobes of the cerebrum are most commonly involved, although the entire cerebrum and cerebellum may be affected (Dohrmann *et al.* 1976).

The neuroimaging appearances are diverse. The circumscribed or diffuse lesions may be solid or cystic with mass effect, edema or hemorrhage, and usually enhance after contrast administration (Barnes *et al.* 1992).

Optic pathway glioma

Optic pathway gliomas account for 3 to 6 per cent of brain tumors in infants and children, occurring with equal frequency in males and females (Koos and Miller 1971, Hoffman 1983). They occur most commonly in children under 10 years of age, with a peak incidence between 4 and 6 years (Russell and Rubinstein 1989). They are the most common primary brain abnormalities in neurofibromatosis (Farwell *et al.* 1977, Diebler and Dulac 1987). Variable combinations of involvement of the optic chiasm, hypothalamus, third ventricle and optic tracts occur more commonly than prechiasmatic location alone (Tenny *et al.* 1982, Hoffman 1983, Alvord and Lofton 1988).

CT has traditionally been the modality of choice for the detection of optic pathway gliomas. CT permits excellent demonstration of the tumors surrounded by orbital fat. There is usually fusiform dilatation of the optic nerves, although the enlargement may occasionally be eccentric (Barkovich and Edwards 1990). MRI is especially appealing in infants and children because of the lack of exposure of ionizing radiation to the eyes. The MRI appearances are described in conjunction with neurofibromatosis in Chapter 4.

Benign intrinsic tectal glioma

A specific group of intrinsic midbrain tumors has been identified with the presentation of raised intracranial pressure due to hydrocephalus resulting from obstruction of the aqueduct of Sylvius. May *et al.* (1991) made a report of six cases. CT revealed transient focal enhancement in only two patients. Serial scanning subsequently revealed that enhancement became less prominent as the lesions became progressively more calcified.

The MRI appearances of the masses are variable. The signal intensity may be hypo- or isointense with respect to surrounding structures (Fig. 8.10), or may be initially or subsequently increased in intensity. The hyperintensity on T_1-weighted images correlates with the increased density within the tectum on CT scans. There is no contrast enhancement following gadolinium administration. Hyperintensity of the mass on T_2-weighted images has been observed in all cases.

Gliomatosis cerebri

The term 'gliomatosis cerebri' was originally proposed by Nevin (1938) to describe gliomatous tumors of the CNS with diffuse neoplastic elements. The tumor is associated with widespread overgrowth of glial elements, mainly astrocytomal (Yanaka *et al.* 1992). Gliomatosis cerebri occurs, and may predominate, in children or young adults (Barnes *et al.* 1992).

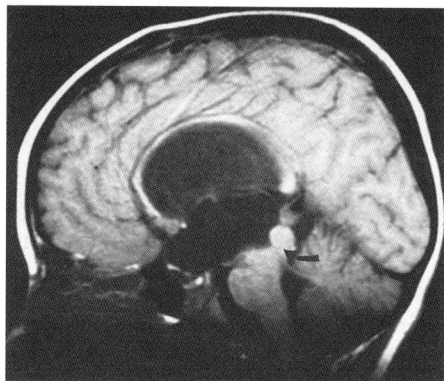

Fig. 8.10. Tectal glioma. T_1-weighted spin echo sagittal scan demonstrates a solid tectal mass *(arrow)*. There was no contrast enhancement on a subsequent contrast enhanced scan.

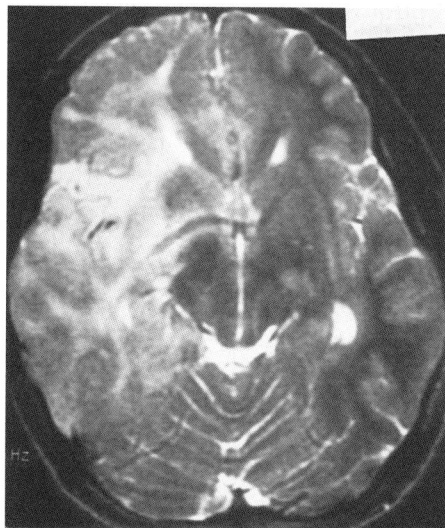

Fig. 8.11. Gliomatosis cerebri. T_2-weighted spin echo axial scan demonstrates diffuse areas of high signal intensity in several locations within the right cerebral hemisphere.

Clinical signs and symptoms are disproportionately mild, usually nonspecific and nonfocal despite the diffuse parenchymal involvement. CT shows diffuse lesions, usually isodense to surrounding brain, which usually do not enhance following intravenous administration of contrast medium. MRI also reveals diffuse lesions, with contiguous areas of high signal intensity areas on T_2-weighted images (Yanaka *et al.* 1992) (Fig. 8.11). Contrast enhancement was not noted in the case described by Yanaka and co-workers, nor in a 3-year-old boy at our hospital.

Ependymal tumors

Ependymal tumors of childhood are more commonly located infratentorially within the posterior fossa than supratentorially (Naidich and Zimmerman 1984, Russell and Rubinstein 1989). Supratentorial ependymomas arise from ependymal cell rests within white matter or from ependyma of the ventricle. This tumor is similar in appearance to PNETs and choroid plexus carcinoma (Maroldo and Barkovich 1992).

Supratentorial ependymomas have a very varied appearance on both CT and MRI (Barkovich 1992). The mass is usually of low signal intensity on T_1-weighted images, with variable signal intensity on proton density and T_2-weighted images (Zimmerman 1990*b*). The major characteristic of an ependymoma on MRI is heterogeneity, due to the presence of intratumoral calcification, cysts and occasional hemorrhage (Barkovich 1992). Cyst formation or necrosis typically occurs in 70–80 per cent of supratentorial ependymomas, with calcification in 50 per cent of cases (Pfleger and Gerson 1993).

178

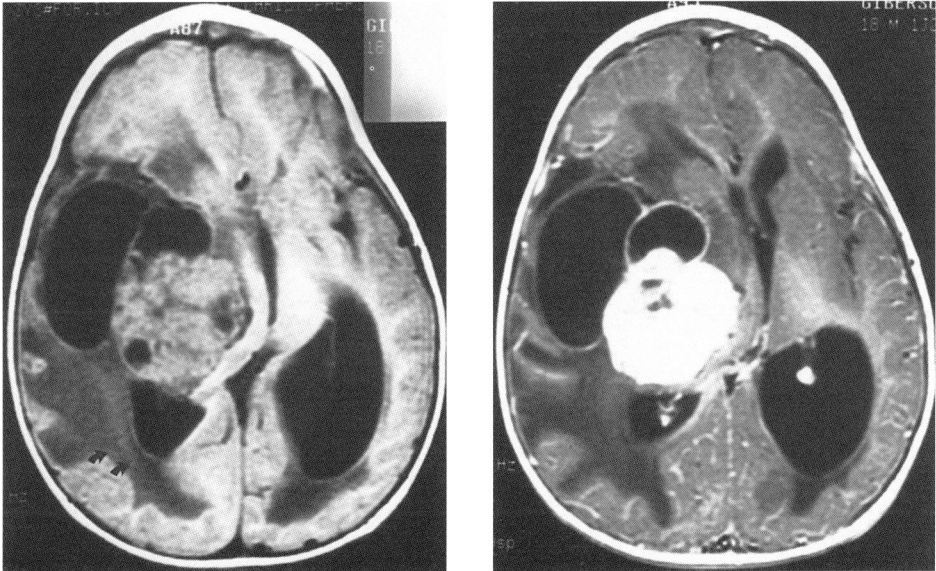

Fig. 8.12. Choroid plexus papilloma. T_1-weighted spin echo non-contast *(left)* and contrast enhanced *(right)* axial scans demonstrate hydrocephalus and a large intraventricular contrast enhancing mass. There is a large cystic component. Peritumoral edema is present.

Supratentorial ependymomas less commonly are homogeneous on MRI, appearing indistinguishable from a hemispheric astrocytoma (Barkovich 1992).

Choroid plexus tumors
Papillomas and carcinomas are the two common tumors of the choroid plexus in childhood. Papillomas arise from epithelial cells from any site of choroid plexus within the cranial cavity.

Choroid plexus tumors comprise approximately 5 per cent of supratentorial tumors in children (Barkovich and Edwards 1990). They may occur at any age but are mainly tumors of childhood. The majority occur in infants or children under 5 years of age (Ambrosino *et al.* 1988, Radkowski *et al.* 1988). Papillomas are usually discovered in the first year of life whereas carcinomas present at a later age but usually within the first five years (Barkovich and Edwards 1990). There is a marked male preponderance for both papilloma and carcinoma (Duffner and Cohen 1986, Tomita *et al.* 1988).

While the fourth ventricle is affected most in adults, the lateral ventricle, especially the trigone, is most commonly involved in children. Most series have shown a left-sided predominance (Hopper *et al.* 1987, Tomita *et al.* 1988), although in one large series slightly greater frequency on the right side was reported (Rovit *et al.* 1970). Extension of a lateral ventricle papilloma through the choroidal fissure into the quadrigeminal cistern and the contralateral ventricle has been reported (Bohm and Strang 1961, Raimondi and

179

Gutierrez 1975). The third and fourth ventricles are less commonly affected in children (Pascual–Castroviejo *et al.* 1983).

Tumoral calcification is infrequent, occurring in up to one fifth of cases (Rovit *et al.* 1970, Kendall *et al.* 1983).

Papillomas are usually well defined and separate from surrounding brain, whereas some carcinomas show anaplastic change with invasion of the adjacent brain (Barkovich and Edwards 1990).

Hydrocephalus is almost invariably associated with these tumors. This may result from CSF overproduction, obstruction of CSF pathway by tumor, or impaired CSF absorption from hemorrhage (Barnes *et al.* 1992).

The MRI appearance is of a large intraventricular mass that is iso- or hypointense on T_1-weighted images and iso- to hyperintense on T_2-weighted images (Fig. 8.12). Invasive papillomas or carcinomas may display heterogeneous signal intensity with irregular contrast enhancement, hemorrhage or cyst formation (Barnes *et al.* 1992). Choroid plexus carcinomas usually invade surrounding brain inciting vasogenic edema. They may be difficult to diagnose because of similarity in appearance to PNETs (Barkovich and Edwards 1990).

Craniopharyngioma

Craniopharyngiomas arise from embryonic squamous cell rests following incomplete closure of the hypophyseal or craniopharyngeal duct. The rests may occur at numerous sites along the entire craniopharyngeal duct from the floor of the third ventricle inferiorly to the body of the sphenoid bone and retropharyngeal space (Duffy 1920).

This tumor accounts for about 50 per cent of the sellar and intrasellar tumors of infancy and childhood (Banna 1976, Fitz *et al.* 1978). They generally occur in childhood but may occur at all ages from the neonatal period on (Majd *et al.* 1971). There is a second peak between the fourth and sixth decades of life that has led to speculation that they may represent metaplasia of anterior pituitary cells (Hunter 1955). Males are more commonly affected than females (Barkovich and Edwards 1990).

The majority of craniopharyngiomas (70 per cent) arise within the sella, with the remainder located in the suprasellar region (Matson 1969). They may rarely arise entirely within the third ventricle (Matthews 1983), sphenoid bone or sinus, or present as tumors of the clivus. They may become large and extend into the anterior, middle or posterior cranial fossae (Harwood-Nash and Fitz 1976).

Craniopharyngiomas may be cystic, solid or mixed to varying degrees. Calcification may be present in the form of a circumferential rim or solid pieces within the tumor.

The MRI appearances are characteristic, appearing as multilobular masses that extend superiorly from the diaphragma sellae (Barkovich and Edwards 1990). The solid portion of the tumor is iso- or hypointense on T_1-weighted images and iso- to hyperintense on T_2-weighted images. Gadolinium enhancement of the tumor or cyst wall is commonly noted (Barnes *et al.* 1992). The cystic component is commonly of high signal intensity on all pulse sequences because of the aqueous cholesterol, hemorrhage (methemoglobin) or proteinaceous fluid (Barnes *et al.* 1992) (Fig. 8.13). Increased signal intensity of the

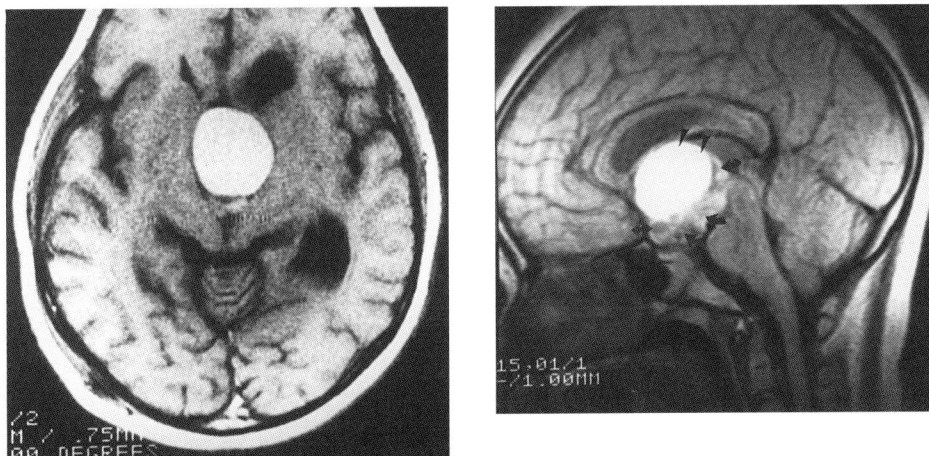

Fig. 8.13. Craniopharyngioma. Predominantly T_1-weighted spin echo non-contrast axial *(left)* and sagittal *(right)* scans demonstrate a suprasellar mass of mainly high signal intensity. There are both cystic and solid *(arrow)* components within the tumor mass.

cystic fluid on T_1-weighted images has been correlated with a protein concentration $\geq 90\,g/L$, free methemoglobin, or both (Ahmadi *et al.* 1992). Hypointense signal characteristics of the cyst may reflect predominance of keratin, calcium or iron (Barnes *et al.* 1992).

Rathke's cleft cyst

Rathke's cleft cyst represents a remnant of the apical portion of Rathke's pouch which persists into postnatal life between the pars distalis and pars nervosa of the pituitary (Russell and Rubinstein 1989). The cyst may be entirely confined to the sella turcica or may project beneath the optic chiasm. The contents of the cyst may be fluid, or may be inspissated and brown from old hemorrhage. Remnants of the compressed pituitary gland are flattened and incorporated into the outer part of the cyst wall (Russell and Rubinstein 1989). The MRI appearance of the mass is of high signal intensity on T_1-weighted images (Barkovich and Edwards 1990). The differential diagnosis of this lesion includes craniopharyngioma, arachnoid cyst, pituitary cyst and adenoma (Barnes *et al.* 1992).

Pituitary tumors

Pituitary adenomas have long been considered to be rare in infancy and childhood, accounting for 0.7 per cent of intracranial tumors in the series of Harwood-Nash and Fitz (1976) and 1.5 per cent in the series of Koos and Miller (1971). With earlier detection the frequency has increased in infants and children. Richmond and Wilson (1978) reported a 33 per cent incidence of pituitary adenomas in the 74 parasellar tumors detected in patients under 20 years of age.

The traditional classification of pituitary adenomas into chromophobe, chromophile

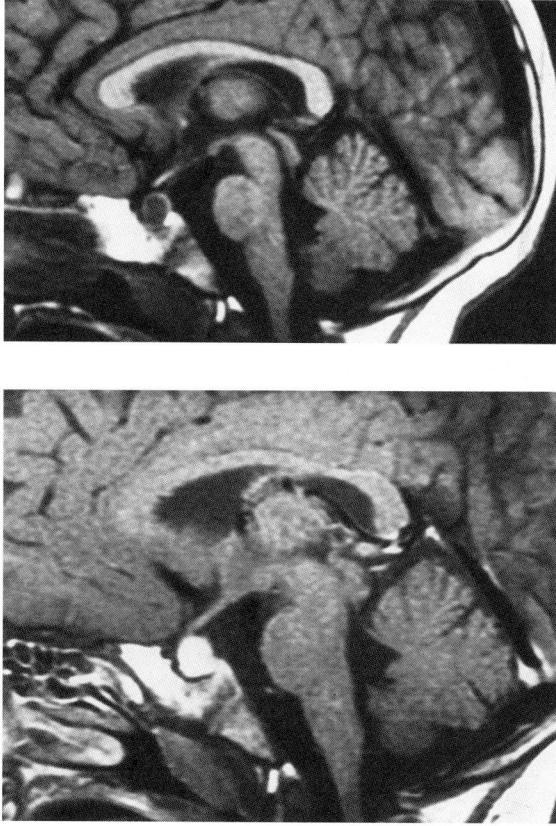

Fig. 8.14. Pituitary adenoma. T$_1$-weighted spin echo non-contrast *(top)* and contrast enhanced *(bottom)* sagittal scans demonstrate enlargement of the pituitary, enhancing with contrast.

(eosinophilic and basophilic) and mixed cell tumors has now been superseded by functional classification according to endocrine activity.

Endocrinologically active adenomas account for 75 per cent of adenomas (Russell and Rubinstein 1989). These include the prolactin-secreting prolactinoma, growth hormone (somatotrophic), corticotrophic, thyrotrophic, gonadotrophic and mixed secretory types. In a large series of 76 pituitary tumors in children, 57 per cent were prolactinomas, 25 per cent corticotrophic, and 12 per cent somatotrophic (Laws *et al.* 1987). The remaining 25 per cent of adenomas are endocrinologically inactive. They are termed null-cell adenomas (Kovacs *et al.* 1980).

Macroadenomas are more common than microadenomas in children, the reverse of the situation in adults (Rutka *et al.* 1992).

They are usually hypo- or isointense on T$_1$-weighted images, and are iso- to hyperintense on proton density and T$_2$-weighted images (Davis *et al.* 1987) (Fig. 8.14).

182

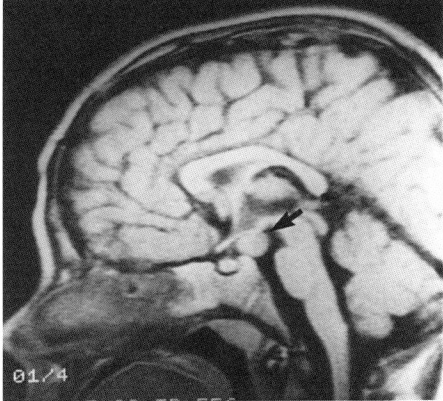

Fig. 8.15. Hypothalamic hamartoma. T_1-weighted spin echo non-contrast sagittal scan demonstrates a well-defined solid mass *(arrow)* in the region of the hypothalamus.

Microadenomas are usually hypointense to the rest of the gland on T_1-weighted images and do not enhance to the same extent as the rest of the pituitary gland on T_1-weighted post-gadolinium images (Pojunas *et al.* 1986, Kulkarni *et al.* 1988).

Suprasellar extension of macroadenomas is best demonstrated by coronal MRI (Zimmerman 1990*a*).

Hypothalamic hamartoma

A hamartoma is a congenital malformation which consists of a tumor-like collection of normal tissue in an abnormal location.

Hypothalamic hamartoma (hamartoma of the tuber cinereum) is a rare entity. The tuber cinereum region includes the small bilateral protuberances of gray matter, the middle hypothalamic nuclei located between the infundibular stalk and the large prominent mamillary bodies (Boyko *et al.* 1991). Axons in the tuberoinfundibular tract leading from these nuclei carry secretory granules that contain releasing hormones. These allow for the modulation of gonadotropin (Carpenter 1985).

Ectopic hamartomas may occur in an extracranial location especially the soft palate or nasal bridge (Davis 1990). Well defined masses of ectopic gray matter in the centrum ovale have been followed by the development of ganglioglioma and gangliocytoma, suggesting a histologic progression (Russell and Rubinstein 1989).

Hypothalamic hamartoma may be associated with growth-hormone-secreting pituitary adenoma, resulting in acromegaly (Asa *et al.* 1980). There is also an association with other multiple congenital abnormalities in the Pallister–Hall syndrome, consisting of abnormal olfactory bulbs, absence of the pituitary gland, hypoplastic thyroid and adrenal glands, cryptorchidism, cardiac and renal anomalies, imperforate anus, syndactyly and short metacarpals (Hall *et al.* 1980).

Males are more commonly affected than females. Precocious puberty is the most common presenting sign, usually manifested under 2 years of age. Gelastic seizures and mental retardation or behavioral disorders may also be present (Zuniga *et al.* 1983, Breningstall 1985).

The MRI appearance of hypothalamic hamartoma is that of a well defined round mass that is suspended from the tuber cinereum or mamillary bodies (Barkovich and Edwards 1990). The mass is usually isointense on T_1-weighted images and hyperintense on T_2-weighted images (Barkovich and Edwards 1990, Davis 1990, Barnes *et al.* 1992) (Fig. 8.15). The isointensity on MRI is comparable to the appearance on CT where the mass is isodense to normal gray matter. Abnormal iodine enhancement on CT or gadolinium enhancement on MRI is usually absent (Barnes *et al.* 1992).

Primitive neuroectodermal tumor
The term 'primitive neuroectodermal tumor' was introduced by Hart and Earle (1973) to describe a rare group of malignant, predominantly undifferentiated (>90 per cent) tumors in the cerebral hemispheres of children. A common neuroepithelial precursor for these tumors was postulated. This concept was subsequently expanded to include those primitive tumors sharing common neuroepithelial precursors in sites other than the cerebrum such as the brainstem, cerebellum, spinal cord, craniofacial structures and extra-CNS locations (Parker *et al.* 1975, Kosnik *et al.* 1978, Becker and Hinton 1983, Rorke *et al.* 1985, Dehner *et al.* 1986). They have been referred to by numerous terms including cerebral or central neuroblastoma, PNET of the cerebrum and cerebral medulloblastoma (Dehner 1981, Rorke 1983).

Rubinstein (1975) proposed that these tumors were independent entities recognized by distinctive patterns of differentiation from a unique cell of origin. Rorke (1983) contended that numerous tumors named on the basis of morphology and location, with similar clinical and pathologic characteristics, should be considered variants of a single cell type, the PNET. The tumors are thus classified by phenotypic characteristics (Rorke 1983). This classification addresses undifferentiated neuroepithelial round cell tumors, and is included in the proposed modification of the WHO classification of pediatric CNS tumors (Rorke *et al.* 1985).

Supratentorial PNETs occur from the neonatal period to adulthood, but predominate in the first decade of life. The median age of presentation is 8 years, with a peak incidence evenly distributed between birth and 5 years of age (Heideman *et al.* 1989). Males and females are equally affected.

The vast majority of supratentorial PNETs are located in the cerebral hemispheres, with 90 per cent occurring in the frontal, parietal, temporal and occipital lobes in order of increasing frequency. Fewer than 10 per cent of these tumors occur in midline structures (Heideman *et al.* 1989).

The appearances of supratentorial PNET on CT and MRI correlate with the gross pathologic findings (Robles *et al.* 1992). Both CT and MRI demonstrate sharply circumscribed, expansile masses in the deep white matter (Kingsley and Harwood-Nash 1984, Figueroa *et al.* 1989, Robles *et al.* 1991).

They often have a cystic component that may correspond to necrosis and/or hemorrhage (Figueroa *et al.* 1989, Robles *et al.* 1991). Edema is not a prominent feature and is usually minimal, localized to the immediate vicinity of the tumor. Non-contrast CT is helpful in demonstrating the calcification that occurs in slightly over one half of all cases and is superior to MRI in identifying calvarial asymmetries or bone erosion (Robles *et al.* 1992).

MRI is superior to CT for evaluating these tumors because of its multiplanar capability which better demonstrates tumor morphology, edema and tumor nodules (Robles *et al.* 1992). The MRI appearance is variable to hypointense or even hyperintense on T_1-weighted images and iso-, hypo- or hyperintense on T_2-weighted images (Davis 1990, Barnes *et al.* 1992, Robles *et al.* 1992). The higher protein content of the cystic components is responsible for a slightly higher signal than CSF on all pulse sequences (Robles *et al.* 1992). Gadolinium-enhanced MRI best demonstrates tumor nodules and meningeal or subarachnoid involvement.

The differential diagnosis of a large supratentorial PNET includes other expansile tumors such as ependymomas which may be extraventricular, teratomas, large mesenchymal tumors and abscesses (Hinshaw *et al.* 1983, Zimmerman 1990*b*, Robles *et al.* 1992).

Pineal region tumors
The numerous pineal region tumors have been classified by Russell and Rubinstein (1989) into several major groups: (1) pineoblastoma: (2) pineocytoma; (3) glial tumors (astrocytoma, glioblastoma); (4) germ cell tumors; (5) other tumors such as meningiomas arising from the tela choroidea or tentorium, melanomas and non–neoplastic cysts. These tumors account for around 3–8 per cent of intracranial tumors in children (Hoffman *et al.* 1983).

The pineal parenchymal tumors, pineoblastoma and pineocytoma, account for 20–40 per cent of pineal region tumors (Heideman *et al.* 1989). Pineoblastomas mostly affect children in the first decade of life. There is a 2:1 male–female ratio (Russell and Rubinstein 1989). There is an association with bilateral retinoblastomas (Bader *et al.* 1982, Brownstein *et al.* 1984). The cases are usually hereditary. Pineocytomas occur mostly in adults but children may also be affected during the first decade of life. There is no particular sex predilection (Russell and Rubinstein 1989).

Pineoblastomas and pineocytomas are iso- or hypodense on non-contrast CT scans, with marked uniform enhancement following intravenous administration of iodinated contrast media (Barkovich and Edwards 1990). Pineoblastomas contain cystic non-enhancing foci and are larger and more irregularly shaped than pineocytomas or germinomas (Barkovich and Edwards 1990). There is frequent inferior extension into the posterior fossa and there may also be anterior extension into the third ventricle.

MRI provides excellent anatomic definition of masses in the pineal region and may demonstrate small lesions in children with hydrocephalus that may be missed by CT (Edwards *et al.* 1988, Davis 1990). The appearance of these tumors on MRI is non-specific (Davis 1990). They are usually iso- to hypointense on T_1-weighted images and iso- to hyperintense on T_2-weighted images (Barkovich and Edwards 1990, Davis 1990, Barnes *et al.* 1992). Heavily calcified masses may appear hypointense. Gadolinium enhancement is useful in the detection of CSF metastases as these may not be detected on T_1- and T_2-weighted images prior to enhancement, and also in the follow-up examinations after surgery or moderation (Barkovich and Edwards 1990, Davis 1990).

185

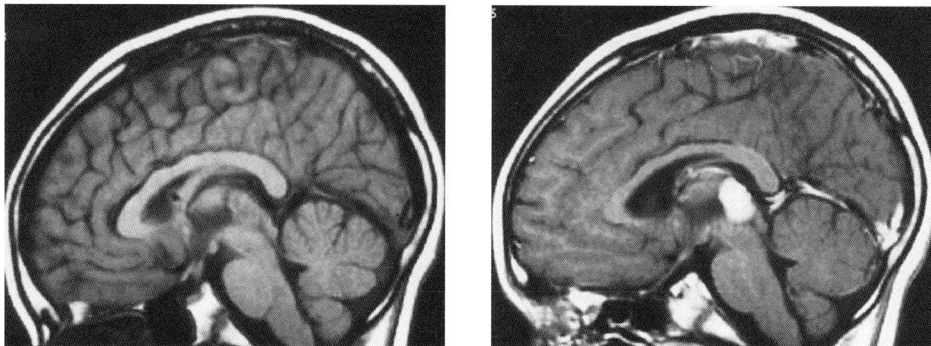

Fig. 8.16. Pineal germinoma. T_1-weighted spin echo non-contrast *(left)* and contrast enhanced *(right)* sagittal scans demonstrate homogeneous enhancement within a pineal mass.

Germ cell tumors

Germinoma

Germinoma is the most common variety of intracranial germ cell tumor. Originally termed pinealoma, it is the most common tumor arising in the pineal region (Russell and Rubinstein 1989). Germinoma in the suprasellar type was originally termed ectopic pinealoma.

There is a marked male preponderance for germinomas in the pineal region (Russell and Rubinstein 1989); however, the sex distribution has been noted to be equal in the suprasellar region (Takeuchi *et al.* 1978, Russell and Rubinstein 1989).

The CT appearance of a germinoma is an iso- or hyperdense mass that enhances after intravenous iodinated contrast media. The MRI appearance is of an iso- or hypointense mass on T_1-weighted images with gadolinium enhancement. The tumor is iso- or hypointense, or occasionally hyperintense, on T_2-weighted images (Kilgore *et al.* 1986, Barkovich and Edwards 1990, Tien *et al.* 1990) (Fig. 8.16). The tumors may occasionally be of low signal intensity on T_2-weighted images. This appearance is attributed to the high nuclear to cytoplasmic ratio in these tumors with a resulting diminished free water content (Barkovich and Edwards 1990).

Meningioma

Meningiomas are rare in children and adolescents, accounting for 1–2 per cent of all intracranial tumors (Huh 1964, Medline *et al.* 1968). Drake *et al.* (1986) reported a marked male preponderance in their series, although this conclusion was not supported by Barkovich and Edwards (1990).

Meningiomas arise in close relationship to the arachnoid villi which are most commonly located in the parasagittal region, followed in decreasing frequency by the cavernous and parasellar regions, tuberculum sellae, lamina cribrosa, foramen magnum and torcular Herophili (Russell and Rubinstein 1989). A small number of meningiomas have no dural attachment, arising from the velum interpositum or tela choroidea to grow

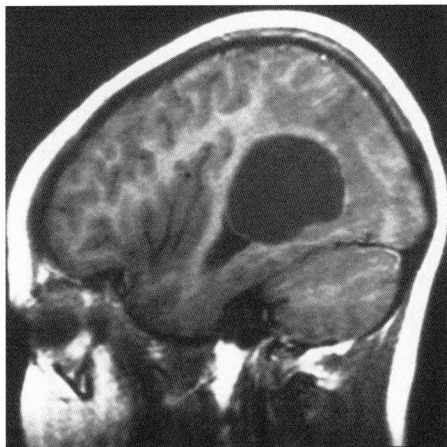

Fig. 8.17. Meningioma. T_1-weighted spin echo sagittal scan demonstrates a large low signal intensity mass within the lateral ventricle.

within the lateral, third and fourth ventricles (Schaerer and Woolsey 1960, Gassel and Davies 1961, Lee *et al.* 1979).

In children, meningiomas are more commonly located within the ventricles and the posterior fossa (Merten *et al.* 1974). Approximately a quarter of meningiomas occur in association with neurofibromatosis (Davis 1990).

Meningiomas mostly arise from the inner dural surface growing toward the brain in the form of bulky masses termed global meningiomas (Naidich 1990). Other forms are sessile, pedunculated, and meningioma-en-plaque. Osseous changes include mild pressure erosion from the mass, bone destruction, and focal or diffuse hyperostosis (Naidich 1990). Distal metastases are uncommon.

The histologic types of meningioma have been divided into five main subgroups: syncytial, transitional, fibrous, angioblastic and sarcomatous (Courville 1930, Russell 1950).

Two rare forms of meningioma in children are malignant meningioma and meningosarcoma (Russell and Rubinstein 1989). Malignancy is reported to occur in 7–16 per cent of meningiomas in children (Herz *et al.* 1980, Davidson and Hope 1989, Ferrante *et al.* 1989). The incidence of malignancy decreases with age.

The MRI appearances of meningioma are variable (Naidich 1990). The mass is usually isointense to gray matter on T_1-weighted images (Fig. 8.17), while on T_2-weighted images it may be isointense (Barkovich and Edwards 1990), show a slight difference in signal intensity (Naidich 1990) or be hyperintense (Zimmerman *et al.* 1985, Elster *et al.* 1989). When a meningioma is isointense on a noncontrast MRI study, the presence of such a mass may be inferred by (i) reduced signal from the diploë of adjacent bone which would suggest hyperostosis, (ii) a thin rim of reduced signal intensity from CSF at the brain–tumor interface or capsular veins, or (iii) mottled signal intensity due to calcification (Zimmerman *et al.* 1985). Densely calcified areas are of low signal intensity. The signal intensity on T_2-weighted images has been shown to correlate with the histologic type of meningioma (Elster *et al.* 1989). Fibroblastic or transitional types were found to be

187

hypointense to the cerebral cortex, whereas angioblastic and syncytial meningiomas demonstrated marked hyperintensity on T_2-weighted images.

Uniform intense enhancement within the solid portion of the mass is usually seen after gadolinium enhancement (Barkovich and Edwards 1990). Heterogenous enhancement of an intraventricular mass should suggest that the tumor is a malignant meningioma rather than a benign one (Greenberg *et al.* 1993).

Leukemia

Leukemia may involve the CNS in three forms (Russell and Rubinstein 1989): (i) diffuse leptomeningeal infiltration, often accompanied by invasion of cranial and spinal nerve roots; (ii) impaction of leukemic cells within cerebral white matter; and (iii) rarely, solid masses in the extradural spaces and craniospinal bones.

Leptomeningeal infiltration by leukemia is common. The CNS is the most frequent site of initial relapse in cases of acute lymphocytic leukemia of childhood (Aur *et al.* 1972). Dural infiltration was found in 70 per cent of patients with lymphocytic leukemia (Moore *et al.* 1960). Meningeal leukemia is infrequently demonstrated by either CT or MRI (Barnes *et al.* 1992).

Leukemic masses, designated chloromas, are granulocytic sarcomas that represent a subtype of myelogenous leukemia. They are extramedullary foci of malignant granulopoiesis (Liu *et al.* 1973). They occur most commonly in children and young adults, with a peak incidence between 4 and 5 years of age (Atkinson 1939, Liu *et al.* 1973).

Leukemic masses are iso- or hyperdense on CT. The MRI appearance is of a mass that is iso- or hypointense on T_1-weighted images, and iso-, hypo- or occasionally hyperintense on T_2-weighted images. Marked enhancement is expected following iodine or gadolinium administration for CT and MRI respectively (Barnes *et al.* 1992).

Malignant lymphoma

Primary malignant lymphomas of the CNS are now generally classified with the systemic non-Hodgkin lymphomas, with almost all cases composed of lymphoid cells of B origin (Russell and Rubinstein 1989). They can occur at any age. Primary cerebral lymphomas are rare, accounting for fewer than 1 per cent of all intracranial tumors (Jellinger *et al.* 1975) and 2 per cent of all malignant lymphomas (Henry *et al.* 1974).

Congenital and acquired immunodeficiency disorders are associated with the development of malignant lymphomas. The congenital group includes Wiskott–Aldrich syndrome and other dysglobulinemias associated with T-lymphocyte depression (Bale *et al.* 1977). Acquired disorders of the immune system include iatrogenic complications following cardiac and renal transplantation (Shneck and Penn 1971) and infection, *e.g.* HTLV III/ LAV or HIV (Lehrich and Hedley-Whyte 1983, Snider *et al.* 1983).

Cerebral lymphomas have also been reported in association with systemic lupus erythematosus treated with immunosuppression (Lipsmeyer 1972), Epstein–Barr virus infection (Hochberg *et al.* 1983), and Sjögren syndrome (Lehrich and Richardson 1978).

The cerebrum is area most often affected. The tumor may be located in any lobe or in the basal ganglia (Russell and Rubinstein 1989). Other sites described are the brain-

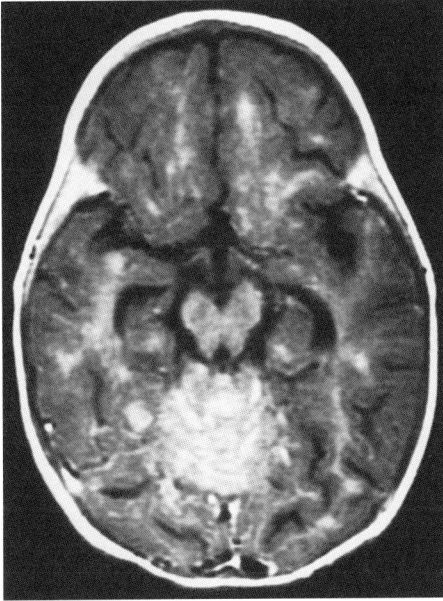

Fig. 8.18. Lymphomatoid granulomatosis. Axial, T$_1$-weighted contrast enhanced scan demonstrates multifocal areas of tumoral enhancement.

stem and cerebellum (Henry *et al.* 1974).

The CT appearance of lymphoma is of an iso- or hyperdense lesion with moderate to marked contrast enhancement. The corresponding MRI appearance is of a tumor mass that is iso- or slightly hypointense on T$_1$-weighted images (Schwaighofer *et al.* 1989, Zimmerman 1990*c*) and iso- to hypointense (Zimmerman 1990*a*) or slightly hyperintense (Schwaighofer *et al.* 1989) on proton density and T$_2$-weighted images. Gadolinium enhancement may be homo- or heterogeneous, with mild edema and minimal or absent mass effect (Barnes *et al.* 1992).

Lymphomatoid granulomatosis
Lymphomatoid granulomatosis was first described by Liebow *et al.* (1972) as an angio-centric and angiodestructive lymphoreticular proliferative and granulomatous disease. As there has been subsequent evidence that this disease is a distinctive type of lymphoma, it should be viewed as part of a larger family of peripheral T-cell lymphomas (Myers 1990).

Although the disease mainly affects older adults, it has been found in children and young adults from 7 to 20 years of age (Katzenstein *et al.* 1979).

The lungs are predominantly involved. Other sites include the CNS in at least 20 per cent of patients, kidneys and skin (Liebow 1972). The CNS is usually only involved after well-established disease in the lungs and other sites; however, primary lymphomatoid granulomatosis of the CNS can rarely occur as the first or sole manifestation (Schmidt *et al.* 1984). There are numerous forms of CNS lesions including necrotic cavitary masses, solid tumor masses, parenchymal and leptomeningeal infiltration, infarction, hemorrhage and aneurysm (Verity and Wolfson 1976, Pena 1977, Sackett *et al.* 1979, Kapila *et al.*

189

1988). The lesions may be unifocal or bifocal in either supratentorial or infratentorial location. Unifocal lesions are more common (Kerslake *et al.* 1991).

The CT appearances of this disease are variable. Some lesions may be of decreased density with poorly defined borders on the non-contrast scan, followed by slight enhancement after contrast administration (Sackett 1979), while others may demonstrate solid enhancement (Ironside *et al.* 1984). Parenchymal hemorrhages in the absence of coagulopathy have been demonstrated in the frontal and temporal lobes (Kapila *et al.* 1988).

MRI shows low signal intensity on T_1-weighted images, and high signal intensity on T_2-weighted spin echo images (Kerslake *et al.* 1991) (Fig. 8.18). Differential diagnosis from inflammatory and other neoplastic conditions by MRI is limited.

Metastatic disease

Metastatic involvement of the CNS may result from distant tumors and systemic diseases, from leptomeningeal seeding in the intracranial space, or from direct extension.

Metastatic tumors arising from non–CNS primary tumors are usually hematogenous in origin. The most common primary tumors are sarcomas, including osteogenic sarcoma, Ewing sarcoma and rhabdomyosarcoma (Lewis 1988). Other tumors noted rarely for cerebral metastases are Wilm's tumor (Hammock and Milhorat 1981) and hepatoblastoma (Exelby *et al.* 1975). These metastases to brain parenchyma may be single or multiple lesions of variable size, with or without vasogenic edema and mass effect (Davis 1990). The diagnosis is suggested by multiplicity, with a tendency to be aggregated in middle cerebral artery territory and the gray–white matter junction. Hemorrhage and pronounced enhancement are most common, while necrosis, calcification and cyst formation are uncommon (Pedersen *et al.* 1989).

Leptomeningeal seeding in the intracranial space may result from primary CNS tumors such as medulloblastoma, ependymoma, PNET, germinoma, high grade astrocytoma, malignant choroid plexus papilloma and pineoblastoma (Kun *et al.* 1985) and systemic disorders such as lymphoma and leukemia.

Skull metastases to the bone and adjacent dura arise from lymphoma, leukemia and neuroblastoma.

The CT appearance of a parenchymal metastatic lesion is a low density mass that displays moderate to marked contrast enhancement (Pedersen *et al.* 1989). Lesions adjacent to dense bone may not be detected, however, due to artifactual interference (Davis 1990).

MRI shows slightly hypointense lesions on T_1-weighted pulse sequences and iso- or hyperintense signal on T_2-weighted pulse sequences (Barkovich and Edwards 1990). Parenchymal lesions may be missed on non-contrast MRI, especially if they are small with little mass effect, adjacent to CSF interfaces or other CNS abnormalities (Claussen *et al.* 1985, Russell *et al.* 1987).

Gadolinium enhanced T_1-weighted pulse sequences are essential for the detection of hematogenous and leptomeningeal metastases (Russell *et al.* 1987, Davis 1990). Masses containing hemorrhage or fat can be readily differentiated by use of a non-contrast T_1-weighted pulse sequence (Davis 1990).

REFERENCES

Ahmadi, J., Destian, S., Apuzzo, M.L.J., Segall, H.D., Zee, C-S. (1992) 'Cystic fluid in craniopharyngiomas: MR imaging and quantitative analysis.' *Radiology*, **182**, 783–785.

Albright, A.L. (1992) 'Posterior fossa tumors.' *Neurosurgery Clinics of North America*, **3**, 881–891.

—— Price, R.A., Guthkelch, A.N. (1983) 'Brainstem gliomas of children. A clinicopathological study.' *Cancer*, **52**, 2313–2319.

—— Wisoff, J.H., Zelzter, P.M., Deutsch, M., Finlay, J., Hammond, D. (1989) 'Current neurosurgical treatment of medulloblastomas in children.' *Pediatric Neuroscience*, **15**, 276–282.

Alvord, E.C., Lofton, S. (1988) Gliomas of the optic nerve or chiasm. Outcome by patients' age, tumor site, and treatment.' *Journal of Neurosurgery*, **68**, 85–98.

Amador, L.V. (1983) *Brain Tumors in the Young.* Springfield, IL: Charles C. Thomas.

Ambrosino, M.M., Hernanz-Schulman, M., Genieser, N.B., Wisoff, J., Epstein, F. (1988) 'Brain tumors in infants less than a year of age.' *Pediatric Radiology*, **19**, 6–8.

Armington, W.G., Osborn, A.G., Cubberly, D.A., Harnsberger, H.R., Boyer, R., Naidich, T.P., Sherry, R.G. (1985) 'Supratentorial ependymoma: CT appearance.' *Radiology*, **157**, 367–372.

Asa, S.L., Bilbao, J.M, Kovacs, K., Linfoot, J.A. (1980) 'Hypothalamic neuronal hamartoma associated with pituitary growth hormone cell adenoma and acromegaly.' *Acta Neuropathologica*, **52**, 231–234.

Asai, A., Hoffman, H.J., Hendrick, E.B., Humphreys, R.P., Becker, L.E. (1989) 'Primary intracranial neoplasms in the first year of life.' *Child's Nervous System*, **5**, 230–233.

Atkinson, F.R.B. (1939) 'Chloroma in children.' *British Journal of Children's Diseases*, **36**, 18–34.

Aur, R.J.A., Simon, J.V., Hustu, H.O., Verzosa, M.S. (1972) 'A comparative study of central nervous system irradiation and intensive chemotherapy early in remission of childhood acute lymphocytic leukemia.' *Cancer*, **29**, 381–391.

Bader, J.L., Meadows, A.T., Zimmerman, L.E., Rorke, L.B., Voute, P.A., Champion, L.A.A., Miller, R.W. (1982) 'Bilateral retinoblastoma with ectopic intracranial retinoblastoma: bilateral retinoblastoma.' *Cancer Genetics and Cytogenetics*, **5**, 203–213.

Bale, J.F., Wilson, J.F., Hill, H.R. (1977) 'Fatal histiocytic lymphoma of the brain associated with hyperimmuno-globulinemia-E and recurrent infections.' Cancer, 39, 2386–2390.

Banna, M. (1976) 'Craniopharyngioma: based on 160 cases.' *British Journal of Radiology*, **49**, 206–223.

Barkovich, A.J. (1992) 'Neuroimaging of pediatric brain tumors.' *Neurosurgery Clinics of North America*, **3**, 739–769.

—— Edwards, M. (1990) 'Brain tumors of childhood.' *In:* Barkovich, A.J. (Ed.) *Pediatric Neuroimaging.* New York: Raven Press, pp. 149–203.

Barnes, P.D. (1990) 'Magnetic resonance in pediatric and adolescent neuroimaging.' *Neurologic Clinics*, **8**, 741–757.

—— Kupsky, W.J., Strand, R.D. (1992) 'Cranial and intracranial tumors.' *In:* Wolpert, S.M., Barnes, P.D. (Eds.) *MRI in Pediatric Neuroradiology.* St. Louis: Mosby–Year Book, pp. 204–298.

Becker, L.E., Hinton, D. (1983) 'Primitive neuroectodermal tumors of the central nervous system.' *Human Pathology*, **14**, 538–550.

Benitez, W.I., Glasier, C.M., Husain, M., Angtuaco, E.J.C., Chadduck, W.M. (1990) 'MR findings in childhood gangliogliomas.' *Journal of Computer Assisted Tomography*, **14**, 712–716.

Bilaniuk, L.T., Zimmerman, R.A., Littman, P., Gallo, E., Rorke, L.B., Bruce, D.A., Schut, L. (1980) 'Computed tomography of brainstem gliomas in children.' *Radiology*, **134**, 89–95.

Bird, C.R., Drayer, B.P., Medina, M., Rekate, H.L., Flom, R.A., Hodak, J.A. (1988) 'Gd-DTPA-enhanced MR imaging in pediatric patients after brain tumor resection.' *Radiology*, **169**, 123–126.

Bohm, E., Strang, R. (1961) 'Choroid plexus papillomas.' *Journal of Neurosurgery*, **18**, 493–500.

Bonnin, J.M., Rubinstein, L.J., Papasozomenos, S.C.H., Marangos, P.J. (1984) 'Subependymal giant cell astrocytoma. Significance and possible cytogenetic implications of an immunohistochemical study.' *Acta Neuropathologica*, **62**, 185–193.

Boyko, O.B., Curnes, J.T., Oakes, W.J., Burger, P.C. (1991) 'Hamartomas of the tuber cinereum: CT, MR and pathologic findings.' *American Journal of Neuroradiology*, **12**, 309–314.

Breningstall, G.N. (1985) 'Gelastic seizures, precocious puberty and hypothalamic hamartoma.' *Neurology*, **35**, 1180–1183.

Brody, A.S. (1991) 'New perspectives in CT and MR imaging.' *Neurologic Clinics*, **9**, 273–286.

Brownstein, S., de Chadarevian, J–P., Little, J.M. (1984) 'Trilateral retinoblastoma. Report of two cases.'

191

Archives of Ophthalmology, **102**, 257–262.

Brant-Zawadzki, M. (1988) 'MR imaging of the brain.' *Radiology*, **166**, 1–10.

Buetow, P.C., Smirniotopoulos, J.G., Done, S. (1990) 'Congenital brain tumors: a review of 45 cases.' *American Journal of Neuroradiology*, **11**, 793–799.

Carpenter, M.B. (1985) *Core Text of Neuroanatomy. 3rd Edn.* Baltimore: Williams & Wilkins.

Castillo, M., Davis, P., Takei, Y., Hoffman, J.C. (1990) 'Intracranial ganglioglioma: MR, CT and clinical findings in 18 patients.' *American Journal of Neuroradiology*, **11**, 109–114.

Claussen, C., Laniado, M., Schorner, W. (1985) 'Gadolinium-DTPA in MR imaging of glioblastomas and intracranial metastases.' *American Journal of Neuroradiology*, **6**, 669–674.

Cohen, M., Duffner, P. (1989) 'Tumors of the brain and spinal cord.' *In:* Swaiman, K. (Ed.) *Pediatric Neurology.* St. Louis: Mosby–Year Book, pp. 661–714.

Courville, C.B. (1930) 'Ganglioglioma: tumor of the central nervous system. Review of literature and report of two cases.' *Achieves of Neurology and Psychiatry*, **24**, 439–491.

Cramer, F., Kimsey, W. (1952) 'Cerebellar hemangioblastomas. Review of 53 cases, with special reference to cerebellar cysts and the association of polycythemia.' *Archives of Neurology and Psychiatry*, **67**, 237–252.

Davidson, G.S., Hope, J.K. (1989) 'Meningeal tumors of childhood.' *Cancer*, **63**, 1205–1210.

Davis, P.C. (1990) 'Tumors of the brain.' *In:* Cohen, M.D., Edwards, M.K. (Eds.) *Magnetic Resonance Imaging of Children.* Philadelphia: B.C. Decker, pp. 155–220.

—— Hoffman, J.C., Spenser, T. (1987) 'MR imaging of pituitary adenoma: CT, clinical and surgical correlation.' *American Journal of Neuroradiology*, **8**, 107–112.

Dehner, L.P. (1981) 'Primitive neuroectodermal tumors of the central nervous system in childhood: retrospective and review.' *In:* Humphrey, G.B., Dehner, L.P., Grindey, G.B. (Eds.) *Pediatric Oncology.* The Hague: Martinus, pp. 277–288.

—— (1986) 'Peripheral and central primitive neuroectodermal tumors. A nosologic concept seeking a consensus.' *Archives of Pathology and Laboratory Medicine*, **110**, 997–1105.

Demierre, B., Stichnoth, F.A., Hori, A., Spoerri, O. (1986) 'Intracerebral ganglioglioma.' *Journal of Neurosurgery*, **65**, 177–182.

Diebler, C., Dulac, O. (1987) 'Neurocutaneous syndromes.' *In: Pediatric Neurology and Neuroradiology.* New York: Springer–Verlag, pp. 85–109.

Dohrmann, G.J., Farwell, J.R. (1976) 'Intracranial neoplasms in children: a comparison of North America, Europe, Africa and Asia.' *Diseases of the Nervous System*, **37**, 696–697.

—— —— Flannery, J.T. (1976) 'Glioblastoma multiforme in children.' *Journal of Neurosurgery*, **44**, 442–448.

Dorne, H., O'Gorgman, A.M., Melanson, D. (1988) 'Computed tomography of intracranial gangliogliomas.' *American Journal of Neuroradiology*, **7**, 281–285.

Drake, J.M., Hendrick, E.B., Becker, L.E., Chuang, S.H., Hoffman, S.J., Humphreys, R.P. (1986) 'Intracranial meningiomas in children.' *Pediatric Neuroscience*, **12**, 134–139.

Duffner, P.K., Cohen, M.E. (1986) 'Treatment of brain tumors in babies and very young children.' *Pediatric Neuroscience*, **12**, 304–310.

—— —— Freeman, A.I. (1985) 'Pediatric brain tumors: an overview.' *CA: A Cancer Journal For Clinicians*, **35**, 287–301.

Duffy, W.C. (1920) 'Hypophyseal duct tumors; a report of three cases and a fourth case of cyst of Rathke's pouch.' *Annals of Surgery*, **72**, 537–555.

Edwards, M.S.B., Hudgins, R.J., Wilson, C.B., Levin, V.A., Wara, W.M. (1988) 'Pineal region tumors in children.' *Journal of Neurosurgery*, **68**, 689–697.

Elster, A.D., Arthur, D.W. (1988) 'Intracranial hemangioblastomas: CT and MR findings.' *Journal of Computer Assisted Tomography*, **12**, 736–739.

—— Challa, V.R., Gilbert, T.H., Richardson, D.N., Contento, J.C. (1989) 'Meningiomas: MR and histopathologic features.' *Radiology*, **170**, 857–862.

Exelby, P.R., Filler, R.M., Grosfeld, J.L. (1975) 'Liver tumors in children in the particular reference to hepatoblastoma and hepatocellular carcinoma: American Academy of Pediatrics Surgical Section Survey—1974.' *Journal of Pediatric Surgery*, **10**, 329–337.

Farwell, J.R., Dohrmann, G.J., Flannery, J.T. (1977) 'Central nervous system tumors in children.' *Cancer*, **40**, 3123–3132.

Favier, J., Pizzolato, G.P., Berney, J. (1985) 'Oligodendroglial tumors in childhood.' *Child's Nervous System*, **1**, 33–38.

Ferrante, L., Acaui, M., Artico, M., Mastronardi, L., Fortuna, A. (1989) 'Pediatric intracranial meningiomas.'

British Journal of Neurosurgery, **3**, 189–196.

Figueroa, R.E., El Gammal, T., Brooks, B.S., Holgate, R., Miller, W. (1989) 'MR findings in primitive neuro-ectodermal tumors.' *Journal of Computer Assisted Tomography*, **13**, 773–778.

Fitz, C.R., Wortzman, G., Harwood-Nash, D.C., Holgate, R.C., Barry, J.F., Boldt, D.W. (1978) 'Computed tomography in craniopharyngiomas.' *Radiology*, **127**, 687–691.

Fortuna, A., Celli, P., Palma, L. (1980) 'Oligodendrogliomas of the spinal cord.' *Acta Neurochirurgica*, **52**, 305–329.

Garrido, E., Becker, L.F., Hoffman, L.J., Hendrick, E.B., Humphreys, R. (1978) 'Gangliogliomas in children: a clinicopathological study.' *Child's Brain*, **4**, 339–46.

Gassel, M.M., Davies, H. (1961) 'Meningiomas in the lateral ventricles.' *Brain*, **84**, 605–607.

Gjerris, F. (1978) 'Clinical aspects and long-term prognosis in supratentorial tumors of infancy and childhood.' *Acta Neurologica Scandinavica*, **57**, 445–470.

—— Klinken, L. (1978) 'Long-term prognosis in children with benign cerebellar astrocytoma.' *Journal of Neurosurgery*, **49**, 179–184.

Gol, A., McKissock, W. (1959) 'The cerebellar astrocytomas: a report on 98 verified cases.' *Journal of Neurosurgery*, **16**, 287–296.

Greenberg, S.B., Schneck, M., Faerber, E.N., Kanev, P.M., de Chadarevian, J.P. (1993) 'Meningiosarcoma.' *American Journal of Roentgenology*, **160**, 1111–1112.

Gusnard, D.A. (1990) 'Cerebellar neoplasms in children.' *Seminars in Roentgenology*, **25**, 263–278.

Hall, J.G., Pallister, P.D., Clarrister, P.D., Clarren, S.K., Beckwith, J.B., Wiglesworth, F.W., Fraser, F.C., Cho, S., Benke, P.J., Reed, S.D. (1980) 'Congenital hypothalamic hamartoblastoma, hypopituitarism, imperforate anus and post-axial polydactyly—a new syndrome? Clinical, causal, and pathogenic considerations.' *American Journal of Medical Genetics*, **7**, 47–74.

Hammock, M.K., Milhorat, T.H. (1981) *Cranial Computed Tomography in Infancy and Childhood.* Baltimore: Williams & Wilkins.

Hart, M.N., Earle, K.M. (1973) 'Primitive neuroectodermal tumors of the brain in children.' *Cancer*, **32**, 890–896.

Harwood-Nash, D.C. (1991) 'Primary neoplasms of the central nervous system in children.' *Cancer*, **67**, 1223–1228.

—— Fitz, C.R. (1976) *Neuroradiology in Infants and Children.* St. Louis: C.V. Mosby.

Heideman, R.L., Packer, R.J., Albright, L.A., Freeman, C.R., Rorke, L.B. (1989) 'Tumors of the central nervous system.' *In:* Pizzo, P.A., Poplack, D.G. (Eds.) *Principles and Practice of Pediatric Oncology.* Philadelphia: J.B. Lippincott, pp. 505–553.

Henry, J.M., Heffner, R.R., Dillard, S.H., Earle, K.M., Davis, R.L. (1974) 'Primary malignant lymphomas of the central nervous system.' *Cancer*, **34**, 1293–1302.

Herz, D.A., Shapiro, K., Shulman, K. (1980) 'Intracranial meningiomas of infancy, childhood and adolescence.' *Child's Brain*, **7**, 43–56.

Hinshaw, P.B., Ashwal, S., Thompson, D.R., Hasso, A.N. (1983) 'Neuroradiology of primitive neuroectodermal tumors.' *Neuroradiology*, **25**, 87–92.

Hochberg, F.H., Miller, G., Schooley, R.T. (1983) 'Central nervous system lymphoma related to Epstein–Barr virus.' *New England Journal of Medicine*, **309**, 745–748.

Hoffman, H.J. (1983) 'Optic pathway gliomas.' *In:* Amador, L. (Ed.) *Brain Tumors in the Young.* Springfield, IL: Charles C. Thomas, pp. 622–633.

—— Yoshida, M., Becker, L.E., Hendrick, E.B., Humphreys, R.P. (1983) 'Pineal region tumors in childhood. Experiences at the Hospital for Sick Children.' *Concepts in Pediatric Neurosurgery*, **4**, 360–386.

Honda, E., Hayashi, T., Kuramoto, S. (1984) 'A case of choroid plexus papilloma in the lateral ventricle complicated by a neuroepithelial cyst in the posterior fossa in a new born infant.' *Kurume Medical Journal*, **31**, 115–124.

Hopper, K.D., Foley, L.C., Nieves, N.L., Smirniotopoulos, J.G. (1987) 'The interventricular extension of choroid plexus papillomas.' *American Journal of Neuroradiology*, **8**, 469–472.

Huh, K. (1964) 'A study of the incidence of calcification in a histological survey of surgical biopsies of meningiomas.' *Journal of Neurosurgery*, **21**, 751–757.

Hunter, I.J. (1955) 'Squamous metaplasia of cells of the anterior pituitary gland.' *Journal of Pathology and Bacteriology*, **69**, 141–145.

Ironside, J.W., Martin, J.F., Timperly, R.J. (1984) 'Lymphomatoid granulomatosis with cerebral involvement.' *Neuropathology and Applied Neurobiology*, **10**, 397–406.

193

Jellinger, J., Sunder-Plassmann, M. (1973) 'Connatal intracranial tumors.' *Neuropediatrics*, **4**, 46–53.

Jellinger, K., Radaszkiewcz, T., Slowik, F. (1975) 'Primary malignant lymphomas of the central nervous system in man.' *Acta Neuropathologica*, Suppl. 6, 95–102.

Jooma, R., Kendall, B.E. (1982) 'Intracranial tumors in the first year of life.' *Neuroradiology*, **23**, 267–274.

Kapila, A., Gupta, K.L., Garcia, J.H. (1988) 'CT and MR of lymphomatoid granulomatosis of the CNS: report of four cases and review of the literature.' *American Journal of Neuroradiology*, **9**, 1139–1143.

Katzenstein, A-Z., Carrington, C.B., Liebow, A.A. (1979) 'Lymphomatoid granulomatosis. A clinicopathologic study of 152 cases.' *Cancer*, **43**, 360–373.

Kendall, B., Reider-Grosswater, I., Valentine, A. (1983) 'Diagnosis of masses presenting within the ventricles on computed tomography.' *Neuroradiology*, **25**, 11–22.

Kerslake, R., Rowe, D., Worthington, B.S. (1991) 'CT and MR imaging of CNS lymphomatoid granulomatosis.' *Neuroradiology*, **33**, 269–271.

Kingsley, D.P.E., Harwood-Nash, D.C.F. (1984) 'Radiological features of neuroectodermal tumors of childhood.' *Neuroradiology*, **26**, 463–467.

Kilgore, D.P., Strother, C.M., Starshak, R.J., Haughton, V.M. (1986) 'Pineal germinoma: MR imaging.' *Radiology*, **158**, 435–438.

Koos, W.T., Miller, M.H. (1971) *Intracranial Tumors of Infants and Children.* St. Louis: C.V. Mosby.

Kosnik, E.J., Boesel, C.P., Bay, J., Sayers, M.P. (1978) 'Primitive neuroectodermal tumors of the central nervous system in children.' *Journal of Neurosurgery*, **48**, 741–746.

Kovacs, K., Horvath, E., Ryan, N., Ezrin, C. (1980) 'Null cell adenoma of the human pituitary.' *Virchows Archiv. A. Pathological Anatomy and Histopathology*, **387**, 165–174.

Kulkarni, M.V., Lee, K.F., McArdle, C.B., Yeakley, J.W., Haar, F.L. (1988) 'MR imaging of pituitary microadenomas: technical considerations and CT correlation.' *American Journal of Neuroradiology*, **9**, 5–11.

Kun, L.E., D'Souza, B., Tefft, M. (1985) 'The value of surveillance testing in childhood brain tumors.' *Cancer*, **56**, 1818–1823.

—— Kovner, E.H., Sanford, R.A. (1988) 'Ependymomas in children.' *Pediatric Neuroscience*, **14**, 57–63.

Laws, E.R., Scheithaver, B.W., Groover, R.V. (1987) 'Pituitary tumors in childhood and adolescence.' *Progress in Experimental Tumor Research*, **30**, 359–361.

Lee, S.R., Sanches, J., Mark, A.S., Dillon, W.P., Norman, D., Newton, T.H. (1989) 'Posterior fossa hemangioblastomas: MR imaging.' *Radiology*, **171**, 463–468.

Lee, Y., Lin, S., Horner, F.A. (1979) 'The third ventricle meningioma mimicking a colloid cyst in a child.' *American Journal of Roentgenology*, **132**, 669–671.

—— Van Tassel, P., Bruner, M., Moser, R.P., Share, J.C. (1989) 'Juvenile pilocystic astrocytomas: CT and MR characteristics.' *American Journal of Neuroradiology*, **10**, 363–370.

Lehrich, J.R., Hedley-Whyte, E.T. (1983) 'Malignant lymphoma, immunoblastic type, and acquired immunodeficiency syndrome. Case records of the Massachusetts General Hospital. Case 32, 1983.' *New England Journal of Medicine*, **309**, 359–369.

—— Richardson, E.P. (1978) 'Malignant lymphoma, histiocytic type, with Sjogren's syndrome. Case records of the Massachusetts General Hospital. Case 49, 1978.' *New England Journal of Medicine*, **299**, 1349–1359.

Lewis, A.J. (1988) 'Sarcoma metastatic to the brain.' *Cancer*, **61**, 593–601.

Liebow, A.A., Carrington, C.R.B., Friedman, P.J. (1972) 'Lymphomatoid granulomatosis.' *Human Pathology*, **3**, 457–558.

Lipsmeyer, E.A. (1972) 'Development of malignant cerebral lymphoma in a patient with systemic lupus erythematosus treated with immunosuppression.' *Arthritis and Rheumatism*, **15**, 183–186.

Liu, P.I., Ishimaru, T., McGregor, D.H., Ckada, H., Steer, A. (1973) 'Autopsy study of granulocytic sarcoma (chloroma) in patients with myelogenous leukemia. Hiroshima–Nagasaki 1949–1969.' *Cancer*, **31**, 948–955.

Lizak, P.F., Woodruff, W.W. (1992) 'Posterior fossa neoplasms: multiplanar imaging.' *Seminars in Ultrasound, CT and MRI*, **13**, 182–206.

Majd, M., Farkas, J., Lopresti, J.M., Chandra, R., Hung, W., Lussenhop, A.J. (1971) 'A large calcified craniopharyngioma in the newborn.' *Radiology*, **99**, 399–400.

Maroldo, T.V., Barkovich, A.J. (1992) 'Pediatric brain tumors.' *Seminars in Ultrasound, CT and MRI*, **13**, 412–448.

Matson, D.D. (1969) *Neurosurgery of Infancy and Childhood, 2nd Edn.* Springfield, IL: C.C. Thomas.

Matthews, P.D. (1983) 'Intraventricular craniopharyngioma.' *American Journal of Neuroradiology*, **4**, 984–985.

May, P.L., Blaser, S.I., Hoffman, H.J., Humphreys, R.P., Harwood-Nash, D.C. (1991) 'Benign intrinsic tectal "tumors" in children.' *Journal of Neurosurgery*, **74**, 867–871.

McKeran, R.O., Thomas, D.G.T. (1980) 'The clinical study of gliomas.' *In:* Thomas, D.G.T., Graham, D.I. (Eds.) *Brain Tumors: Scientific Basis, Clinical Investigation and Current Therapy.* London: Butterworths, pp. 194–230.

Medline, N.M., Kay, R.W., Robertson, D.M. (1968) 'Intraventricular meningioma; discussion of malignant features.' *Archives of Pathology*, **35**, 562–566.

Merten, D.F., Gooding, C.A., Newton, T.H., Malamud, N. (1974) 'Meningiomas of childhood and adolescence.' *Journal of Pediatrics*, **84**, 696–700.

Meyers, S.P., Kemp, S.S., Tarr, R.W. (1992) 'MR imaging features of medulloblastomas.' *American Journal of Roentgenology*, **158**, 859–865.

Moore, E.W., Thomas, L.B., Shaw, R.K., Freireich, E.J. (1960) 'The central nervous system in acute leukemia.' *Archives of Internal Medicine*, **105**, 451–468.

Mueller, B.A., Gurney, J.A. (1992) 'Epidemiology of pediatric brain tumors.' *Neurosurgery Clinics of North America*, **3**, 715–721.

Myers, J.L. (1990) 'Lymphomatoid granulomatosis: past, present, future?' *Mayo Clinic Proceedings*, **65**, 274–278.

Naidich, T.P. (1990) 'Imaging evaluation of meningiomas. Categorical course. Neoplasms of the central nervous system.' *Paper presented at the 25th Annual Meeting of the American Society of Neuroradiology, Los Angeles, March 17–18, 1990.*

—— Zimmerman, R.A. (1984) 'Primary brain tumors in children.' *Seminars in Roentgenology*, **19**, 100–114.

Nelson, M., Diebler, C., Forbes, W. (1991) 'Pediatric medulloblastoma: atypical CT features at presentation in the SIOP II trial.' *Neuroradiology*, **33**, 140–142.

Nevin, S. (1938) 'Gliomatosis cerebri.' *Brain*, **6**, 170–191.

Packer, R.J., Nicholson, H.S., Vezina, L.G., Johnson, D.L. (1992) 'Brainstem gliomas.' *Neurosurgery Clinics of North America*, **3**, 863–879.

Panitch, H.S., Berg, B.O. (1970) 'Brainstem tumors of childhood and adolescence.' *American Journal of Diseases of Children*, **119**, 465–472.

Parker, J., Mortara, R., McCloskey, J. (1975) 'Biological behavior of primitive neuroectodermal tumors. Significant supratentorial childhood gliomas.' *Surgical Neurology*, **4**, 383–388.

Pascual-Castroviejo, I., Villarejo, F., Perez-Higueras, A., Morales, C., Pascual-Pascual, S.T. (1983) 'Childhood chronic plexus neoplasms: a study of 14 cases less than 2 years old.' *European Journal of Pediatrics*, **140**, 51–56.

Pedersen, H., McConnell, J., Harwood–Nash, D.C., Fitz, C.R., Chuang, S.H. (1989) 'Computed tomography in intracranial supratentorial metastases in children.' *Neuroradiology*, **21**, 19–23.

Pena, C.E. (1977) 'Lymphomatoid granulomatosis with cerebral involvement.' *Acta Neuropathologica*, **37**, 193–197.

Pfleger, M.J., Gerson, L.P. (1993) 'Supratentorial tumors in children.' *Neuroimaging Clinics of North America*, **3**, 671–687.

Pinto, R.S., Kricheff, I.I. (1984) 'Neuroradiology of intracranial neuromas.' *Seminars in Roentgenology*, **19**, 44–52.

Pojunas, K.W., Daniels, D.L., Williams, A.L. (1986) 'MR imaging of prolactin-secreting microadenomas.' *American Journal of Neuroradiology*, **7**, 209–213.

Raaf, J., Kernohan, J.W. (1944) 'Relation of abnormal collections of cells in posterior medullary velum of the cerebellum to origin of medulloblastoma.' *Archives of Neurology and Psychiatry*, **52**, 163–169.

Radkowski, M.A., Naidich, T.P., Tomita, T., Byrd, S.E., McLone, D.G. (1988) 'Neonatal brain tumors: CT and MR findings.' *Journal of Computer Assisted Tomography*, **12**, 10–20.

Raimondi, A.J., Gutierrez, F.A. (1975) 'Diagnosis and surgical treatment of choroid plexus papillomas.' *Child's Brain*, **1**, 81–115.

Richmond, I.L., Wilson, C.B. (1978) 'Pituitary adenomas in childhood and adolescence.' *Journal of Neuro-surgery*, **49**, 163–168.

Ringertz, N., Nordenstam, H. (1951) 'Cerebellar astrocytoma.' *Journal of Neuropathology and Experimental Neurology*, **10**, 343–367.

Robles, H.A., Smirniotopoulos, J.G., Bryan, R.N. (1991) 'Intracranial primitive neuroectodermal tumors: a radiologic–pathologic correlation of supratentorial and infratentorial PNETs.' *Paper presented at the 29th Annual Meeting of the American Society of Neuroradiology, Washington, DC, 1991.*

—— —— Figueroa, R.E. (1992) 'Understanding the radiology of intracranial primitive neuroectodermal

195

tumors from a pathological perspective: a review.' *Seminars in Ultrasound, CT and MRI*, **13**, 170–181.

Rollins, N., Mendelsohn, D., Mulne, A., Barton, R., Diehl, J., Reyes, N., Sklar, F. (1990) 'Recurrent medullo-blastoma: frequency of tumor enhancement on Gd–DTPA MR imaging.' *American Journal of Neuroradiology*, **11**, 583–587.

Rorke, L.B. (1983) 'The cerebellar neuroblastoma and its relationship to primitive neuroectodermal tumors.' *Journal of Neuropathology and Experimental Neurology*, **42**, 1–15.

—— Gilles, F.H., Davis, R.L., Becker, L.E. (1985) 'Revision of the World Health Organization classification of brain tumors for childhood brain tumors.' *Cancer*, **56**, 1869–1886.

Rovit, R.L., Schecter, M.M., Chodroff, P. (1970) 'Choroid plexus papillomas: observations on radiographic diagnosis.' *American Journal of Roentgenology*, **110**, 608–617.

Rubinstein, L.J. (1975) 'The cerebellar medulloblastoma: its origin, differentiation, morphological variants, and clinical behavior'. *In:* Vincken, P.J., Bruyn, G.W. (Eds.) *Tumors of the Brain and Skull. Part III.* New York, Elsevier, pp 167–194.

Russell, D.S. (1950) 'Meningeal tumors: a review.' *Journal of Clinical Pathology*, **3**, 191–211.

—— Rubinstein, L.J. (1989) *Pathology of Tumors of the Nervous System. 5th Edn.* Baltimore: Williams & Wilkins.

Russell, E.J., Geremia, G.K., Johnson, C.E., Huckman, M.S., Ramsey, R.G., Washburn-Bleck, J., Turner, D.A., Norusis, M. (1987) 'Multiple cerebral metastases: detectability with Gd-DTPA-enhanced MR imaging.' *Radiology*, **165**, 609–617.

Rutka, J.T., Hoffman, H.J., Drake, J.M., Humphreys, R.P. (1992) 'Suprasellar and sellar tumors in childhood and adolescence.' *Neurosurgery Clinics of North America*, **3**, 803–820.

Sackett, J.F., Zurhein, G.M., Bhimani, S.M. (1979) 'Lymphomatoid granulomatosis involving the central nervous system: radiologic–pathologic correlation.' *American Journal of Roentgenology*, **132**, 823–826.

Sato, O., Tamura, A., Saro, K. (1975) 'Brain tumors of early infants.' *Child's Brain*, **1**, 121–125.

Schaerer, J.P., Woolsey, R.D. (1960) 'Intraventricular meningiomas of the fourth ventricle.' *Journal of Neurosurgery*, **17**, 337–341.

Schmidt, B.J., Meagher-Villemure, K., Carpio, J.D. (1984) 'Lymphomatoid granulomatosis with isolated involvement of the brain.' *Annals of Neurology*, **15**, 478–481.

Schneck, S.A., Penn, I. (1971) 'De-novo brain tumors in renal transplant recipients.' *Lancet*, **1**, 983–986.

Schwaighofer, B.W., Hesselink, J.R., Press, G.A., Wolf, R.L., Healy, M.E., Berhoty, D.P. (1989) 'Primary intracranial CNS lymphoma: MR manifestations.' *American Journal of Neuroradiology*, **10**, 725–729.

Simon, J., Szumowski, J., Totterman, S. (1988) 'Fat suppression MR imaging of the orbit.' *American Journal of Neuroradiology*, **9**, 961–968.

Smith, R.R. (1990) 'Brainstem tumors.' *Seminars in Roentgenology*, **25**, 249–262.

—— Zimmerman, R.A., Packer, R.J., Bilaniuk, L.T., Hackney, D.B., Goldberg, H.I., Grossman, R.I. (1987) 'Pediatric brainstem gliomas: comparison of evaluation by CT and MRI.' *American Journal of Neuroradiology*, **8**, 954. *(Abstract.)*

Snider, W.D., Simpson, W.D., Aronyk, K.E., Nielsen, S.L. (1983) 'Primary lymphoma of the nervous system associated with acquired immunodeficiency syndrome.' *New England Journal of Medicine*, **308**, 45. *(Letter.)*

Spoto, G.P., Press, G.A., Hesselink, J.R., Solomon, M. (1990) 'Intracranial ependymoma and subependymoma: MR manifestations.' *American Journal of Neuroradiology*, **11**, 83–97.

Steinberg, G.K., Shuer, L.M., Conley, .FK., Hanbery, J.W. (1985) 'Evolution and outcome in malignant astro-glial neoplasms of the cerebellum.' *Journal of Neurosurgery*, **62**, 9–17.

Sutton, L.N., Packer, R.J., Rorke, L.B., Bruce, D.A., Schut, L. (1983) 'Cerebral gangliogliomas during child-hood.' *Neurosurgery*, **13**, 124–128.

Takaku, A., Kodama, N., Ohaɪa, N., Hori, S. (1978) 'Brain tumor in newborn babies.' *Child's Nervous System*, **38**, 365–375.

Takeuchi, J., Handa, H., Nagata, I. (1978) 'Suprasellar germinoma.' *Journal of Neurosurgery*, **49**, 41–48.

Tenny, R.T., Laws, E.R., Younge, B.R. Rush, J.A. (1982) 'The neurosurgical management of optic glioma. Results in 104 patients.' *Journal of Neurosurgery*, **57**, 452–458.

Tice, H., Barnes, P.D., Goumnerova, L., Scott, R.M., Tarbell, N.J. (1993) 'Pediatric and adolescent oligo-dendrogliomas.' *American Journal of Neuroradiology*, **14**, 1293–1300.

Tien, R., Barkovich, A.J., Edwards, M.S.B. (1990) 'MR imaging of pineal tumours.' *American Journal of Neuroradiology*, **11**, 557–565.

Tomita, T., McLone, D. (1985) 'Brain tumors during the first 24 months of life.' *Neurosurgery*, **17**, 913–919.

—— —— Flannery, A.M. (1988) 'Choroid plexus papillomas of neonates, infants and children.' *Pediatric Neuroscience*, **14**, 23–30.

Van Eys, J. (1984) 'Malignant tumors of the central nervous system.' *In:* Sutow, W.W., Fernback, D.J., Vietti, T.J. (Eds.) *Clinical Pediatric Oncology. 3rd Edn.* St. Louis: C.V. Mosby, pp. 516–538.

Verity, M.A., Wolfson, W.L. (1976) 'Cerebral lymphomatoid granulomatosis. A report of two cases, with disseminated necrotizing leukoencephalography in one.' *Acta Neuropathologica*, **36**, 117–124.

Vion-Drury, J., Vincentelli, F., Jiddane, M. (1987) 'MR imaging of epidermoid cysts.' *Neuroradiology*, **29**, 333–338.

Wacker, M.R., Cogen, P.H., Etzell, J.E., Daneshvar, L., Davis, R.L., Prados, M.D. (1992) 'Diffuse leptomeningeal involvement by a ganglioglioma in a child. Case report.' *Journal of Neurosurgery*, **77**, 302–306.

Yanaka, K., Kamezaki, T., Kobayashi, E., Matsueda, K., Yoshii, Y., Nose, T. (1992) 'MR imaging of diffuse glioma.' *American Journal of Neuroradiology*, **13**, 349–351.

Zee, C.S., Segall, H.D., Ahmadi, J., Becker, T.S., McComb, J.G., Miller, J.H. (1983) 'Computed tomography of posterior fossa ependymomas in childhood.' *Surgical Neurology*, **20**, 221–226.

—— —— Nelson, M., Destian, S., Ahmadi, J. (1993) 'Infratentorial tumors in children.' *Neuroimaging Clinics of North America*, **3**, 705–713.

Zimmerman, R.A. (1990a) 'Imaging of intrasellar, suprasellar and parasellar tumors.' *Seminars in Roentgenology*, **25**, 174–197.

—— (1990b) 'Pediatric supratentorial tumors.' *Seminars in Roentgenology*, **25**, 225–248.

—— (1990c) 'Central nervous system lymphoma.' *Radiologic Clinics of North America*, **28**, 697–721.

—— Bilaniuk, L.T., Pahlajani, H. (1978) 'Spectrum of medulloblastomas demonstrated by computed tomography.' *Radiology*, **126**, 137–141.

—— Fleming, C.A., Saint-Louis, L.A., Lee, B.C.P., Manning, J.J., Deck, M.D.F. (1985) 'Magnetic resonance imaging of meningiomas.' *American Journal of Neuroradiology*, **6**, 149–157.

Zulch, K.J. (1979) *Histological Typing of Tumours of the Central Nervous System.* Geneva: World Health Organization.

Zuniga, O.F., Tanner, S.M., Wild, W.O., Mosier, H.D. (1983) 'Hamartoma of CNS associated with precocious puberty.' *American Journal of Diseases of Children*, **137**, 127–133.

9
METABOLIC AND DEGENERATIVE DISORDERS

Benjamin C.P. Lee

The white matter is involved in many metabolic and degenerative disorders. The role of MRI is to demonstrate rather than to diagnose white matter abnormalities (Golden 1987). Although a specific diagnosis is seldom made on MRI appearances alone, a basic knowledge of the clinical, pathological and biochemical nature of these disorders is helpful in understanding these changes (Young *et al.* 1985, Nowell *et al.* 1989, Swaiman 1989*a*). The pertinent MR appearances of the commoner types of white matter disorders will be presented.

MRI features of gray/white matter disorders
MR techniques
Spin echo techniques with short and long TR and TE are routinely used as T_1- and T_2-weighted images. When more heavy T_1 weighting is desired an inversion recovery sequence is added to the spin echo T_1 sequence. The myelin of the white matter in children over 9 months of age is easily detected on T_2-weighted images, and the increased signal of abnormalities is apparent. Although T_1-weighted images may help determine the presence or absence of myelin there is no good method of detecting white matter abnormalities in infants up to this age. The higher water content of unmyelinated fibers in younger infants imparts an increased signal in T_2-weighted images and renders this technique ineffective for detecting white matter abnormalities (Holland *et al.* 1986, Barkovich *et al.* 1988, Dietrich *et al.* 1988, Valk and van der Knaap 1989). Contrast enhancement is seen in the acute stages of primary white matter disorders and is probably nonspecific, as it is also observed in other diseases such as infarcts and brain necrosis.

Metabolic disorders may affect any region of the brain but abnormal signals are more readily seen in the white matter. The gray matter may be involved, although changes in these regions may not be readily apparent on MRI. White matter lesions are seen as areas of increased signal on T_2-weighted images. Although the same lesions may occasionally be detected on T_1-weighted images this technique is much less sensitive (Fig. 9.1). The following features are important in evaluation of white matter disorders: (a) location of the white matter abnormalities (whether these are generalized or localized); (b) basal ganglia involvement; (c) cortical gray matter involvement; (d) macrocephaly (without hydrocephalus); (e) presence of decreased signal; (f) hydrocephalus; and (g) contrast enhancement (Tables 9.1, 9.2) (Figs. 9.2–9.5). Secondary changes such as abnormal signal of the pyramidal tracts, hypoplastic corpus callosum, increased perineural spaces,

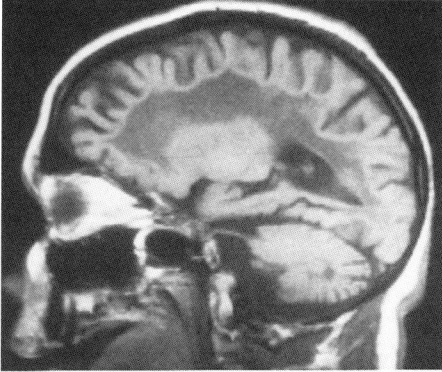

Fig. 9.1. Metachromatic leukodystrophy. T_1-weighted image shows decreased signal diffusely in the white matter.

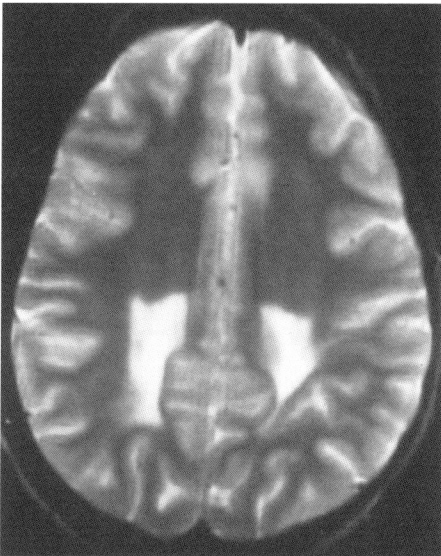

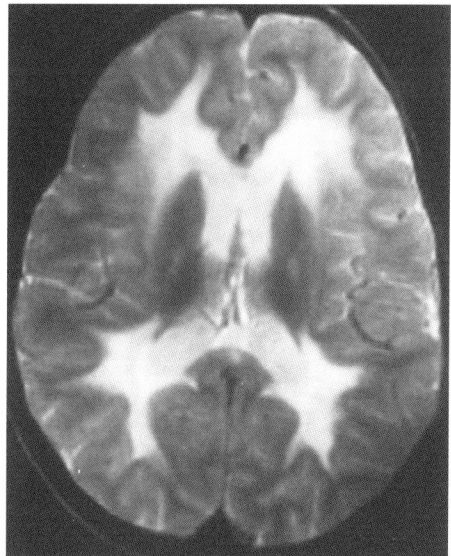

Fig. 9.2. Metachromatic leukodystrophy. T_2-weighted image shows increased signal posteriorly (Krabbe disease) *(left)*, and throughout the white matter *(right)*.

cortical atrophy and ventricular dilatation signify the severity of the neurological damage and should also be noted (Figs. 9.6–9.9).

White matter disorders

The white matter is affected in disorders of (a) peroxisomes, (b) lysosomes, (c) mitochondria, and (d) amino acid and carbohydrate metabolism (Stam 1970, Valk and van der Knaap 1989, Wolpert *et al*. 1992) (Table 9.3). In other cases the mechanism of the white matter appearances is unclear. Although many of these disorders affect the CNS, only the more common ones will be considered here. Primary white matter diseases are generally

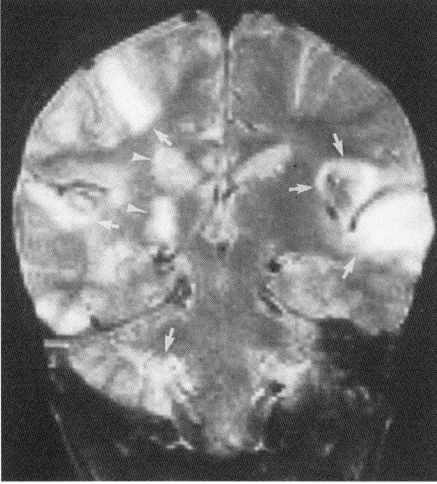

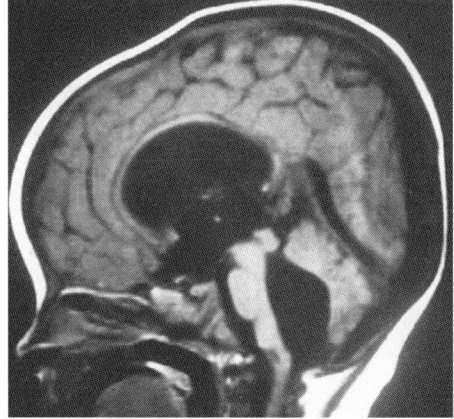

Fig. 9.4. Hurler's disease. T_1-weighted image shows hydrocephalus involving the lateral, third and fourth ventricles.

Fig. 9.3. MELAS syndrome. T_2-weighted image shows increased signal involving the white and gray matter *(arrows)* and the basal ganglia *(arrowheads)*.

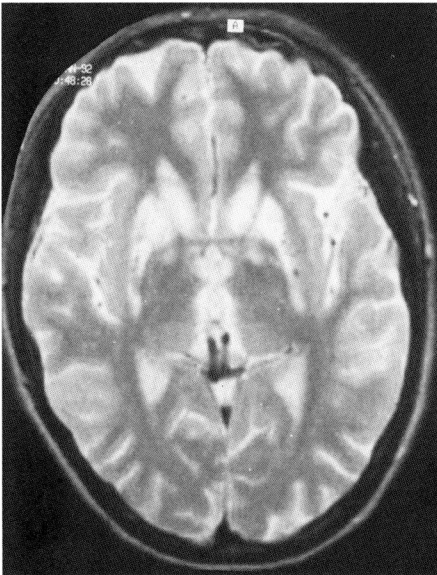

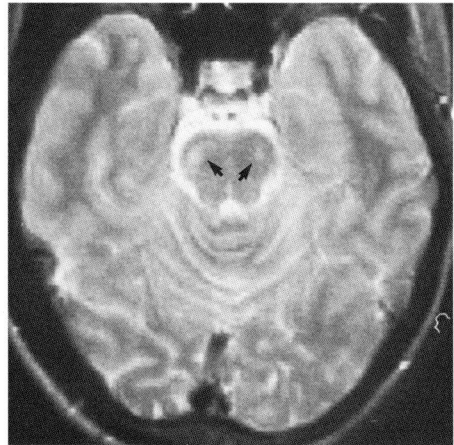

Fig. 9.6. Krabbe's disease. T_2-weighted image shows increased signal in the pyramidal tracts *(arrows)*.

Fig. 9.5. Leigh's disease. T_2-weighted image shows increased signal in the putamen, head of caudate and a portion of the globus pallidus.

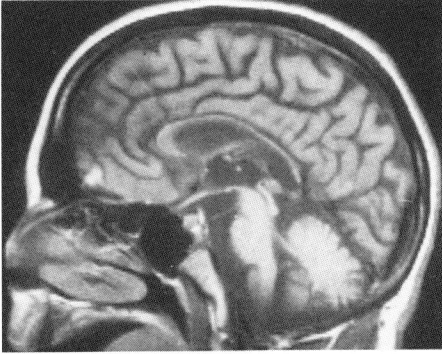

Fig. 9.7. Metachromatic leukodystrophy. T$_1$-weighted image shows atrophic corpus callosum.

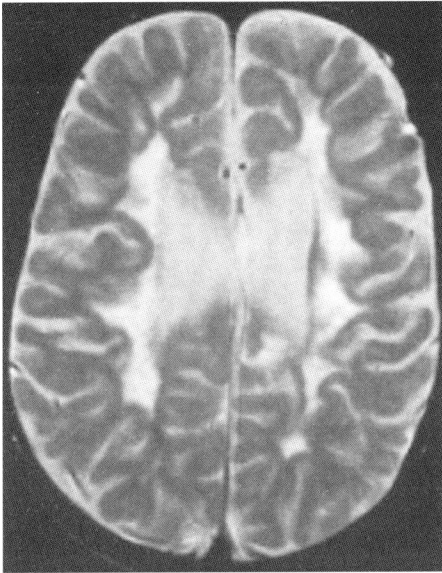

Fig. 9.8. Neonatal adrenoleukodystrophy. T$_2$-weighted image shows cortical atrophy and diffuse white matter disease.

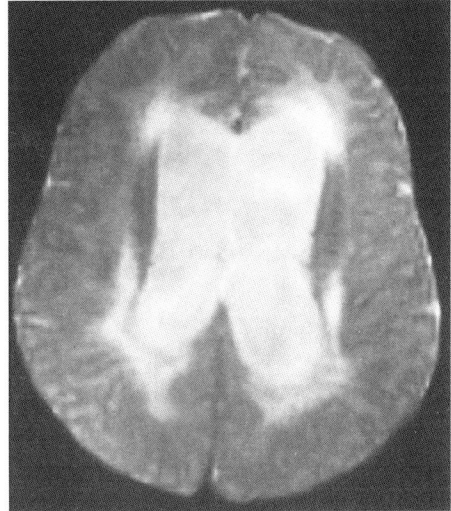

Fig. 9.9. Krabbe's disease. T$_2$-weighted image shows ventricular dilatation and diffuse white matter disease.

dysmyelinating, with defective formation or maintenance of myelin. Additional demyelination of formed myelin occurs concurrently in many instances (Poser 1961, 1987). Clinically, the common denominators of all white matter disorders are psychomotor retardation, spasticity and focal neurological defects which depend on the location affected. Seizures may occur in primary white matter disorders but are more commonly the presenting feature of gray matter abnormalities (Swick 1989). The sex, age of onset and clinical course are important factors which should be considered in the diagnosis of specific disorders.

TABLE 9.1
MRI features of metabolic and neurodegenerative disorders

A. Location of lesion: generalized or focal
B. Evidence of hypomyelination
C. Cavitation changes
D. Basal ganglia involvement
E. Cortical gray matter involvement
F. Cerebellar involvement
G. Macrocephaly
H. Configuration of the cranium
I. Hydrocephalus
J. Regions of decreased signal: blood or calcium
K. Contrast enhancement
L. Secondary changes
  • Abnormal signal of internal capsule pyramidal tracts
  • Atrophy of cerebral peduncles
  • Hypoplastic corpus callosum
  • Cortical atrophy
  • Ventricular dilatation
  • Increased perineuronal spaces in the white matter

TABLE 9.2
Disorders with specific MRI features

Macrocephaly: Krabbe's disease, Hurler's disease, Alexander's
    disease, Canavan's disease

Location of white matter changes:
    Posterior: X-linked adrenoleukodystrophy
    Anterior: Alexander's disease

Basal ganglia involvement: Leigh's disease, Kearn–Sayre
    syndrome, glutaric acidemia I, methylmalonic acidemia,
    Fabry's disease, Cockayne's disease

'Infarcts' ± white matter involvement: MELAS, MERFF,
    Leighs's disease, homocystinuria, Fabry's disease

Peroxisomal disorders
Peroxisomes are cell organelles responsible for peroxidation and metabolism of long chain
fatty acids. Disorders may involve single or multiple enzymes. Adrenoleukodystrophy is
associated with accumulation of very long chain and other fatty acids (Moser 1986,
Schutgens *et al.* 1986, Fishman 1989).

  X-linked adrenoleukodystrophy presents in boys usually between the ages of 4 and 8
years. Visual problems occur early and precede adrenocortical hormone deficiency
(Swaiman 1989*c*). Very long chain fatty acids are found in the blood and skin fibroblasts.
The MRI appearances are characterized by predominant and early involvement of the

TABLE 9.3
Common causes of white matter disease

A. PEROXISOMAL DISORDERS
 X-linked adrenoleukodystrophy
 Neonatal adrenoleukodystrophy
 Zellweger syndrome

B. LYSOSOMAL DISORDERS
 Lipidosis
 • Krabbe's disease (globoid cell leukodystrophy)
 • Metachromatic leukodystrophy
 • Fabry's disease
 • Tay–Sachs disease
 • Niemann–Pick disease
 • Gaucher's disease
 Mucopolysaccharidosis
 • Type I Hurler's disease
 • Type II Hunter's disease
 • Type III Sanfilippo's disease
 • Type IV Morquio's disease
 • Type VI Maroteaux–Lamy disease

C. MITOCHONDRIAL DISORDERS
 Leigh's disease (subacute necrotizing leukoencephalopathy)
 Kearns–Sayre syndrome
 MELAS syndrome (mitochondrial myopathy, encephalopathy, lactic
  acidosis, strokes)
 MERRF syndrome (myclonic epilepsy with ragged red fibers)

D. AMINOACIDOPATHIES/AMINOACIDURIAS
 Aminoacidopathies—phenylketonuria
 (Enzyme defect)
 • Tyrosinemia
 • Maple syrup urine disease
 • Homocystinuria
 • Methylmalonic acidemia
 • Glutaric acidemia type I
 Aminoaciduria—Lowe (oculocerebrorenal) syndrome
 (Transport defect)

E. PRIMARY WHITE MATTER DISORDERS
 Alexander's disease
 Canavan's disease
 Perlizaeus–Merzbacher disease
 Cockayne's disease

F. DIFFERENTIAL DIAGNOSIS
 Hypoxia–ischemia—periventricular leukomalacia
 ADEM (acute disseminated encephalomyelopathy)
 Demyelination
 PML
 Infection—AIDS
 Therapy
 • Radiation
 • Methotrexate

occipital lobes and visual pathway (Schaumberg *et al.* 1975, Young *et al.* 1983, Bewe-meyer *et al.* 1985, Cherryman and Smith 1985, Nishio *et al.* 1985, Huckman *et al.* 1986, Kumar *et al.* 1987, Volkow *et al.* 1987, van der Knaap and Valk 1989*b*). These changes eventually become generalized throughout the hemispheres. A variant of this disease involves the spinal cord and peripheral nerves (adrenomyeloneuropathy) (Griffin *et al.* 1977, Fishman 1989).

Neonatal adrenoleukodystrophy, which presents at birth, is quite distinct from X-linked adrenoleukodystrophy and is caused by defects in multiple enzymes (Goldfischer *et al.* 1985, Kelly *et al.* 1986). The MRI abnormalities are distributed throughout the white matter, with no predilection for the occipital lobes (van der Knaap and Volk 1991) (see Fig. 9.8).

Lysosomal disorders
Myelin is made up of large quantities of lipids and some lipoproteins. The former consist of cholesterol, glyco- and phospholipids synthesized from substrate material by enzymatic activity (Svennerholm 1964, Norton 1981). Lysosomal defects involving specific enzymes result in accumulation of phospho-/glycolipids, mucopolysaccharide and glycoprotein derivatives, and profoundly affect myelination (Scriver 1989, Swaiman 1989*c*). Cholesterol, which is not involved in these processes, and glycoprotein defects which rarely affect the white matter will not be considered in this discussion.

Lipidosis is the generic term for accumulation of various phospho- and glycolipids. The complex metabolism involves degradation of cerebroside, ganglioside, sulfatide and sphingomyelin into fatty acids and sphingosine. Deficiency of the appropriate enzymes results in accumulation of these substances (Swaiman 1989*c*) (Fig. 9.10). Cerebral involvement occurs with sulfatides, cerebrosides and some of the gangliosides, and is less common with sphingomyelin disorders.

Krabbe's disease (globoid cell leukodystrophy) is an autosomal recessive disorder due to a deficiency of the enzyme galactocerebroside β-galactosidase which results in accumulation of galactocerebroside. Characteristic globoid cells are present in the white matter, and there is much associated lack of myelin and severe gliosis. Macrocephaly is common. The disease, which is manifest by 3 to 6 months, is rapidly progressive, and most patients are dead by the second year. A late onset form which presents in adolescence is less common (Suzuki and Suzuki 1970, Swaiman 1989*c*).

On MRI the periventricular distribution of the white matter changes are nonspecific (Baram *et al.* 1986). The infantile form, which is rapidly progressive, results in severe dilatation of the lateral and third ventricles early in the course of the disease. These end-stage appearances, together with clinical macrocephaly, resemble hydrocephalus (Laxdal and Hallgrimsson 1974) (see Fig. 9.9). It has been postulated that the excessive amounts of galactocerebroside produce a cytoxic metabolic psychosine which inhibits myelination and is responsible also for demyelination (Igisu and Suzuki 1984). The late-onset disease has a milder and less progressive course and may show increased signal only in the posterior portions of the hemispheres (see Fig. 9.2*a*) (Kurokawa *et al.* 1987).

Metachromatic leukodystrophy is an autosomal recessive disorder due to deficiency

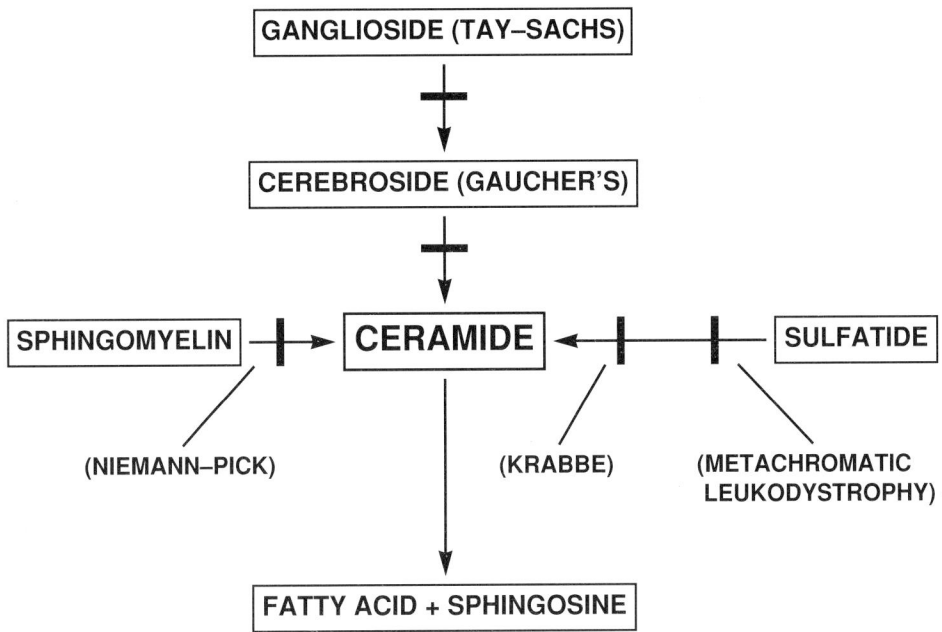

Fig. 9.10. Lipidosis (sphingosine) metabolic pathway.

of arylsulfatase A (cerebroside sulfatase A) which results in accumulation of sulfatides. The deficiency is systemic and affects other organs in addition to the nervous system. Onset of symptoms is early in the infantile form, but is later with the juvenile and adult forms (Suzuki 1984, Swaiman 1989c).

MRI appearances of the severe end-stage disease are indistinguishable from other forms of white matter disorders. The degree of ventricular enlargement is in general less than that in Krabbe's disease, reflecting a less unremitting course. MRI of the later-onset form shows no particular predisposition to any part of the cerebral hemispheres (Reider-Grosswasser and Bornstein 1987, Waltz et al. 1987). A striking feature is the increased T_2 signal in the cerebellar hemispheres seen in many cases (Nowell et al. 1988) (Fig. 9.11).

Fabry's disease (angiokeratoma corporis diffusum) is a rare disorder due to deficiency of the enzyme α-galactosidase A which results in accumulation of glycosphingolipids. The diagnosis is usually made by the presence of characteristic cutaneous and corneal lesions. Neurological lesions thought to be the result of thromboses of small cerebral vessels may be seen on MRI (Maisey and Cosh 1980, Moumdjian et al. 1989, Swaiman 1989c). Basal ganglia infarcts occur when these vessels are involved (Fig. 9.12).

Tay–Sachs disease is an uncommon disorder occurring in Ashkenazi Jews due to

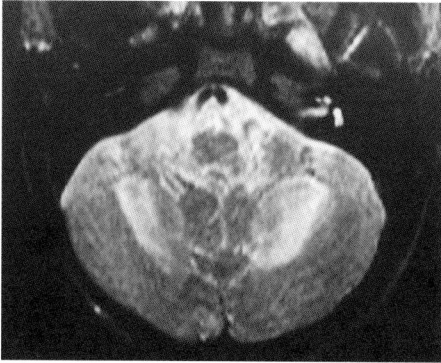

Fig. 9.11. Metachromatic leukodystrophy. T$_2$-weighted image shows increased signal in the cerebellar hemispheres.

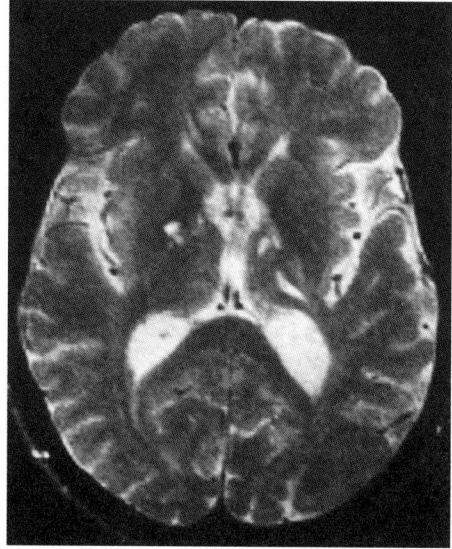

Fig. 9.12. Fabry's disease. T$_2$-weighted image shows multiple small regions of increased signal in the basal ganglia and internal capsules due to infarcts.

deficiency in the enzymes responsible for the breakdown of gangliosides (Crocker 1961, Swaiman 1989c). Nonspecific increased white matter signal has been described in this and other rare gangliosidoses (Wolpert *et al.* 1992).

Niemann–Pick disease is due to deficiency of the enzyme sphingomyelinase which results in accumulation of sphingomyelin. The disorder is systemic, and clinical diagnosis is usually obvious; occasionally cerebral involvement results in intellectual and motor deterioration (Swaiman 1989c).

Gaucher's disease is due to deficiency of the enzyme glucocerebrosidase which results in accumulation of cerebroside. Since the amount of glucocerebroside in the brain is very small, neurologic involvement is less common and severe than systemic manifestations (Swaiman 1989c).

Mucopolysaccharidoses are caused by deficiency of enzymes involved in degradation of heparan, dermatan or keratan sulfate (Lindsay *et al.* 1948, McKusick and Neufeld 1983). Six major types of abnormalities involving the skeletomuscular and nervous systems have been identified. The neurological deficits are most pronounced in type I (Hurler's), where there is excessive deposition of sulfates in the CNS; the defect is less severe in types II (Hunter), III (Sanfilippo) and VI (Maroteaux–Lamy), and least, if at all, in the type IV (Morquio) syndrome (Henderson 1952, Dekaban and Constantopoulos 1977, Swaiman 1989c). In general, the clinical status of the neurological impairment is somewhat related to the severity of the MRI abnormalities.

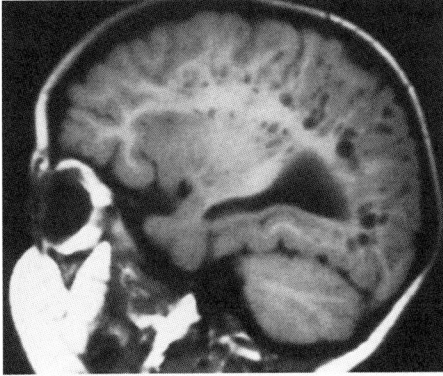

Fig. 9.13. Hurler's disease. T_1-weighted image shows multiple lacunae-like lesions in the white matter.

MRI appearances range from subtle loss of gray/white matter distinction, to markedly increased T_2 signal associated with extreme dilatation of the ventricles (Johnson *et al.* 1984, Eggli and Dorst 1986). Multiple lacunar defects throughout the white matter, visible on T_1- and sometimes on T_2-weighted images are dilated perineuronal spaces filled with mucopolysaccharide 'gargoyle' cells (Henderson *et al.* 1952, Norman *et al.* 1959, Murata *et al.* 1989, Rauch *et al.* 1989) (Fig. 9.13). Although these lesions are common in Hurler's mucopolysaccharidosis, they cannot be differentiated from nonspecific dilatation of the perineuronal spaces which occurs when the brain is severely affected by other types of white matter disorder.

Communicating hydrocephalus occurs in Hurler's syndrome and mucopolysaccharidoses which affect the brain, and is due to blockage of cerebrospinal fluid (CSF) absorption at the sagittal sinus (Shinnar *et al.* 1982) (see Fig. 9.4). It is often impossible to determine whether this or severe atrophy is responsible for the extreme ventricular dilatation seen. Since periventricular CSF absorption occurs with hydrocephalus, it may be impossible to differentiate the abnormal signal of such periventricular fluid from the increased signal of demyelination.

Amino-acidurias
These autosomal recessive enzymatic defects involve the pathways of amino acid metabolism. A specific enzyme deficiency is recognized in most cases but the mechanism of cerebral involvement is unclear (Moser 1977, Swaiman 1989*b*). The MRI changes reported in a number of these disorders are nonspecific and may involve the basal ganglia (Berman 1969, Uziel *et al.* 1988, Brismar *et al.* 1990*a*). It is important to document the abnormalities, as some of these lesions improve with the appropriate replacement therapies.

Phenylketonuria and maple syrup urine disease are the two relatively common disorders with significant cerebral involvement. Defects resulting in accumulation of intermediate amino acids in the urea cycle and other metabolic pathways are uncommon and will not be discussed.

Phenylketonuria is due to defective phenylalanine hydroxylase required for conversion of phenylalanine to tyrosine. Routine screening of blood reveals an incidence of 1/14,000 (Berman 1969). Diagnosis is important as there is often dramatic improvement with dietary therapy. Tyrosinemia is due to a defect of tyrosine breakdown caused by tyrosine hydrolase deficiency (Swaiman 1989b).

Maple syrup urine disease is due to failure to catabolize branch-chained amino acids (valine, leucine and isoleucine) and has an incidence of 1/200,000. In addition to white matter changes, basal ganglia involvement has been reported (Menkes and Solcher 1967, Uziel *et al.* 1988).

Mitochondrial disorders

The mitochondria is involved in the oxidative respiratory cycle. The specific defect responsible for the disorders is unclear, and several enzymes are often involved. These disorders affect cerebral parenchymal and smooth muscle metabolism, and may give rise to lactic acidosis or increased pyruvate levels (Shapira *et al.* 1977, Petty *et al.* 1986). From the radiological point of view these disorders involve the basal ganglia, portions of the brainstem and cortical gray matter, presumably because of their high metabolic activity. The white matter, being metabolically less active, is not involved, unless there has been significant ischemia and infarcts.

MELAS syndrome (mitochondrial *m*yopathy, *e*ncephalopathy, *l*actic *a*cidosis, *s*trokes) is characterized by recurrent strokes and lactic acidosis. The strokes are probably secondary to involvement of the smooth muscles of the peripheral cerebral arteries (Pavlakis *et al.* 1984, Morita *et al.* 1989, Swick 1989). The MRI findings reflect infarcts involving the cortex and the adjacent white matter (Allard *et al.* 1988, Rosen *et al.* 1990) (see Fig. 9.3). A closely related order, *MERRF syndrome* (*m*yoclonic *e*pilepsy with *r*agged *r*ed *f*ibers), also affects cortical gray matter.

Leigh's disease (subacute necrotizing encephalopathy) is an X-linked autosomal defect in pyruvate metabolism, involving deficiencies in pyruvate dehydrogenase and related enzymes (David *et al.* 1976, Robinson *et al.* 1987, van Erven *et al.* 1987, Swaiman 1989b). Increased signal is seen on T_2-weighted images typically in the putamen, caudate and tegmentum, although other portions of the basal ganglia and brainstem as well the white matter may also be involved (Koch *et al.* 1986, Davis *et al.* 1987, Geyer *et al.* 1988, Medina *et al.* 1990) (see Fig. 9.5). The locations and pathological changes are similar to Wernicke's encephalopathy except that the mammillary bodies are spared. Kearns–Sayre syndrome is an autosomal dominant defect with elevated serum pyruvate with pathological changes similar to Leigh's disease (Demange *et al.* 1989).

Disorders of unknown cause

These disorders do not cause any specific biochemical alterations and are diagnosed by the clinical features, and by specific pathological appearances on brain biopsy. The most common disorders are Alexander, Canavan, Cockayne and Perlizaeus–Merzbacher diseases.

Alexander's disease is a rare disorder of unknown cause which presents in infancy or

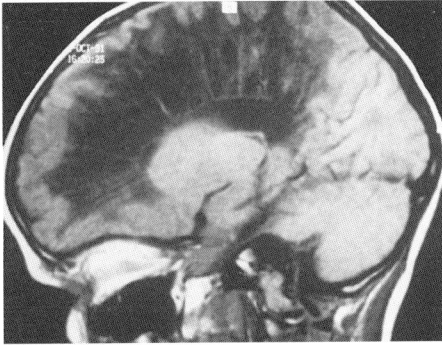

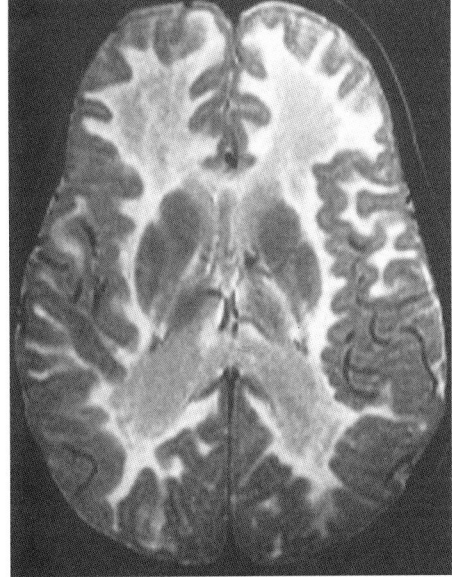

Fig. 9.14. Alexander's disease. *(Above)* T_1-weighted image shows diffuse decreased signal in the white matter, and no ventricular dilation or cortical atrophy. *(Right)* T_2-weighted image images shows diffuse increased signal throughout the white matter. The periventricular regions had intermediate signal similar to the ventricles.

in adolescence, has a progressive course and is characterized by macrocephaly. No known biochemical marker is detected and the histological hallmark is astrocytic eosinophilic Rosenthal fibers (Vogel and Hallervorden 1962, Russo *et al.* 1976, Borrett and Becker 1985, Fishman 1989). On MRI the characteristic frontal lobe location of the abnormal increased T_2 signal in the early stages distinguishes it from other degenerative white matter disorders. The abnormalities progress eventually to involve the entire brain and lead to atrophy (Fig. 9.14). Contrast enhancement has been reported on CT scans, but the significance of this finding is unclear (Holland and Kendall 1962). It probably represents the acute stage of dys- and demyelination and is also seen at this stage of progression in other white matter disorders.

Canavan's disease is an autosomal recessive disorder which presents in infancy or early childhood, and usually has a rapidly fatal course. There is a deficiency of *N*-acetylaspartylase which results in accumulation of *N*-acetylaspartase in the plasma and urine (Hagenfeldt *et al.* 1987, Matalon *et al.* 1988). The characteristic spongy appearance on histological examination is due to vacuoles in the white matter and is responsible for the eponym 'spongiform leukodystrophy' (Adachi 1973). Macrocephaly is pronounced, at least in the initial stage (Fishman 1989). The MRI changes are in general non-specific, with abnormal signal throughout the white matter (Brismar *et al.* 1990*b*, McAdam 1990). Decreased signal from the susceptibility effect of presumed hemorrhage has been reported in one case (Wolpert 1992).

Pelizaeus–Merzbacher disease is an X-linked recessive disorder, with occasional sporadic cases, which usually presents in infancy but may occur rarely in adults. No known biochemical abnormality has been found. Pathologically there are patchy areas of

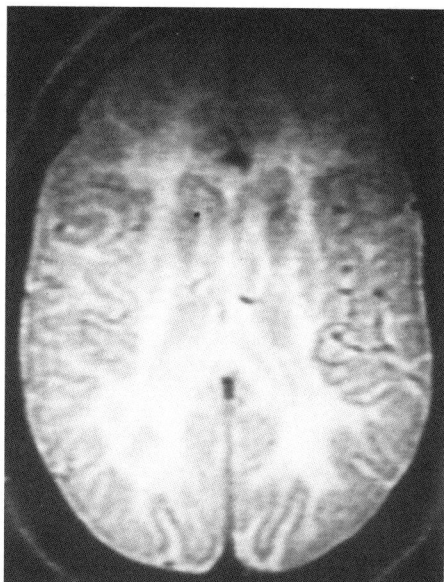

Fig. 9.15. Pelizaeus–Merzbacher disease. T_2-weighted image shows diffuse increased signal in the white matter.

demyelination with normal myelin in the perivascular regions giving rise to the typical 'tigroid' appearance. Although generally considered a demyelination disorder, the lack of myelin breakdown products pathologically lend support to hypomyelination as the cause, at least in the cases presenting in infancy (Watanabe 1969, Seitelberger 1970, Schneck *et al.* 1971). The cases reported on MRI in general show signal changes which suggest diffuse hypomyelination in the cerebral hemispheres and brainstem (Journel *et al.* 1987, Penner *et al.* 1987, Shimomura *et al.* 1988, van der Knaap and Valk 1989*a*) (Fig. 9.15). Scattered regions of hyperintensity on T_2 images reflecting the typical 'tigroid' appearances with normal signal in between are uncommon (Fishman 1989). Decreased T_2 signal presumably due to iron products in the basal ganglia has been reported (Silverstein *et al.* 1990).

Cockayne's disease is a disorder of hypomyelination, similar in some cases to Pelizaeus–Merzbacher disease, with additional involvement of other organs. The disease presents in childhood with a characteristic facies and skin rash. No specific biochemical abnormality is found. Autosomal recessive inheritance is found in some families (Moossy 1967, Joshi *et al.* 1987, Fishman 1989). MRI changes are similar to those of Pelizaeus–Merzbacher disease and show diffuse increased signal on T_2-weighted images compatible with generalized hypomyelination. Focal increased T_2 has been described (Nishio *et al.* 1988, Boltshauser *et al.* 1989). Calcification of the basal ganglia may be seen as decreased signal (Faerber 1986).

Differential diagnosis
Several other diseases result in MRI appearances in the white matter similar to those from the preceding causes (see Table 9.2). These include hypoxia–ischemia, acute dissemin-

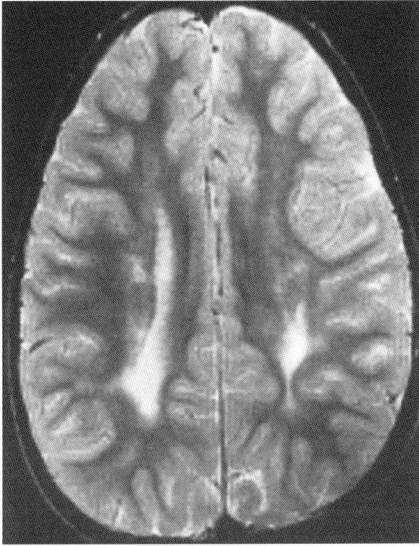

Fig. 9.16. Periventricular leukomalacia of hypoxia–ischemia. T$_2$-weighted image shows areas of decreased signal in the periventricular regions adjacent to the posterior portions of the lateral ventricles which are focally dilated.

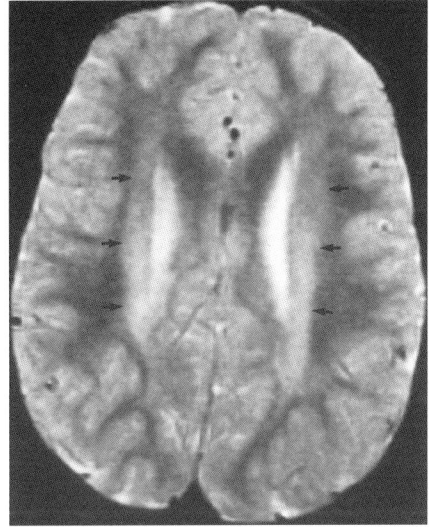

Fig. 9.17. Hypoxia–ischemia. T$_2$-weighted image shows increased signal throughout the entire periventricular white matter *(arrows)*.

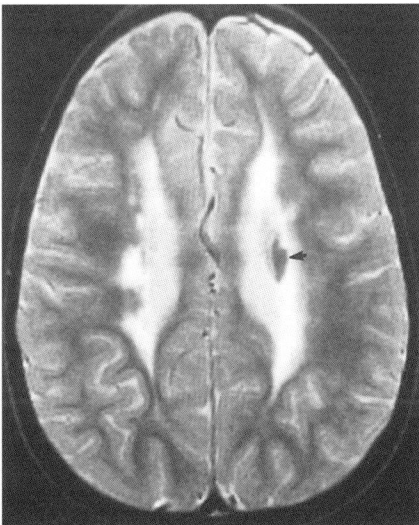

Fig. 9.18. Hemorrhagic periventricular leuko-malacia. T$_2$-weighted image shows periventricular increased signal and a region of decreased signal due to hemosiderin *(arrow)*.

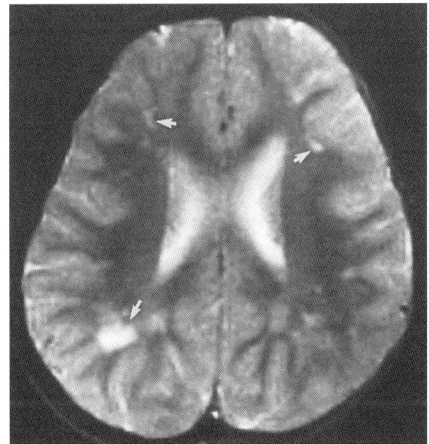

Fig. 9.19. Hypoxia–ischemia. T$_2$-weighted image shows multiple small regions of increased signal close to the gray/white junction *(arrows)*.

211

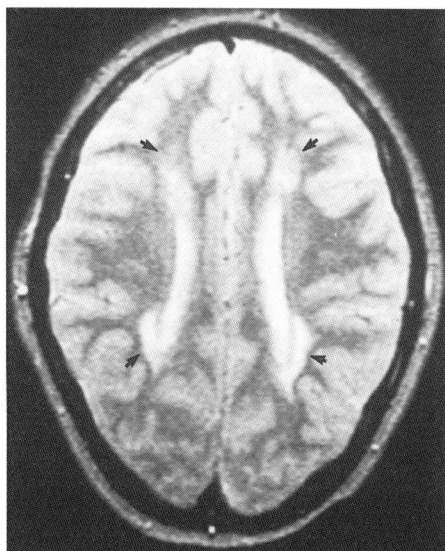

Fig. 9.20. Methotrexate therapy. T_2-weighted image shows increased signal in the periventricular regions posteriorly and anteriorly *(arrows)*.

ated encephalomeningitis, infections, progressive multifocal leukomalacia, demyelination, trauma, radiation and chemotherapy. The clinical history is pertinent in diagnosing many of these disorders.

Hypoxia–ischemia

Increased periventricular signal on T_2-weighted images are seen after perinatal hypoxia–ischemia. The posterior regions are preferentially affected, and there is usually dilatation of the adjacent lateral ventricles (Fig. 9.16). Sometimes the entire periventricular region is diffusely involved, and the appearances may be indistinguishable from other white matter disorders (Fig. 9.17). The presence of hemosiderin indicating previous hemorrhage is pathognomic and distinguishes these from other causes of periventricular abnormalities (Fig. 9.18). Occasionally multiple regions of increased signal are visible on T_2-weighted images, and can be very confusing (Fig. 9.19). These changes are due to periventricular leukomalacia, and are caused by ischemia in the 'watershed' region between the centrifugal and centripetal arterial blood supply. These abnormalities result eventually in cerebral palsy. Although the clinical history suggests that this is the cause of white matter changes in infants and young children, it is often difficult to ascertain the severity of the hypoxia–ischemia in older children.

Radiation and chemotherapy

The location of white matter changes from radiation therapy depends on the radiation port, but may be generalized, in which case the appearances are indistinguishable from other causes. Chemotherapy, typically using intrathecal agents such as methotrexate, gives rise to periventricular white matter changes (Fig. 9.20). Unless hemorrhage or calcification is present these abnormalities are also nonspecific. Some of the abnormalities are transient, presumably due to edema, and disappear after discontinuing the chemotherapy.

Other disease entities
Other causes of white matter changes include ADEM (acute disseminated encephalo-myelopathy), PML (progressive multifocal leukoencephalopathy), demyelination, trauma and infectious disorders such as AIDS. These do not have specific MRI appearances but should be included in the differential diagnosis of all abnormal white matter signals.

Summary
The MRI appearances of white matter disorders are diverse and this modality is used to confirm clinically suspected diseases and to monitor the effects of therapy rather than to make specific diagnoses. Most white matter diseases fall into the following four categories: peroxisomal, lysosomal, mitochondrial, and amino acid/carbohydrate metabolic disorders. Most of these disorders give rise to nonspecific MRI changes, but a few have distinct appearances. Other common causes of similar white matter changes include hypoxia–ischemia, and chemo- and radiation therapy.

REFERENCES

Adachi, M., Schneck, L., Cara, J., Volk, B.W. (1973) 'Spongy degeneration of the central nervous system (Van Bogaert and Bertrand type; Canavan's disease). A review.' *Human Pathology*, **4**, 331–347.

Allard, J.C., Tilak, S., Carter, A.P. (1988) 'CT and MR of MELAS syndrome.' *American Journal of Neuroradiology*, **9**, 1234–1238.

Baram, T.Z., Goldman, A.M., Percy, A.K. (1986) 'Krabbe disease: specific MRI and CT findings.' *Neurology*, **36**, 111–115.

Barkovich, A.J., Kjos, B.O., Jackson, D.E., Norman, D. (1988) 'Normal maturation of the neonatal and infant brain: MR imaging at 1.5 T.' *Radiology*, **166**, 173–180.

Berman, J.L., Cunningham, G.C., Day, R.W., Ford, R., Hsia, D.Y.Y. (1969) 'Causes for high phenylalanine with normal tyrosine in newborn screening programs.' *American Journal of Diseases of Children*, **117**, 54–65.

Bewermeyer, H., Bamborschke, S., Ebhardt, G., Hünermann, B., Heiss, W.D. (1985) 'MR imaging in adreno-leukomyeloneuropathy.' *Journal of Computer Assisted Tomography*, **9**, 793–796.

Boltshauser, E., Yalcinkaya, C., Wichmann, W., Reutter, F., Prader, A., Valavanis, A. (1989) 'MRI in Cockayne syndrome type I.' *Neuroradiology*, **31**, 276–277.

Borrett, D., Becker, L.E. '(1985) Alexander's disease. A disease of astrocytes.' *Brain*, **108**, 367–385.

Brismar, J., Aqeel, A., Gascon, G., Ozand, P. (1990a) 'Malignant hyperphenylalaninemia: CT and MR of the brain.' *American Journal of Neuroradiology*, **11**, 135–138.

—— Brismar, G., Gascon, G, Ozand, P. (1990b) 'Canavan disease: CT and MR imaging of the brain.' *American Journal of Neuroradiology*, **11**, 805–810.

Cherryman, G.R., Smith, F.W. (1985) 'Nuclear magnetic resonance in adrenoleukodystrophy: report of a case.' *Clinical Radiology*, **36**, 539–540.

Crocker, A.C. (1961) 'The cerebral defect in Tay–Sachs disease and Niemann–Pick disease.' *Journal of Neurochemistry*, **7**, 69–80.

David, R.B., Mamunes, P., Rosenblum, W.I. (1976) 'Necrotizing encephalomyelopathy (Leigh).' *In:* Vinken, P.J., Bruyn, G.W. (Eds.) *Handbook of Clinical Neurology. Vol. 28.* Amsterdam: North Holland, pp. 349–363.

Davis, P.C., Hoffman, J.C., Braun, I.F., Ahmann, P., Krawiecki, N. (1987) 'MR of Leigh's disease (subacute necrotizing encephalomyelopathy).' *American Journal of Neuroradiology*, **8**, 71–75.

Dekaban, A.S., Constantopoulos, G. (1977) 'Mucopolysaccharidosis types I, II, IIIA and V. Pathological and biochemical abnormalities in the neural and mesenchymal elements of the brain.' *Acta Neuropathologica*, **39**, 1–7.

Demange, P., Gia, H.P., Kalifa, G., Sellier, M. (1989) 'MR of Kearns–Sayre syndrome.' *American Journal of Neuroradiology*, **10**, S91.

Dietrich, R.B., Bradley, W.G., Zaragoza, E.J., Otto, R.J., Taira, R.K., Wilson, G.H., Kangarloo, H. (1988) 'MR evaluation of early myelination patterns in normal and developmentally delayed infants.' *American Journal of Neuroradiology*, **9**, 69–76.

Eggli, K.D., Dorst, J.P. (1986) 'The mucopolysaccharidoses and related conditions.' *Seminars in Roentgenology*, **21**, 275–294.

Faerber, E.N. (1986) *Cranial Computed Tomography in Infants and Children. Clinics in Developmental Medicine No. 93.* London: Spastics International Medical Publications.

Fishman, M.A. (1989) 'Disorders primarily of white matter.' *In:* Swaiman, K.F. (Ed.) *Pediatric Neurology: Principles and Practice.* St. Louis: C.V. Mosby, 755–775.

Geyer, C.A., Sartor, K.J., Prensky, A.J., Abramson, C.L., Hodges, F.J., Gado, M.H. (1988) 'Leigh disease (subacute necrotizing encephalomyelopathy): CT and MR in five cases.' *Journal of Computer Assisted Tomography*, **12**, 40–44.

Golden, G.S. (1987) 'Metabolic disorders.' *In:* Golden, G.S. (Ed.) *Textbook of Pediatric Neurology.* New York: Plenum.

Goldfischer, S., Collins, J., Rapin, I., Coltoff-Schiller, B., Chang, C-H., Nigro, M., Black, V.H., Javitt, N.B., Moser, H.W., Lazarow, P.B. (1985) 'Peroxisomal defects in neonatal onset and X-linked adrenoleukodystrophies.' *Science*, **227**, 67–70.

Griffin, J.W., Goren, E., Schaumburg, H., Engel, W.K., Loriaux, L. (1977) 'Adrenomyeloneuropathy: a probable variant of adrenoleukodystrophy.' *Neurology*, **27**, 1107–1113.

Hagenfeldt, L., Bollgren, I., Venizelos, N. (1987) 'N-acetylaspartic aciduria due to aspartoacylase deficiency—a new aetiology of childhood leukodystrophy.' *Journal of Inherited Metabolic Disease*, **10**, 135–141.

Henderson, J.L., Macgregor, A.R., Thannhauser, S.J., Holden, R. (1952) 'The pathology and biochemistry of gargoylism. A report of three cases with a review of the literature.' *Archives of Disease in Childhood*, **27**, 230–253.

Holland, I.M., Kendall, B.E. (1980) 'Computed tomography in Alexander's disease.' *Neuroradiology*, **20**, 103–106.

Holland, B.A., Haas, D.K., Norman, D., Brant-Zawadzki, M., Newton, T.H. (1986) 'MRI of normal brain maturation.' *American Journal of Neuroradiology*, **7**, 201–208.

Huckman, M.S., Wong, P.W.K., Sullivan, T., Zeller, P., Geremia, G.K. (1986) 'Magnetic resonance imaging compared with computed tomography in adrenoleukodystrophy.' *American Journal of Diseases of Children*, **140**, 1001–1003.

Igisu, H., Suzuki, K. (1984) 'Progressive accumulation of toxic metabolite in a genetic leukodystrophy.' *Science*, **224**, 753–755.

Johnson, M.A., Desai, S., Hugh-Jones, K., Starer, F. (1984) 'Magnetic resonance imaging of the brain in Hurler syndrome.' *American Journal of Neuroradiology*, **5**, 816–819.

Joshi, R.M., Kallapur, S.G., Gandhi, R.K., Ketkar, D.R., Mohire, M.D., Kulkarni, V.S., Patnekar, P.N. (1987) 'Cockayne syndrome. (A case report.)' *Journal of Postgraduate Medicine*, **33**, 43–44.

Journel, H., Roussey, M., Gandon, Y., Allaire, C., Carsin, M., le Marec, B. (1987) 'Magnetic resonance imaging in Pelizaeus–Merzbacher disease.' *Neuroradiology*, **29**, 403–405.

Kelley, R.I., Datta, N.S., Dobyns, W.B., Hajra, A.K., Moser, A.B., Noetzel, M.J., Zackai, E.H., Moser, H.W. (1986) 'Neonatal adrenoleukodystrophy: new cases, biochemical studies, and differentiation from Zellweger and related peroxisomal polydystrophy syndromes.' *American Journal of Medical Genetics*, **23**, 869–901.

Koch, T.K., Yee, M.H.C., Hutchinson, H.T., Berg, B.O. (1986) 'Magnetic resonance imaging in subacute necrotizing encephalomyelopathy (Leigh's disease).' *Annals of Neurology*, **19**, 605–607.

Kumar, A.J., Rosenbaum, A.E., Naidu, S., Wener, L., Citrin, C.M., Lindenberg, R., Kim, W.S., Zinreich, S.J., Molliver, M.E., *et al.* (1987) 'Adrenoleukodystrophy: correlating MR imaging with CT.' *Radiology*, **165**, 497–504.

Kurokawa, T., Chen, Y-J., Nagata, M., Hasuo, K., Kobayashi, T., Kitaguchi, T. (1987) 'Late infantile Krabbe leukodystrophy: MRI and evoked potentials in a Japanese girl.' *Neuropediatrics*, **18**, 182–183.

Laxdal, T., Hallgrimsson, J. (1974) 'Krabbe's globoid cell leucodystrophy with hydrocephalus.' *Archives of Disease in Childhood*, **49**, 232–235.

Lindsay, S., Reilly, W.A., Gotham, T.J., Skahen, R. (1948) 'Gargoylism. II. Study of pathologic lesions and clinical review of twelve cases.' *American Journal of Diseases of Children*, **76**, 239–306.

214

McAdams, H.P., Geyer, C.A., Done, S.L., Deigh, D., Mitchell, M., Ghaed, V.N. (1990) 'CT and MR imaging of Canavan disease.' *American Journal of Neuroradiology*, **11**, 397–399.

McKusick, V.A., Neufeld, E.F. (1983) 'The mucopolysaccharide storage diseases.' *In:* Stanbury, J.B., Wyngaarden, J.B., Fredrickson, D.S., Goldstein, J.L., Brown, M.S. (Eds.) *The Metabolic Basis of Inherited Disease. 5th Edn.* New York: McGraw–Hill, pp. 751–777.

Maisey, D.N., Cosh, J.A. (1980) 'Basilar artery aneurysm and Anderson–Fabry disease.' *Journal of Neurology, Neurosurgery and Psychiatry*, **43**, 85–87.

Matalon, R., Michals, K., Sebesta, D., Deanching, M., Gashkoff, P., Casanova, J. (1988) 'Aspartoacylase deficiency and *N*-acetylaspartic aciduria in patients with Canavan disease.' *American Journal of Medical Genetics*, **29**, 463–471.

Medina, L., Chi, T.L., De Vivo, D.C., Hilal, S.K. (1990) 'MR findings in patients with subacute necrotizing encephalomyelopathy (Leigh syndrome): correlation with biochemical defect.' *American Journal of Neuroradiology*, **11**, 379–384.

Menkes, J.H., Solcher, H. (1967) 'Maple syrup disease. Effects of dietary therapy on cerebral lipids.' *Archives of Neurology*, **6**, 486–491.

Moossy, J. (1967) 'The neuropathology of Cockayne's syndrome.' *Journal of Neuropathology and Experimental Neurology*, **26**, 654–660.

Morita, K., Ono, S., Fukunaga, M., Yasuda, T., Higashi, Y., Terao, A., Morita, R. (1989) 'Increased accumulation of N-isopropyl-p-(^{123}I)-iodoamphetamine in two cases with mitochondrial encephalomyopathy with lactic acidosis and strokelike episodes (MELAS).' *Neuroradiology*, **31**, 358–361.

Moser, H.W. (1977) 'Brain amino acid metabolism. (Emphasis on aspects relevant to the pathophysiology of genetically determined disorders.)' *In:* Vinken, P.J., Bruyn, G.W. (Eds.) *Handbook of Clinical Neurology, Vol. 29.* Amsterdam: North Holland, pp. 17–28.

—— (1986) 'Peroxisomal disorders.' *Journal of Pediatrics*, **108**, 89–91.

Moumdjian, R., Tampieri, D., Melanson, D., Ethier, R. (1989) 'Anderson–Fabry disease: a case report with MR, CT, and cerebral angiography.' *American Journal of Neuroradiology*, **10**, S69–S70.

Murata, R., Nakajima, S., Tanaka, A., Miyagi, N., Matsuoka, O., Kogame, S., Inoue, Y. (1989) 'MR imaging of the brain in patients with mucopolysaccharidosis.' *American Journal of Neuroradiology*, **10**, 1165–1170.

Nishio, H., Kodama, S., Tsobuta, T., Takumi, T., Takahashi, T., Yokoyama, S., Matsuo, T. (1985) 'Adreno-leukodystrophy without adrenal insufficiency and its magnetic resonance imaging.' *Journal of Neurology*, **232**, 265–270.

—— —— Matsuo, T., Ichihashi, M., Ito, H., Fujiwara, Y. (1988) 'Cockayne syndrome: magnetic resonance images of the brain in a severe form with early onset.' *Journal of Inherited Metabolic Disease*, **11**, 88–102.

Norman, R.M., Urich, H., France, N.E. (1959) 'Perivascular cavitation of the basal ganglia in gargoylism.' *Journal of Mental Science*, **105**, 1070–1077.

Norton, W.T. (1981) 'Formation, structure and biochemistry of myelin.' *In:* Siegel, G.J., Albers, R.W., Agranoff, B.V., Katzman, R. (Eds.) *Basic Neurochemistry. 3rd Edn.* Boston: Little, Brown, pp. 63–92.

Nowell, M.A., Grossman, R.I., Hackney, D.B., Zimmerman, R.A., Goldberg, H.I., Bilaniuk, L.T. (1988) 'MR imaging of white matter disease in children.' *American Journal of Neuroradiology*, **9**, 503–509.

Pavlakis, S.G., Phillips, P.C., DiMauro, S., De Vivo, D.C., Rowland, L.P. (1984) 'Mitochondrial myopathy, encephalopathy, lactic acidosis, and strokelike episodes: a distinctive clinical syndrome.' *Annals of Neurology*, **16**, 481–488.

Penner, M.W., Li, K.C., Gebarski, S.S., Allen, R.J. (1987) 'MR imaging of Pelizaeus–Merzbacher disease.' *Journal of Computer Assisted Tomography*, **11**, 591–593.

Petty, R.K.H., Harding, A.E., Morgan-Hughes, J.A. (1986) 'The clinical features of mitochondrial myopathy.' *Brain*, **109**, 915–938.

Poser, C.M. (1961) 'Leukodystrophy and the concept of dysmyelination.' *Archives of Neurology*, **4**, 323–332.

—— (1987) 'The dysmyelinating diseases.' *In:* Baker, A.B., Joynt, R.J. (Eds.) *Clinical Neurology. Vol. 3.* Philadelphia: Harper & Row.

Rauch, R.A., Frilous, L.A., Lott, I.T. (1989) 'MR imaging of cavitary lesions in the brain with Hurler/Scheie.' *American Journal of Neuroradiology*, **10**, S1–S3.

Reider-Grosswasser, I., Bornstein, N. (1987) 'CT and MRI in late-onset metachromatic leukodystrophy.' *Acta Neurologica Scandinavica*, **75**, 64–69.

Robinson, B.H., De Meirleir, L., Glerum, M., Sherwood, G., Becker, L. (1987) 'Clinical presentation of mitochondrial respiratory chain defects in NADH-coenzyme Q reductase and cytochrome oxidase: clues to pathogenesis of Leigh disease.' *Journal of Pediatrics*, **110**, 216–222.

215

Rosen, L., Phillips, S., Enzmann, D. (1990) 'Magnetic resonance imaging in MELAS syndrome.' *Neuroradiology*, **32**, 168–171.

Russo, L.S., Aron, A., Anderson, P.J. (1976) 'Alexander's disease: a report and reappraisal.' *Neurology*, **26**, 607–614.

Schaumburg, H.H., Powers, J.M., Raine, C.S., Suzuki, K., Richardson, E.P. (1975) 'Adrenoleukodystrophy. A clinical and pathological study of 17 cases.' *Archives of Neurology*, **32**, 577–591.

Schneck, L., Adachi, M., Volk, B.W. (1971) 'Congenital failure of myelinization: Pelizaeus–Merzbacher disease?' *Neurology*, **21**, 817–824.

Schutgens, R.B.H., Heymans, H.S.A., Wanders, R.J.A., van den Bosch, H., Tager, J.M. (1986) 'Peroxisomal disorders: a newly recognized group of genetic diseases.' *European Journal of Pediatrics*, **144**, 430–440.

Scriver, C.R., Beaudet, A.L., Sly, W.S., Valle, D. (Eds.) (1989) *The Metabolic Basis of Inherited Disease. 5th Edn.* New York: McGraw–Hill.

Seitelberger, F. (1970) 'Pelizaeus–Merzbacher disease.' *In:* Vinken, P.J., Bruyn, G.W. (Eds.) *Handbook of Clinical Neurology. Vol. 10.* Amsterdam: North Holland; New York: Elsevier, pp. 150–202.

Shapira, Y., Harel, S., Russell, A. (1977) 'Mitochondrial encephalomyopathies: a group of neuromuscular disorders with defects in oxidative metabolism.' *Israel Journal of Medical Sciences*, **13**, 161–164.

Shimomura, C., Matsui, A., Choh, H., Funahashi, M., Suzuki, Y., Tsuchiya, K. (1988) 'Magnetic resonance imaging in Pelizaeus–Merzbacher disease.' *Pediatric Neurology*, **4**, 124–125.

Silverstein, A.M., Hirsh, D.K., Trobe, J.D., Gebarski, S.S. (1990) 'MR imaging of the brain in five members of a family with Pelizaeus–Merzbacher disease.' *American Journal of Neuroradiology*, **11**, 495–499.

Shinnar, S., Singer, H.S., Valle, D. (1982) 'Acute hydrocephalus in Hurler's syndrome.' *American Journal of Diseases of Children*, **136**, 556–557.

Stam, F.C. (1970) 'Concept, classification and nosology of the leukodystrophies.' *In:* Vinken, P.J., Bruyn, G.W. (Eds.) *Handbook of Clinical Neurology. Vol. 10.* Amsterdam: North Holland, pp. 1–42.

Suzuki, K. (1984) 'Biochemical pathogenesis of genetic leukodystrophies: comparison of metachromatic leukodystrophy and globoid cell leukodystrophy (Krabbe's disease).' *Neuropediatrics*, **15** (Suppl.), 32–36.

—— Suzuki, Y. (1970) 'Globoid cell leucodystrophy (Krabbe's disease): deficiency of galactocerebroside β-galactosidase.' *Proceedings of the National Academy of Sciences of the USA*, **66**, 302–309.

Svennerholm, L. (1964) 'The distribution of lipids in the human nervous system—I. Analytical procedure. Lipids of foetal and newborn brain.' *Journal of Neurochemistry*, **11**, 839–853.

Swaiman, K.F. (Ed.) (1989*a*) *Pediatric Neurology: Principles and Practice.* St Louis: C.V. Mosby.

—— (1989*b*) 'Aminoacidopathies resulting from deficiency of enzyme activity.' *In:* Swaiman, K.F. (Ed.) *Pediatric Neurology: Principles and Practice.* St. Louis: C.V. Mosby, pp. 931–958.

—— (1989*c*) 'Lysosomal diseases.' *In:* Swaiman, K.F. (Ed.) *Pediatric Neurology: Principles and Practice.* St Louis: C.V. Mosby, pp. 1017–1066.

Swick, H.M. (1989) 'Diseases of gray matter.' *In:* Swaiman, K.F. (Ed.) *Pediatric Neurology: Principles and Practice.* St Louis: C.V. Mosby, pp. 777–794.

Uziel, G., Savoiardo, M., Nardocci, N. (1988) 'CT and MRI in maple syrup urine disease.' *Neurology*, **38**, 486–488.

Valk, J., van der Knaap, M.S. (1989) *Magnetic Resonance of Myelin, Myelination, and Myelin Disorders.* Berlin: Springer Verlag.

van der Knaap, M.S., Valk, J. (1989*a*) 'The reflection of histology in MR imaging of Pelizaeus–Merzbacher disease.' *American Journal of Neuroradiology*, **10**, 99–103.

—— —— (1989*b*) 'MR of adrenoleukodystrophy: histopathologic correlations.' *American Journal of Neuroradiology*, **10**, S12–S14.

—— —— (1991) 'The MR spectrum of peroxisomal disorders.' *Neuroradiology*, **33**, 30–37.

van Erven, P.M.M., Cillessen, J.P.M., Eekhoff, E.M.W., Gabreëls, F.J.M., Doesburg, W.H., Lemmens, W.A.J.G., Stooff, J.L., Renier, W.O., Ruitenbeek, W. (1987) 'Leigh syndrome, a mitochondrial encephalo(myo)pathy. A review of the literature.' *Clinical Neurology and Neurosurgery*, **89**, 217–230.

Vogel, F.S., Hallervorden, J. (1962) 'Leukodystrophy with diffuse Rosenthal fiber formation.' *Acta Neuropathologica*, **2**, 126–143

Volkow, N.D., Patchell, L., Kulkarni, M.V., Reed, K., Simmons, M. (1987) 'Adrenoleukodystrophy: imaging with CT, MRI, and PET.' *Journal of Nuclear Medicine*, **28**, 524–527.

Waltz, G., Harik, S.I., Kaufman, B. (1987) 'Adult metachromatic leukodystrophy. Value of computer tomographic scanning and magnetic resonance imaging of the brain.' *Archives of Neurology*, **44**, 225–227.

Watanabe, I., McCaman, R., Dyken, P., Zeman, W. (1969) 'Absence of cerebral myelin sheaths in a case of presumed Pelizaeus–Merzbacher disease. Electron microscopic and biochemical studies.' *Journal of Neuropathology and Experimental Neurology*, **28**, 243–248.

Wolpert, S.M., Anderson, M.L., Kaye, E.M. (1992) 'Metabolic and degenerative disorders.' *In:* Wolpert, S.M., Barnes, P.D. (Eds.) *MRI in Pediatric Neuroradiology.* St. Louis: C.V. Mosby, pp. 4–15.

Young, I.R., Randell, C.P., Kaplan, P.W., James, A., Bydder, G.M., Steiner, R.E. (1983) 'Nuclear magnetic resonance (NMR) imaging in white matter disease of the brain using spin-echo sequences.' *Journal of Computer Assisted Tomography*, **7**, 290–294.

Young, R.S.K., Osbakken, M.D., Alger, P.M., Ramer, K.C., Weidner, W.A., Daigh, J.D. (1985) 'Magnetic resonance imaging in leukodystrophies in children.' *Pediatric Neurology*, **1**, 15–19.

10
THE ORBIT

Kenneth D. Hopper, John L. Sherman, Danielle K. Boal and Kathleen D. Eggli

The increasing application of orbital MRI has had a dramatic impact in pediatric ophthalmology, especially in evaluating the orbital neural pathways and cerebral cortex. This chapter presents a review of congenital anomalies and orbital pathology in the pediatric patient (Table 10.1). Because congenital diseases and tumors are frequently better evaluated by MRI than by CT, these areas are stressed. Diseases of the globe, or pseudogliomas, and inflammatory and infectious diseases of the orbit are also reviewed.

MR imaging techniques

The orbits are well imaged by 3–4 mm spin echo T_1-weighted images in the axial and coronal planes using either a 192×256 or a 256×256 matrix. Gradient echo images obtained as either a volume (1 mm slice thickness) or with stacked 3 mm slices are frequently useful. A fat-suppression technique should be used on at least one of these sequences. T_2-weighted images are usually obtained in the axial planes with a 3–4 mm slice thickness. Occasionally, oblique sagittal T_1-weighted images orientated along the course of the optic nerve (Fig. 10.1) are helpful. Most orbital imaging should be accompanied by a routine brain MRI scan.

Fat-suppression MRI

The large amount of fat in the orbit is useful on T_1-weighted MRI because it increases the signal-to-noise ratio for most anatomic structures, except the lacrimal gland. However, the presence of high-intensity fatty tissue limits the visibility on enhancing orbital lesions after gadolinium-DTPA administration. A variety of lipid-suppression techniques have been developed to overcome this problem (Simon *et al.* 1988).

The short-inversion-time inversion recovery (STIR) sequence suppresses signal from fat (Fig. 10.2) based on relaxation time rather than chemical constituency (Atlas *et al.* 1988). This method is useful to screen for orbital pathology before gadolinium administration because tissues with prolonged T_1 and T_2 relaxation times (*e.g.* most masses, inflammation, demyelination) have high signal intensity and are sharply contrasted against the null signal of fat. This technique is not as reliable with the use of gadolinium, as substances with short T_1 relaxation times (*e.g.* both fat and areas of gadolinium enhancement) will undergo some degree of signal nulling.

The Dixon method and its variations depend on two separate data sets for calculation of water-only or fat-only images (Dixon 1984). The chemical shift effect between the resonant frequencies of fat and water has been taken advantage of to produce lipid signal suppression. The 'fat-sat' method (Fig. 10.2) is a technique that uses a frequency-

TABLE 10.1
Common pediatric orbital abnormalities*

Orbital cellulitis (frequently from sinusitis)
Penetrating trauma
Pseudotumors (idiopathic inflammations)
Dermoid and epidermoid cysts
Capillary hemangiomas
Lymphangiomas
Rhabdomyosarcomas
Optic nerve gliomas
Neurofibromas
Leukemias
Metastatic tumors (frequently neuroblastoma)

*Listed in order of decreasing frequency.

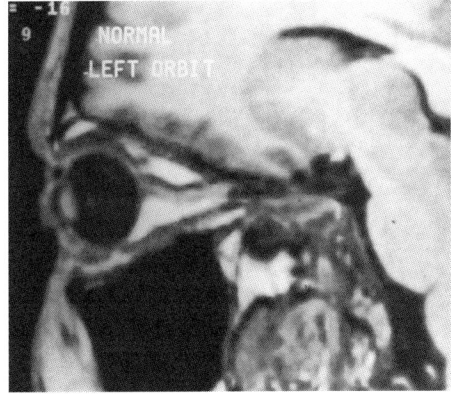

Fig. 10.1. In addition to evaluating the orbit by coronal and axial images, occasionally oblique sagittal images along the course of the optic nerve are useful. This image demonstrates a T_1-weighted oblique sagittal image through a normal left globe and left optic nerve.

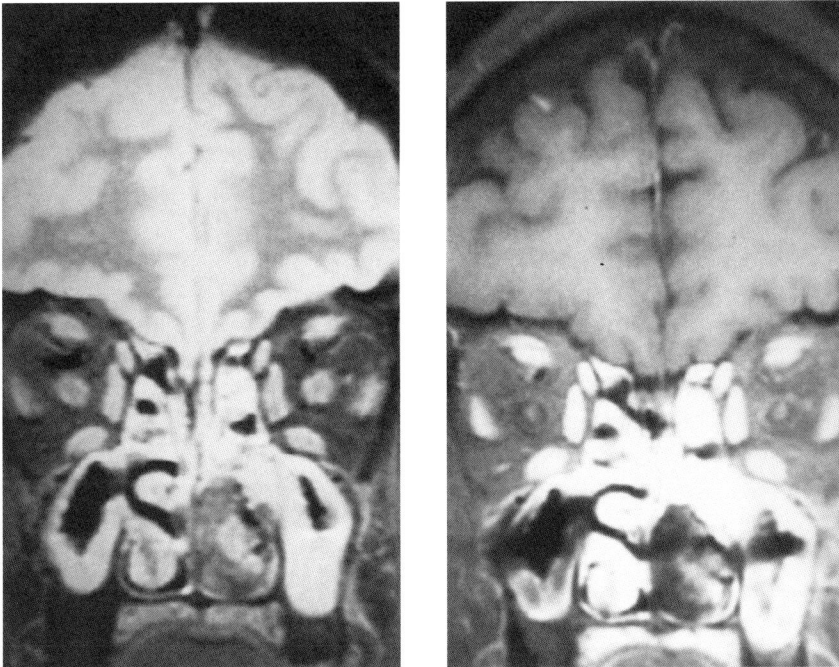

Fig. 10.2. Fat suppression orbital imaging with MRI. The figure on the left demonstrates fat suppression utilizing STIR, while that on the right utilizes a dedicated fat-only suppression technique ('fat sat').

219

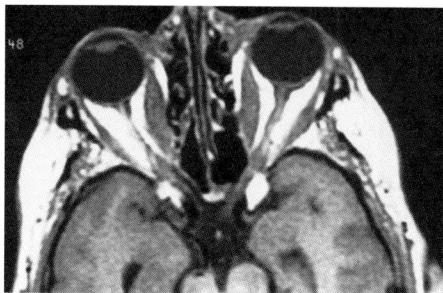

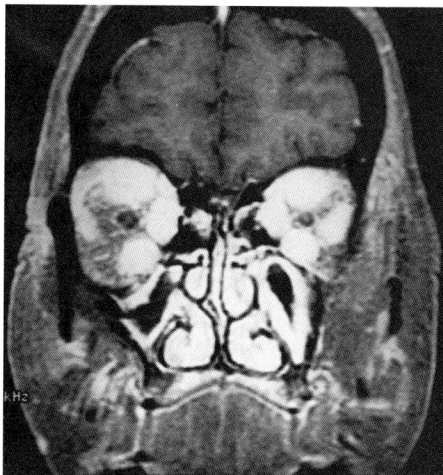

Fig. 10.3. Graves' disease. This young female has extensive enlargement of all extraocular muscles as demonstrated on the axial T_1-weighted image *(above)* and fat suppressed coronal T_1-weighted image *(right)*.

selective presaturation pulse centered on the spectral fat peak for each individual patient (Keller *et al.* 1987). This technique achieves high-level lipid suppression without increasing imaging time or image post-processing (Fig. 10.3).

The slice select gradient reversal (SSGR) technique is another popular chemical shift technique. SSGR scans achieve fat-suppression without chemical shift artifact by selectively refocusing water protons while leaving fat protons defocused (Hinks and Quencer 1988).

Fat-suppression combined with gadolinium enhancement improves lesion conspicuity compared to post-contrast T_1-weighted spin-echo images because high signal intensity enhancing lesions are contrasted against suppressed (low signal) fat rather than non-suppressed (high-signal) fat. Intraorbital and paraorbital lesions can be distinguished easily from intraorbital fat that is suppressed. Because of sharp contrast between tissue planes, this technique is helpful for detecting any intraorbital invasion from paraorbital lesions (Tien *et al.* 1991). The enhanced fat-suppressed images are superior to T_2-weighted images (Barakos *et al.* 1991).

Fat-suppression artifacts or fat-suppression failure may occur at air–fat interfaces due to magnetic susceptibility, spatial misregistration and resonant frequency shift (Anzai *et al.* 1992). These artifacts can be clinically confusing, especially if pre-contrast fat-suppression images are not available for comparison.

Primary congenital abnormalities (Table 10.2)
Anophthalmia, or congenital absence of the eye(s), is a rare sporadically occurring abnormality usually associated with 13–15 (D) trisomy, Klinefelter syndrome, and complex craniofacial malformations. Imaging of children with anophthalmia reveals a poorly formed, shallow orbit with only rudimentary orbital tissue (Fig. 10.4). Primary anophthalmia occurs when the optic vesicle does not form (Mann 1957, Walsh and Hoyt 1969,

TABLE 10.2
Primary congenital diseases of the orbit

Defects in orbital formation
Anophthalmia
Microphthalmia
Cyclopia and synophthalmia
Coloboma
Septo-optic dysplasia and hypoplasia of the optic nerve
Anencephaly
Myelomeningocele and encephalocele
Craniosynostosis: plagiocephaly
Craniofacial anomalies
• Acrocephalosyndactyly (Apert syndrome)
• Craniofacial dysostosis (Crouzon's disease)
• Mandibulofacial dysostosis
• Hypertelorism
• Trigonocephaly
Neurofibromatosis
• Optic nerve glioma, meningioma, schwannoma
• Optic nerve hemangioblastoma
• Plexiform neurofibroma
• Sphenoid wing dysplasia
Tuberous sclerosis
Diseases of the globe (leukokoria: see Table 10.3)
Congenital tumors

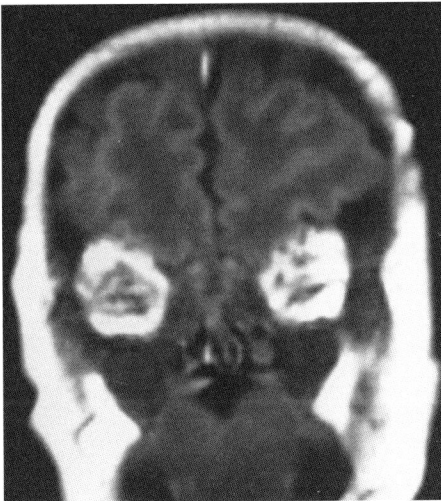

Fig. 10.4. Bilateral anophthalmia in a 1-day-old female. Coronal T$_1$-weighted MRI. While there is some rudimentary right orbital tissue remaining, little is seen on the left. (Reproduced by permission from Hopper *et al.* 1992.)

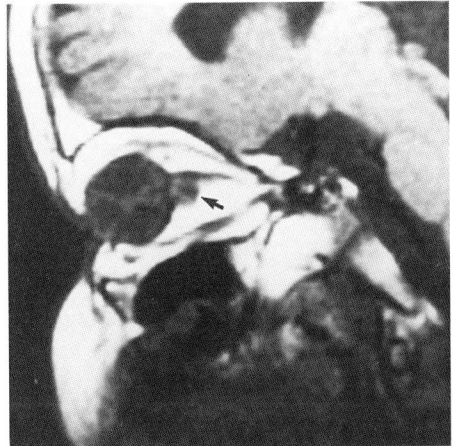

Fig. 10.5. Coloboma. This 2-year-old female with seizures has a posterior optic coloboma *(arrow)*. A small cyst is seen adjacent to the insertion of the optic nerve. Microphthalmos and persistent hyperplastic primary vitreous are also present. (Reproduced by permission from Hopper *et al.* 1988.)

221

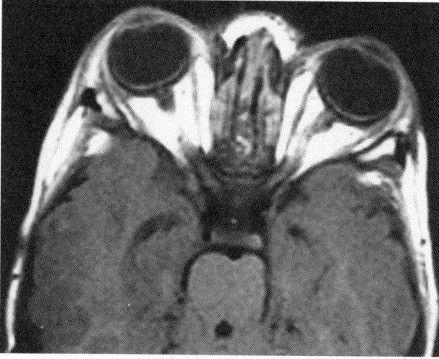

Fig. 10.6. Crouzon's disease. This 1-year-old male with known Crouzon's disease presented with bilateral extensive exophthalmos and papilledema. Axial T$_1$-weighted image demonstrates the shallow orbits with prominent exophthalmos which has resulted from the facial hypoplasia.

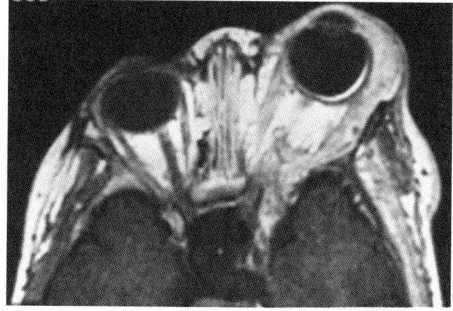

Fig. 10.7. Neurofibromatosis. This plexiform neurofibroma in a 1-year-old girl extends extra-coronally into the orbit as shown on this contrast-enhanced T$_1$-weighted axial image. (Reproduced by permission from Hopper et al. 1991.)

Dash et al. 1984, Shukla 1984). Anophthalmia may be difficult to differentiate from severe microphthalmos or orbital hypoplasia. However, unlike in anophthalmia, children with microphthalmos will have a formed eyeball with a lens (Slamovits et al. 1989). Imaging of these children reveals not only a small globe, but a small, poorly formed orbit as well.

Coloboma refers to any congenital or acquired notch, gap or fissure in any of the ocular structures. Typically, the term describes an incomplete closure of the primitive choroidal fissure of the optic stalk (Mafee et al. 1987b). On CT and MRI, a small cyst is found along the posterior globe at the head of the optic nerve (Fig. 10.5). Colobomas are usually transmitted as an autosomal dominant trait and are bilateral in 60 per cent of patients.

Septo-optic dysplasia is a rare anomaly associated with decreased vision and hypo-plasia of the optic nerves (see Chapter 4, pp. 13–15). A prominent anterior recess of the third ventricle and a small optic canal are typical. Absence or defects in the septum pellucidum and pituitary insufficiency are also present. A number of patients with septo-optic dysplasia will have schizencephaly and seizures (Barkovich et al. 1989).

Congenital craniofacial anomalies which affect the orbits can be classified into two clinical categories: craniosynostoses and the clefting syndromes' (Cohen 1975, Linder et al. 1987, Fries and Katowitz 1990). Craniosynostoses, or premature cranial suture closures, may be classified into three groups: simple craniosynostosis, craniofacial dysostosis (Crouzon syndrome), and acrocephalosyndactyly (Apert syndrome) (Fries and Katowitz 1990). Simple craniostenosis is a diverse group of disorders that can affect the orbit and cause hypertelorism, exophthalmos, exotropia (divergent strabismus) or esotropia (convergent strabismus). Coronal synostosis causes a harlequin appearance of the orbits. Craniofacial anomalies such as Crouzon and Apert syndromes are associated with mid-face hypoplasia, orbital hypertelorism and proptosis (Fig. 10.6). The clefting syndromes are a complex group of disorders which include not only surface defects in the facial soft tissues but usually anomalies in the underlying facial skeleton as well (Fries and Katowitz 1990). Frontal, nasal, and orbital myelomeningoceles and encephaloceles are the most common clefting anomalies affecting the orbit. The Treacher–Collins syndrome, another clefting abnormality, is an inherited hypoplasia of the mandible, zygoma and ear which is associated with drooping of the outer inferior orbital rim.

Neurofibromatosis type I is an autosomal dominant disease of variable penetrance occurring in approximately one in every 3000 births (see Chapter 4, pp. 32–36). This diverse disorder is characterized by multiple cutaneous café-au-lait spots, mental retardation, and neurofibromas of the peripheral, spinal, cranial and sympathetic nerves. Involvement of the eye is common with orbital (Fig. 10.7), optic nerve and eyelid ('bag-of-worms') tumors (Crawford and Morin 1983, Linder *et al.* 1987, Imes and Hoyt 1991). Optic nerve tumors occur in 1–15 per cent of patients with neurofibromatosis and are usually gliomas which can involve any part of the optic nerve, chiasm and optic tracts. The prevalence of neurofibromatosis in children with optic nerve gliomas is 12–38 per cent. Optic nerve meningiomas, retinal hemangioblastomas and schwannomas are occasionally seen. Sphenoid wing dysplasia with enlargement of the superior orbital fissure can lead to pulsatile exophthalmos. Eyelid tumors are usually plexiform neurofibromas and cause ptosis.

Tuberous sclerosis occurs in one in 30,000 births as an autosomal dominant disorder and frequently appears as the classic triad of adenoma sebaceum, mental deficiency and seizures (see Chapter 4, pp. 37–40). Retinal hamartomas are commonly found with tuberous sclerosis, appearing as yellowish, nodular masses near the optic nerve head. Angiomatosis of the retina may be found with von Hippel–Lindau disease. While difficult to discern with CT, small retinal hamartomas and angiomatosis are more easily identified with MRI.

Diseases of the globe
It is frequently difficult to differentiate the most serious intra-ocular pathological process, retinoblastoma, from many other benign mimics (pseudogliomas). Most of these children present with a white, yellow or sometimes pink-white ocular light reflex called leukokoria (Table 10.3). While the differential for leukokoria is long (Sanders 1950, Duke 1958, Hopper *et al.* 1985), CT and MRI can frequently differentiate retinoblastomas from non-malignant pseudogliomas. This differentiation is critical because retinoblastoma is an aggressive cancer and once tumor extends beyond the eye, mortality is always 100 per cent (Abramson 1982).

Retinoblastoma (Shields and Augsburger 1981, Abramson 1982, Mafee 1987*a*) is the primary intra-ocular malignant tumor of childhood, with 90 per cent presenting in children younger than 5 years. Occurring in approximately one in 15,000 to 30,000 births, this neuroectodermal tumor arises from the retina, and characteristic Flexner–Wintersteiner rosettes are seen histologically. While usually presenting as a calcified nodular mass, an occasional tumor is uncalcified. 10 per cent are familial and up to 25 per

TABLE 10.3
Differential diagnosis of leukokoria

Retinoblastoma
Cataracts
Retinopathy of prematurity (ROP)
Coats' disease
Sclerosing endophthalmitis
Long-standing retinal detachment
Persistent hyperplastic primary vitreous (PHPV)
Norrie's disease
Organized vitreous hemorrhage
Retinal dysplasia
Congenital retinal fold
Medulloepithelioma
Phakomatoses

cent are either multifocal within the same eye or are bilateral (Fig. 10.8). Children with bilateral retinoblastomas usually have an automosal dominant genetic transmission with incomplete penetrance. Approximately 1 per cent of retinoblastomas undergo spontaneous regression. Retinomas (or retinocytomas) are considered to be benign variants of retinoblastoma. Bilateral retinoblastomas may occasionally be associated with a pineal neuroectodermal tumor, a so-called 'trilateral' retinoblastoma (Bader *et al.* 1982, Zimmerman 1982).

Coats' disease (retinal telangiectasia) is a primary retinal vascular anomaly characterized by telangiectasia and accumulation of lipoproteinaceous exudate in the retina and subretinal space (Sherman *et al.* 1983). Because Coats' disease can be associated with retinal detachment, these children can present with leukokoria and their disease can be clinically difficult to differentiate from retinoblastoma. On CT and MRI, a unilateral dense vitreous without a focal mass is characteristic, and calcification is only occasionally seen. These findings help differentiate Coats' disease from retinoblastoma, which usually presents as a calcified focal mass. The peak incidence occurs toward the end of the first decade. Two-thirds of patients are male.

Persistent hyperplastic primary vitreous (PHPV) is a persistence and hyperplasia of the embryonic hyaloid vascular system (Mafee *et al.* 1982, Mafee and Goldberg 1987). The friability of these vessels may lead to intravitreal hemorrhage. PHPV is the most common cause of leukokoria after retinoblastoma (Howard and Ellsworth 1965). A cone-shaped central retrolental density is characteristic and is usually caused by the persistent primary hyaloid and infrequently the detached dysplastic retina. Calcification is unusual. The appearance of this central conical structure is well imaged by both CT and MRI (Figs. 10.5, 10.9). Norrie's disease is thought by many to be a congenital form of PHPV (Warburg 1963, Apple *et al.* 1974). In addition to the orbital changes, these children have seizures, hearing loss, mental deficiency and cataracts.

Retinopathy of prematurity (ROP) is seen in very immature infants who develop oxygen toxicity from excessive levels of oxygen. Usually bilateral and asymmetric, the

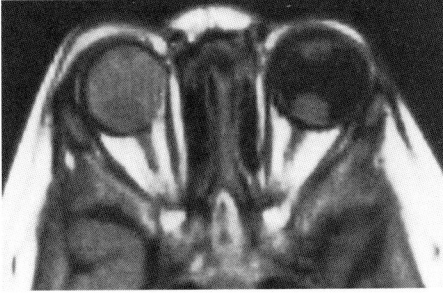

Fig. 10.8. Bilateral retinoblastoma. Bilateral calcified retinoblastomas are visualized by T_1-weighted axial image. The increased signal intensity of the right globe is likely secondary to hemorrhage. Calcification, prominent on CT, is poorly visualized by MRI. (Reproduced by permission from Hopper *et al.* 1992.)

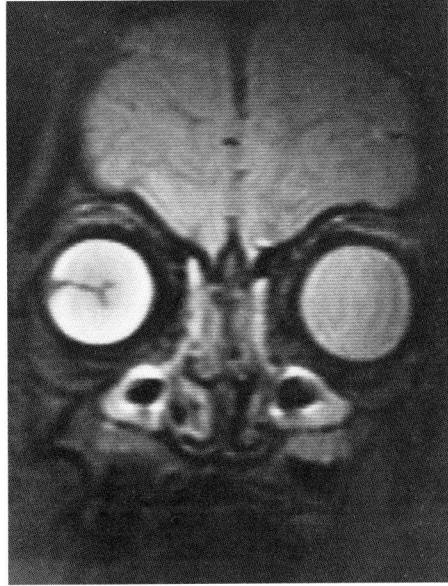

Fig. 10.9. Persistent hyperplastic primary vitreous (PHPV). A cone-shaped, non-calcified central retrolental density is seen in this 3-year-old boy's right eye, visualized best on this coronal T_2-weighted scan. In a child with leukokoria, the imaging of a central cone-shaped density is strongly suggestive of PHPV, although severe retinal detachments cannot be excluded. The increased signal in the right globe is due to hemorrhage. (Reproduced by permission from Magill *et al.* 1990.)

severity of this disorder is dependent upon the birthweight, the amount of oxygen used and the degree of immaturity. In severe cases, these infants develop leukokoria secondary to traction retinal detachments. While ROP was the leading cause of pediatric blindness in the 1950s, its prevalence has since dramatically decreased because of a greater awareness and improved treatment. The retinal detachments where the outer retinal layers are separated by fluid from the underlying retinal pigment epithelial layer are usually easily diagnosed by CT and MRI and differentiated from retinoblastoma.

Sclerosing endophthalmitis is a granulomatous uveitis secondary to a *Toxocara canis* infestation of the eye (Zinkham 1978, Margo *et al.* 1983). Enzyme linked immunosorbent assay for *Toxocara* may be diagnostic. Choroidoretinitis is present in 80 per cent and is bilateral in 85 per cent. Associated convulsions and intracranial calcification are common. A dense vitreous without a discrete mass is usually seen with CT and MRI, a similar pattern as seen with Coats' disease.

Medulloepitheliomas are rare intraocular tumors which occur from the primitive medullary epithelium of the ciliary body and are located anteriorly about the iris (Mafee *et al.* 1985). Occasionally, they may be positioned adjacent to the optic nerve. These children present with leukokoria. On CT and MRI, medulloepitheliomas are usually found to be well-defined, enhance markedly with contrast, and may erode or induce hyperostosis in the orbital wall. The lack of calcification helps differentiate a medullo-epithelioma from a calcified retinoblastoma.

Inflammatory and infectious diseases
Infections and inflammations in and around the eye are the most common orbital disorders of childhood (Weber and Mikulis 1987, Handler *et al.* 1991). While most are superficial (preseptal) and involve the conjunctiva and eyelid (Fig. 10.10), more serious orbital infections are frequently associated with paranasal sinus disease, penetrating trauma, dental or middle ear disease, and as an extension of preseptal disease. In children, three quarters of orbital cellulitis originates as multifocal sinusitis, especially of the ethmoid air cells and the maxillary antrum. As the orbital fat is infiltrated, compression of the superior ophthalmic vein leads to marked eyelid edema. Without prompt treatment, orbital cellulitis can quickly lead to abscess formation and damage to vital orbital struc-tures. CT and MRI are vital in these children in assessing the extent of infection and of abscess formation. A subperiosteal abscess between the periorbita and lamina papyracea usually follows an ethmoid sinusitis. CT and MRI are very useful in helping differentiate preseptal, lacrimal and eyelid infectious processes from true orbital cellulitis.

Thyrotoxicosis (Graves' disease) (Fig. 10.3) is occasionally seen in children. As with affected adults, exophthalmos, a generalized increase in the orbital fat, and diffuse, symmetric and painless enlargement of the extraocular muscles are commonly seen with MRI and CT (Hosten *et al.* 1989, Nugent *et al.* 1990). Because the inferior and medial rectus muscles are most commonly involved with Graves' disease, the orbits should be imaged in the coronal plane. The enlarged muscles typically taper distally at their insertion into the globe, and the muscle edges are regular and sharply defined. There is usually a poor correlation between the amount of orbital involvement and the severity of the patient's hyperthyroidism. The mechanism of Graves' ophthalmopathy is uncertain, with genetics, autoimmune causes, hormones and viruses all having been suggested as possible etiologies. The differential diagnosis for extraocular muscle enlargement includes Graves' disease, lymphoma, orbital pseudotumor, metastatic disease, dural arteriovenous malformation (AVM) and acromegaly.

Orbital pseudotumor, or idiopathic orbital inflammation, is a complex group of painful disorders involving inflammatory infiltration of one or more of the tissues within the bony orbit exclusive of the eyeball (Garner 1973, Curtin 1987, Flanders *et al.* 1989). Frequently, like Graves' disease, patients with pseudotumor present with exophthalmos and extraocular muscle enlargement. However, unlike Graves' disease, the muscle involvement is more asymmetric, the muscle edges are more ill-defined, tapering of the distal muscles is unusual, and the proptosis is painful. Pathologically, an idiopathic inflammation of the orbital structures is usually seen, though any reactive process which

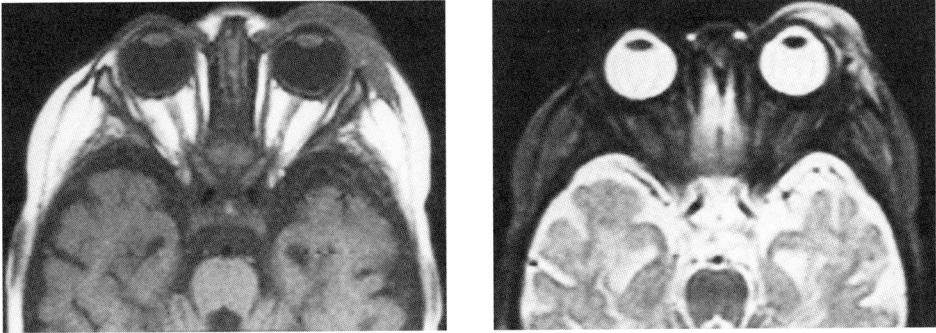

Fig. 10.10. Periorbital cellulitis. This 1-year-old male with Down syndrome and acute lymphocytic leukemia presented with papilledema and a left eyelid cellulitis. The non-contrast axial T_1- *(left)* and T_2-weighted *(right)* images demonstrate marked periorbital swelling with some focal fluid compatible with periorbital cellulitis. The orbital pathology responded promptly to appropriate treatment.

expands the retro-orbital tissues can be considered a pseudotumor. Orbital pseudotumors may be associated with several systemic diseases including Wegener's granulomatosis, sarcoidosis, vasculitis, and lymphoma. Occasionally, orbital pseudotumors are associated with bony destruction (Frohman *et al.* 1986).

Optic neuritis can occur in children. As with adults, the sudden onset of a central vision deficit and orbital pain is common. Axial CT and MR imaging demonstrates diffuse swelling of the optic nerve which usually enhances markedly with contrast administration. While many older patients with optic neuritis have multiple sclerosis, the cause in children is frequently unknown. Occasionally optic neuritis may accompany other infectious, inflammatory and granulomatous processes.

Orbital trauma

Because the facial bones and orbital walls are more elastic in young children, the pediatric facial skeleton is less prone to fracture. In addition, the increased calvarium/face ratio is larger in children, which allows the calvarium to absorb a greater proportion of the blow (Crockett *et al.* 1989). For these reasons, the types of orbital injury from trauma in young children differ from those in adults and even in older children.

Hemorrhage into the anterior chamber is among the most common ocular injuries in children. Penetrating eye injuries are generally more serious than blunt trauma, with infection and orbital foreign bodies as serious sequelae. More serious blunt trauma can cause orbital fractures of the wall, floor and/or roof, optic nerve avulsion, orbital hematomas, retinal tears, and even rupture of the globe itself. In these cases, CT is generally superior in evaluating the bony integrity of the orbit and face as well as in detecting metallic foreign bodies. MRI, on the other hand, detects ocular and optic nerve injuries better than CT.

Fractures of the orbital walls or floor may occur as an isolated event, such as a blow-out fracture from a blow to the eye. Orbital fractures may also be associated with

TABLE 10.4
**Primary and secondary malignant tumors of
the pediatric orbit: experience of the Toronto
Hospital for Sick Children 1919–1981**

Primary tumors	N
Retinoblastoma	148
Rhabdomyosarcoma	14
Uveal melanoma	4
Sarcoma, unclassified	3
Fibrosarcoma	1
Basal cell sarcoma	2
Medulloepithelioma	0
Total cases	172

Secondary tumors (N = 4,384)	%
Acute leukemia	35.9
Chronic leukemia	0.8
Neuroblastoma	9.2
All sarcomas	14.3
Histocytosis	3.9
Hodgkin's lymphoma	11.0
Non-Hodgkin's lymphoma	5.6
Wilm's tumor	6.7
Medulloblastoma	3.5
Other	9.2

fractures of the walls of the maxillary sinus and of the zygomatic arch (tripod fracture). Complex facial fractures which involve the maxilla and pterygoid plates (LeFort I, II and III fractures) usually involve complex fractures of the orbit. While axial and coronal CT better evaluate the bony orbit, MRI may be useful in the assessment of soft-tissue involvement and post-traumatic sequelae (Tonami *et al.* 1991).

Primary tumors

There is a diverse spectrum of benign and malignant tumors which can affect the pediatric orbit (Crawford and Morin 1983, Mafee *et al.* 1987*c*, Stefanyszyn *et al.* 1988) (Table 10.4). Rhabdomyosarcoma (Fig. 10.11) is the most common primary malignant tumor of the orbit in children. However, it is only one tenth as common as retinoblastoma of the globe. Of all pediatric rhabdomyosarcomas, 10 per cent occur primarily in the orbit and another 10 per cent metastasize to or invade the orbit. The median age at presentation is 6 years, and the child presents with rapidly progressing exophthalmos and proptosis of the upper lid. These tumors are highly malignant and invasive and usually originate in the superior orbit. The differential diagnosis includes hemangioma, lymphangioma, dermoid and leiomyoma.

Dermoids and epidermoids are the most common benign orbital tumors of childhood and are found in the upper temporal or upper nasal quadrants. Dermoids are slow growing, can cause adjacent bony erosion, and usually do not cause visual symptoms. The fat content of these tumors aids in their diagnosis.

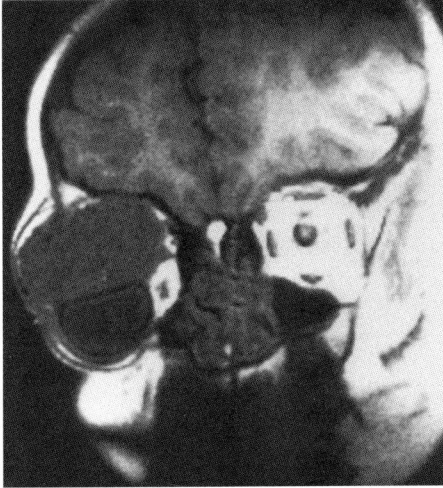

Fig. 10.11. Orbital rhabdomyosarcoma. This young child has a large superior right orbital mass which has compressed and displaced the globe anteriorly and inferiorly. This mass is hypointense on this coronal T_1-weighted image, becoming hyperintense on T_2-weighted images. (Reproduced by permission from Hopper *et al.* 1992.)

There are several orbital vascular abnormalities that can affect the child including orbital varices, AVMs, carotid-cavernous fistulas, capillary and cavernous hemangiomas, blood cysts, arterial malformation, glomus tumors and hemangiopericytomas. Orbital varices are venous dilatations that may cause intermittent proptosis. Typically located along the superior orbit, anterior bony erosions of the roof are characteristic. Superior tortuous dilated vessels are seen on CT and MRI. Scanning during the Valsalva maneuver may help dilate a small varix and differentiate it from a small tumor.

AVMs involving the orbit are extremely rare and usually originate intracranially and communicate with the orbit via the cavernous sinus. Pulsatile proptosis is a common clinical presentation, with chemosis, lid edema and an audible bruit also present. MRI and contrast CT demonstrate multiple tortuous vessels that usually communicate intracranially.

Capillary hemangiomas (Fig. 10.12) are isolated, usually superficial tumors found in the neonate. These infants present with diffusely dilated capillaries and chemosis (excessive edema) of the lid. Capillary hemangiomas often increase in size for six to ten months and then gradually involute. Occasional involvement of the retro-ocular tissues is seen. Cavernous hemangiomas (Fig. 10.13) are one of the more common adult orbital tumors, but their occurrence in children is not uncommon. These tumors are usually located (83 per cent) in the intraconal region. Cavernous hemangiomas present as a homogeneously enhancing mass which displaces but does not involve the optic nerve. Central intraconal masses include, in addition to the cavernous hemangiomas, lymphangiomas, pseudotumors, lymphoma, periperal nerve tumors (neurofibroma, neurilemoma or schwannoma), hemangiopericytoma, and optic nerve gliomas and meningiomas.

Lymphangiomas (vascular hamartomas) are congenital tumors consisting of dilated lymphatic channels surrounded by lymphoid tissue (Graeb *et al.* 1990). These uncommon pediatric lesions may occur in the conjunctiva and eyelid, in the retrobulbar region, or in both (Fig. 10.14). They are benign, slow-growing, encapsulated tumors that cause in-

229

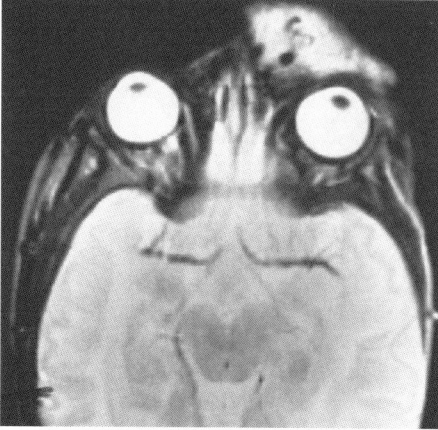

Fig. 10.12. Capillary hemangioma. An axial T$_2$-weighted scan in this 5-month-old female demonstrates a capillary hemangioma superficially and preseptally about the left orbit. Several prominent vessels are noted within the hemangioma. This infant presented with diffusely dilated capillaries and chemosis (excessive edema) of the eyelid. (Reproduced by permission from Hopper *et al.* 1991.)

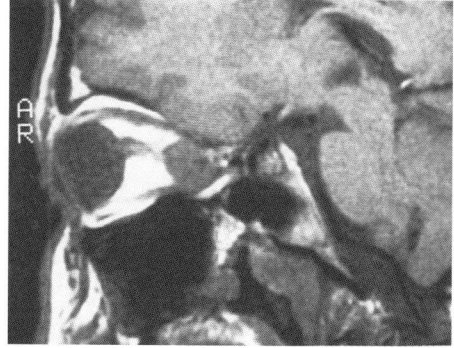

Fig. 10.13. Cavernous hemangioma. A sagittal T$_1$-weighted scan in this 16-year-old male demonstrates an intraconal cavernous hemangioma posteriorly. Cavernous hemangiomas may be differentiated from lymphangioma by their bright enhancement with contrast. (Reproduced by permission from Hopper *et al.* 1992.)

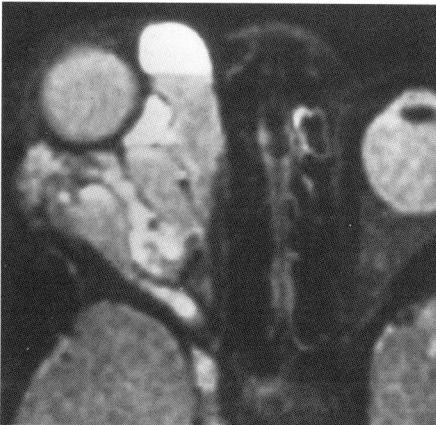

Fig. 10.14. Lymphangioma. This patient experienced sudden proptosis and discoloration about his right eye. T$_2$-weighted MRI demonstrates hemorrhage into a multilocular lymphangioma. The bright methemoglobin is layering anteriorly in each cyst. (By courtesy of Dr Anne Osborn.)

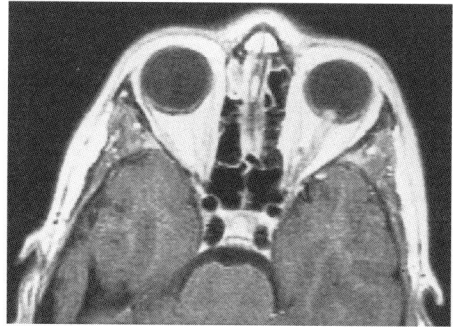

Fig. 10.15. Leukemic infiltration of the optic nerve and retina. This 11-year-old male with acute lymphatic leukemia presented with a mass in the left eye. Axial T$_1$-weighted MRI with gadolinium-DTPA demonstrates diffuse enhancement of the left optic nerve as well as a left retinal enhancing nodule.

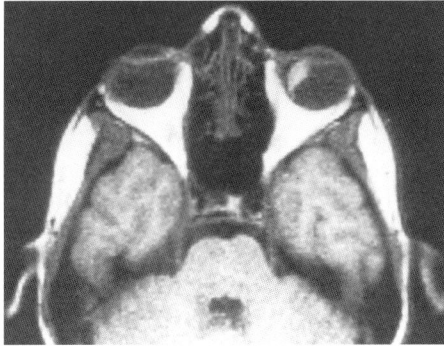

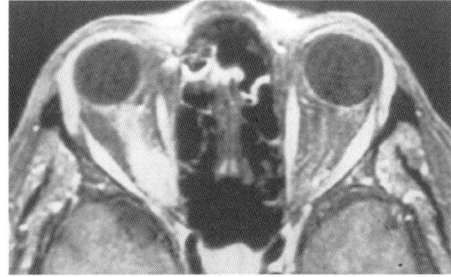

Fig. 10.17. Optic nerve glioma. This 2-year-old male presented with bilateral visual field defects. Contrast enhanced T_1-weighted axial MRI with 'fat-sat' demonstrates a large enhancing mass of the optic chiasm.

Fig. 10.16. Left orbital melanoma. This 17-year-old female presented with a medial right globe mass as seen on this axial T_1-weighted image. This was subsequently proven to be melanoma.

creased exophthalmos and orbital expansion. On CT and MRI, lymphangiomas tend to be less well defined than cavernous hemangiomas, crossing anatomic boundaries such as the conal fascia and orbital septum. While lymphangiomas tend to enhance somewhat with contrast, they do not tend to resemble the dense enhancement of cavernous hemangiomas. Sudden intratumoral hemorrhage is common, resulting in sudden and increased proptosis and the formation of a blood cyst.

Lymphoma of the pediatric orbit may present with either diffuse infiltration or as a focal mass. Nodular lymphoma occurs most commonly about the lacrimal gland, whereas diffuse disease tends to involve the entire intraconal region, encasing the optic nerve and posterior globe. Acute leukemia (Fig. 10.15) can also, in a small percentage of patients, diffusely infiltrate the orbit. More commonly, retinal (13 per cent) and optic nerve (8 per cent) infiltration are seen in conjunction with a swollen, painful eye with proptosis, papilledema, muscle paralysis and retinal hemorrhages. Lymphoid hyperplasia can diffusely infiltrate the orbit and/or involve the lacrimal gland and is usually associated with lymphoma, leukemia, lymphosarcoma, tuberculosis, syphilis and sarcoidosis.

Other less common tumors may primarily involve the orbit. Lacrimal gland tumors may be either epithelial or lymphoid-inflammatory type tumors and present as superficial temporal masses. Childhood orbital melanoma (Fig. 10.16) is rare, with half of the cases occurring about the iris. Melanomas also occur in the ciliary body and posterior choroid. The growth rate of childhood melanoma is the best indicator of malignancy. Osteomas arising within the frontal and ethmoid sinuses may involve the orbit secondarily. Teratomas usually present at or shortly after birth with gross enlargement of the orbit and distortion of the orbital structures and the face. These benign tumors contain multiple types of tissue from all three germ cell layers, and can contain cysts, calcification and areas of fat. Fibroxanthoma is an uncommon focal, encapsulated, benign orbital mass that can be locally invasive. Other mesenchymal tumors such as leiomyoma, leiomyosarcoma,

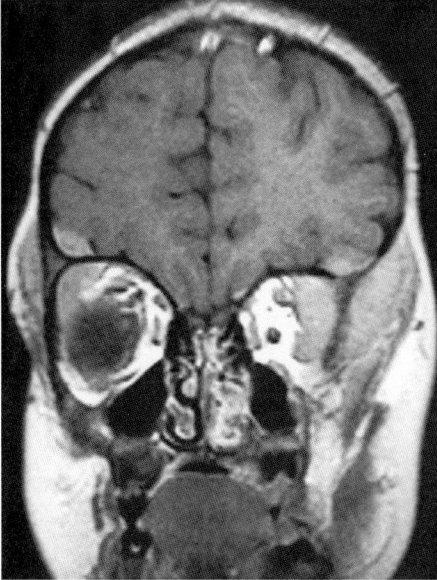

Fig. 10.18. Metastatic neuroblastoma stage 4. This 3½-year-old female presented with a left periorbital soft tissue mass, exophthalmos, and bilateral papilledema. Coronal T$_1$-weighted image with gadolinium-DTPA enhancement demonstrates the left scalp and facial metastatic neuroblastoma infiltrating extraconally into the lateral left orbit and left lacrimal gland. Metastatic disease is also seen in the right orbit, scalp, and epidural region.

lipomas, and liposarcomas are uncommonly seen in the pediatric orbit. Unless associated with neurofibromatosis, optic nerve meningioma is quite rare in the child.

Optic nerve gliomas (juvenile pilocytic astrocytomas) occur primarily in the 2- to 6-year-old child and are associated with neurofibromatosis in 25–50 per cent (Fig. 10.17). There is usually a disparity between the amount of visual loss and the small size of these tumors. Because optic nerve gliomas may remain localized or may extend to and involve the chiasm, MRI is frequently more reliable in determining the tumor's extent. Neural sheath tumors (schwannomas, neurilemomas and neurofibromas) may also involve the orbital nerves. Most schwannomas are associated with neurofibromatosis (10 per cent are malignant) and produce a serpentile thickening of the affected nerve.

Secondary tumors

Unlike in the adult, metastatic involvement of the orbit (see Table 10.4) is less common in children than primary tumors. Intraocular metastases are extremely rare in the pediatric age group whereas adult malignancies commonly metastasize to the ocular choroid. Neuroblastoma (Fig. 10.18) generally occurs in the 2- to 3-year-old child. Secondary orbital involvement is seen in 20 per cent, with metastatic spread of neuroblastoma. Spiculated thickening of the orbital roof, wall or floor is also seen. Histiocytosis involves the orbit in 10 per cent of patients. This involvement may be a focal benign mass, as with eosinophilic granuloma, or a diffuse orbital disease associated with multiple osteolytic bony lesions, as with class I histiocytosis.

A midline granuloma is a destructive inflammatory process that can affect not only the nasal cavity but also adjacent structures. This tumor may represent a localized form of lymphoma, an invasive pseudotumor (Eshaghian and Anderson 1981) or benign sinonasal disease (Som *et al*. 1991). Invasion of the orbit from adjacent tumors is seen with extra-orbital rhabdomyosarcoma, undifferentiated sarcomas, and other anaplastic small, round cell tumors. Mucoceles result from chronic obstruction of a paranasal sinus. Involvement of the frontal and ethmoid sinuses is most common. With the accumulation of secretions, the sinus expands and may encroach upon the orbit. Other benign and malignant masses involving the paranasal sinuses can affect the orbit (Mafee *et al*. 1987*c*).

Conclusion

The advent of CT and MRI has had a dramatic impact upon pediatric ophthalmology. The ability to image the orbit and brain in multiple planes as provided by MRI is of great use in the child with congenital anomalies. Serious inflammatory and infectious diseases are quickly imaged, their extent determined, and appropriate treatment instituted. CT, because it easily evaluates the integrity of the bony orbit and can localize metallic foreign bodies is usually preferred in trauma. Both CT and MRI can differentiate retinoblastoma from other benign mimics (pseudogliomas) in most cases. Finally, orbital imaging in patients with primary or secondary tumors can dramatically improve the detection and localization of lesions and the definition of the extent of invasion.

REFERENCES

Abramson, D.H. (1982) 'Retinoblastoma: diagnosis and management.' *CA: a Cancer Journal for Clinicians*, **32**, 130–140.
Anzai, Y., Lufkin, R.B., Jabour, B.A., Hanafee, W.N. (1992) 'Fat-suppression failure artifacts simulating pathology on frequency-selective fat-suppression MR images of the head and neck.' *American Journal of Neuroradiology*, **13**, 879–884.
Apple, D.J., Fishman, G.A., Goldberg, M.F. (1974) 'Ocular histopathology of Norrie's disease.' *American Journal of Ophthalmology*, **78**, 196–203.
Atlas, S.W., Grossman, R.I., Hackney, D.B., Goldberg, H.I., Bilaniuk, L.T., Zimmerman, R.A. (1988) 'STIR MR imaging of the orbit.' *American Journal of Roentgenology*, **151**, 1025–1030.
Bader, J.L., Meadows, A.T., Zimmerman, L.E., Rorke, L.B., Voute, P.A., Champion, L.A., Miller, R.W. (1982) 'Bilateral retinoblastoma with ectopic intracranial retinoblastoma: trilateral retinoblastoma.' *Cancer Genetics and Cytogenetics*, **5**, 203–213.
Barakos, J.A., Dillon, W.P., Chew, W.M. (1991) 'Orbit, skull base, and pharynx: contrast-enhanced fat suppression MR imaging.' *Radiology*, **179**, 191–198.
Barkovich, A.J., Fram, E.K., Norman, D. (1989) 'Septo-optic dysplasia: MR imaging.' *Radiology*, **171**, 189–192.
Cohen, M.M. (1975) 'An etiologic and nosologic overview of craniosynostosis syndromes.' *Birth Defects*, **11**, 137–189.
Crawford, J.S., Morin, J.D. (1983) *The Eye in Childhood*. New York: Grune & Stratton.
Crockett, D.M., Mungo, R.P., Thompson, R.E. (1989) 'Maxillofacial trauma.' *Pediatric Clinics of North America*, **36**, 1471–1494.
Curtin, H.D. (1987) 'Pseudotumor.' *Radiologic Clinics of North America*, **25**, 583–599.
Dash, R.G., Boparai, M.S., Pai, P. (1984) 'Congenital ectopic encysted eye ball (a case report).' *Indian Journal of Ophthalmology*, **32**, 247–248.
Dixon, W.T. (1984) 'Simple proton spectroscopic imaging.' *Radiology*, **153**, 189–194.
Duke, J.R. (1958) 'Pseudoglioma in children: aspects of clinical and pathological diagnosis.' *Southern Medical Journal*, **51**, 754–759.
Eshaghian, J., Anderson R.L. (1981) 'Sinus involvement in inflammatory orbital pseudotumor.' *Archives of Ophthalmology*, **99**, 627–630
Flanders, A.E., Mafee, M.F., Rao, V.M., Choi, K.H. (1989) 'CT characteristics of orbital pseudotumors and

other orbital inflammatory processes.' *Journal of Computer Assisted Tomography*, **13**, 40–47.

Fries, P.D., Katowitz, J.A. (1990) 'Congenital craniofacial anomalies of ophthalmic importance.' *Survey of Ophthalmology*, **35**, 87–119.

Frohman, L.P., Kupersmith, M.J., Lang, J., Reede, D., Bergeron, R.T., Aleksic, S., Trasi, S. (1986) 'Intracranial extension and bone destruction in orbital pseudotumor.' *Archives of Ophthalmology*, **104**, 380–384.

Garner, A. (1973) 'Pathology of 'pseudotumours' of the orbit: a review.' *Journal of Clinical Pathology*, **26**, 639–648.

Graeb, D.A., Rootman, J., Robertson, W.D., Lapointe, J.S., Nugent, R.A., Hay,. EJ. (1990) 'Orbital lymphangiomas: clinical, radiologic, and pathologic characteristics.' *Radiology*, **175**, 417–421.

Handler, L.C., Davey, I.C., Hill, J.C., Lauryssen, C. (1991) 'The acute orbit: differentiation of orbital cellulitis from subperiosteal abscess by computerized tomography.' *Neuroradiology*, **33**, 15–18.

Hinks, R.S., Quencer, R.M. (1988) 'Multislice chemical shift imaging by slice select gradient reversal (CSI-SSGR).' *Paper presented at the 7th Annual Meeting of the Society of Magnetic Resonance in Medicine, San Francisco.*

Hopper, K.D., Katz, N.N., Dorwart, R.H., Margo, C., Filling-Katz, M., Sherman, J. (1985) 'Childhood leukokoria: computed tomographic appearance and differential diagnosis with histopathologic correlation.' *Radiographics*, **5**, 377–394.

—— Haas, D.K., Sherman, J.L. (1988) 'The radiologic evaluation of congenital and pediatric lesions of the orbit.' *Seminars in Ultrasound, CT and MR*, **9**, 413–427.

—— Sherman, J.L., Boal, D.K.B. (1991) 'Abnormalities of the orbit and its contents in children: CT and MR imaging findings.' *American Journal of Roentgenology*, **156**, 1219–1224.

—— —— —— Eggli, K.D. (1992) 'CT and MR imaging of the pediatric orbit.' *Radiographics*, **12**, 485–503.

Hosten, N., Sander, B., Cordes, M., Schubert, C.J., Schörner, W., Felix, R. (1989) 'Graves ophthalmopathy: MR imaging of the orbits.' *Radiology*, **172**, 759–762.

Howard, G.M., Ellsworth, R.M. (1965) 'Differential diagnosis of retinoblastoma. A statistical survey of 500 children. I. Relative frequency of the lesions which simulate retinoblastoma.' *American Journal of Ophthalmology*, **60**, 610–618.

Imes, R.K., Hoyt, W.F. (1991) 'Magnetic resonance imaging signs of optic nerve gliomas in neurofibromatosis I.' *American Journal of Ophthalmology*, **111**, 729–734.

Keller, P.J., Hunter, W.W., Schmalbrock, P. (1987) 'Multisection fat–water imaging with chemical shift selective presaturation.' *Radiology*, **164**, 539–541.

Linder, B., Campos, M., Schafer, M. (1987) 'CT and MRI of orbital abnormalities in neurofibromatosis and selected craniofacial anomalies.' *Radiologic Clinics of North America*, **25**, 787–802.

Mafee, M.F., Goldberg, M.F. (1987) 'Persistent hyperplastic primary vitreous (PHPV): role of computed tomography and magnetic resonance.' *Radiologic Clinics of North America*, **25**, 683–692.

—— Valvassori, G.E., Capek, V. (1982) 'Computed tomography in the evaluation of patients with persistent hyperplastic primary vitreous (PHPV).' *Radiology*, **145**, 713–717.

—— Peyman, G.A., McKusick, M.A. (1985) 'Malignant uveal melanoma and similar lesions studied by computed tomography.' *Radiology*, **156**, 403–408.

—— Goldberg, M.F., Greenwald, M.J., Schulman, J., Malmed, A., Flanders, A.E. (1987a) 'Retinoblastoma and simulating lesions: role of CT and MR imaging.' *Radiologic Clinics of North America*, **25**, 667–682.

—— Jampol, L.M., Langer, B.G., Tso, M. (1987b) 'Computed tomography of optic nerve colobomas, morning glory anomaly, and colobomatous cyst.' *Radiologic Clinics of North America*, **25**, 693–699.

—— Putterman, A., Valvassori, G.E., Campos, M., Capek, V. (1987c) 'Orbital space-occupying lesions: role of computed tomography and magnetic resonance imaging. An analysis of 145 cases.' *Radiologic Clinics of North America*, **25**, 529–559.

Magill, H.L., Hanna, S.L., Brooks, M.T., Jenkins, J.J., Burton, E.W., Boulden, TF.., Seidel, F.G. (1990) 'Case of the day. Pediatric. Persistent hyperplastic primary vitreous (PHPV).' *Radiographics*, **10**, 515–518.

Mann, I. (1957) *Developmental Abnormalities of the Eye. 2nd Edn.* London: British Medical Association.

Margo, C.E., Katz, N.N.K., Wertz, F.D., Dorwart, R.H. (1983) 'Sclerosing endophthalmitis in children: computed tomography with histopathologic correlation.' *Journal of Pediatric Ophthalmology and Strabismus*, **20**, 180–184.

Nugent, R.A., Belkin, R.I., Neigel, J.M., Rootman, J., Robertson, W.D., Spinelli, J., Graeb, D.M. (1990) 'Graves' orbitopathy: correlation of CT and clinical findings.' *Radiology*, **177**, 675–682.

Sanders, T.E. (1950) 'Pseudoglioma. A clinico-pathologic study of fifteen cases.' *Transactions of the American Ophthalmological Society*, **48**, 575–614.

234

Sherman, J..L, McLean, I.W., Brallier, D.R. (1983) 'Coats' disease: CT–pathologic correlation in two cases.' *Radiology*, **146**, 77–78.

Shields, J.A., Augsburger, J.J. (1981) 'Current approaches to the diagnosis and management of retinoblastoma.' *Survey of Ophthalmology*, **25**, 347–372.

Shukla, Y., Kulshrestha, O.P., Bajaj, K. (1984) 'Congenital cystic eye—a case report.' *Indian Journal of Ophthalmology*, **32**, 249–250.

Simon, J., Szumowski, J., Totterman, S., Kido, D., Ekholm, S., Wicks, A., Plewes, D. (1988) 'Fat-suppression MR imaging of the orbit.' *American Journal of Neuroradiology*, **9**, 961–968.

Slamovits, T.L., Kimball, G.P., Friberg, T.R., Curtin, H.D. (1989) 'Bilateral optic disc colobomas with orbital cysts and hypoplastic optic nerves and chiasm.' *Journal of Clinical Neuro-ophthalmology*, **9**, 172–177.

Som, P.M., Lawson, W., Lidov, M.W. (1991) 'Simulated aggressive skull base erosion in response to benign sinonasal disease.' *Radiology*, **180**, 755–759

Stefanyszyn, M.A., Handler, S.D., Wright, J.E. (1988) 'Pediatric orbital tumors.' *Otolaryngologic Clinics of North America*, **21**, 103–118.

Tien, R.D., Chu, P.K., Hesselink, J.R., Szumowski, J. (1991) 'Intra- and paraorbital lesions: value of fat-suppression MR imaging with paramagnetic contrast enhancement.' *American Journal of Neuroradiology*, **12**, 245–253.

Tonami, H., Yamamoto, I., Matsuda, M., Tamamura, H., Yokota, H., Nakagawa, T., Takarada, A., Okimura, T. (1991) 'Orbital fractures: surface coil MR imaging.' *Radiology*, **179**, 789–794.

Walsh, F.B., Hoyt, W.F. (1969) *Clinical Neuro-ophthalmology. 3rd Edn.* Baltimore: Williams & Wilkins.

Warburg, M. (1963) 'Norrie's disease (atrofia bulborum heriditaria). A report of eleven cases of hereditary bilateral pseudotumour of the retina, complicated by deafness and mental deficiency.' *Acta Ophthalmologica*, **41**, 134–146.

Weber, A.L., Mikulis, D.K. (1987) 'Inflammatory disorders of the paraorbital sinuses and their complications.' *Radiologic Clinics of North America*, **25**, 615–630.

Zimmerman, L.E., Burns, R.P., Wankum, G., Tully, R., Esterly, J.A. (1982) 'Trilateral retinoblastoma: ectopic intracranial retinoblastoma associated with bilateral retinoblastoma.' *Journal of Pediatric Ophthalmology and Strabismus*, **19**, 320–325.

Zinkham, W.H. (1978) 'Visceral larva migrans. A review and reassessment indicating two forms of clinical expression: visceral and ocular.' *American Journal of Diseases of Children*, **132**, 627–633.

11
PEDIATRIC SPINAL DISEASES

Patricia C. Davis

Magnetic resonance studies performed in children have increased in number and complexity in recent years (Barnes *et al.* 1986, Davis *et al.* 1988, Barnes 1992*a,b*). Although plain (X-ray) films and CT remain important for imaging of bony disorders, MRI offers exquisite demonstration of spinal anatomic and pathologic findings without ionizing radiation or the necessity for intrathecal contrast. Growth in clinical indications for pediatric spinal MRI parallels improvements in MRI technology, including faster scanning sequences, tailored spinal surface coils and more reliable monitoring capabilities.

Technical considerations

Factors contributing to image resolution include the field of view, field strength, image matrix, pulse sequence, number of acquisitions, and appropriate matching of surface coil size and configuration to the anatomical area being examined. A variety of spinal surface coil designs may be adapted to advantage in pediatric spinal MRI, especially for small children or those with significant scoliosis. Unfortunately, the geometry and molding of spinal surface coils in general use are sized for adults. If small surface coils are not available, an infant may be placed within an open-ended head coil, an adult knee coil, or feet first in an adult head coil for a spinal examination.

Children, more often than adults, require complete spine or complete spine and brain MRI examinations. Indications for complete spinal examination include scoliosis, meningeal seeding, dysraphism and neurofibromatosis. Timely completion of these complex studies in one sitting without additional appointments or sedation requires efficient selection of pulse sequences, coils, medication and timing of contrast administration. Surface coil technology which facilitates rapid scanning with minimum repositioning of the child is ideal. Creative approaches to this dilemma include technology available on some MRI systems which provides for decoupling of surface coils. This allows simultaneous placement of multiple coils at the start of the procedure, and avoids time-consuming coil exchanges or movement of the sedated child during the study (Davis *et al.* 1993). A flat, license plate shaped spine coil tray or holder can be placed under the patient; this permits precise coil repositioning at measured intervals without disturbing the sedated child. Other options include acquisition of complete spinal images using a body coil and 512×512 matrix images, or sequential spinal column imaging using a long segmented spine coil (Yousem and Schnall 1991).

Most spinal MRI examinations begin with one or more screening spin echo T_1-weighted imaging studies using 3–4mm slice thickness. Sagittal and coronal planes provide screening of long spinal segments with a minimum number of slices. Axial images are added for greater lesion definition at sites of focal disease. Other sequences and planes of imaging depend on the disease suspected or encountered. Multiplanar T_1-weighted imaging provides superb anatomic detail of bone and CSF interfaces. T_2-weighted spin echo imaging provides a myelogram-like image, and aids detection of intramedullary disease, neoplasia, intraspinal cysts, and diastematomyelia. T_2-weighted gradient echo (GRE) pulse sequences may be substituted in some cases to obtain a myelogram-like image or to improve sensitivity for detection of hemorrhage; such imaging has not proved as sensitive for detection of non-hemorrhagic intramedullary disease as conventional T_2-weighted imaging. Spin echo techniques in which multiple echoes can be obtained within a single repetition time (*i.e.* fast spin echo, turbo spin echo, etc.) may be substituted for conventional T_2-weighted imaging in a fraction of the scan time, although the persistent high signal intensity from fat must be considered when bone marrow disorders are suspected. Inversion recovery sequences, such as short tau inversion recovery (STIR) to optimize fat suppression T_1-weighted imaging, or volume acquisition techniques, are used selectively.

Paramagnetic contrast improves imaging of spinal neoplasia or infection/inflammatory diseases. In order to minimize repositioning between pre- and post-contrast sequences, an intravenous catheter is placed in advance. Due to the small doses utilized in children, the paramagnetic contrast dose is carefully flushed through the intravenous tubing in order to ensure adequate administration (Hudgins *et al.* 1991). Contrast enhancement aids characterization and localization of a variety of disorders including: intramedullary neoplasia and demyelinating disease; intradural–extramedullary neoplasia (*i.e.* meningioma, neurofibroma, leptomeningeal neoplasia) or infection; and extradural processes such as diskitis/osteomyelitis, juxtaspinal neoplasia, and postoperative scarring. A preliminary non-contrast T_1-weighted sequence or a fat-suppressed, post-contrast sequence is helpful for differentiation of enhancing from non-enhancing substances which have a short T_1 (*i.e.* fat or methemoglobin).

Normal pediatric spinal MRI
The spinal column in infancy is composed of small incompletely ossified vertebral body centra and relatively large intervening endplate cartilage and intervertebral disks (Ho *et al.* 1988, Sze *et al.* 1991). The small centra appear iso- to hypointense on T_1-weighted, and hypointense on T_2-weighted images in comparison to the adjacent intensity of the disk and endplate cartilage (Fig. 11.1). The intensities of the endplate cartilage and disk are similar on MRI, resulting in poor anatomical differentiation of these structures. By about age 2 years, the increasing mineralization of the vertebrae results in their greater demarcation from the intervening disks and decreased hypointensity on non-contrast T_1- and T_2-weighted images (Fig. 11.2). The normal infant or young child has a straight spinal column or a long, smooth, kyphotic thoracic curve. The cervical and lumbar lordoses and thoracic kyphosis of adulthood develop with weight-bearing in older juveniles and adolescents.

The vertebral body bone marrow is approximately 60 per cent red or hematopoietic marrow during the first decade, and undergoes a progressive transition to a predominantly fatty marrow appearance by young adulthood (Dooms *et al.* 1985). Fatty marrow

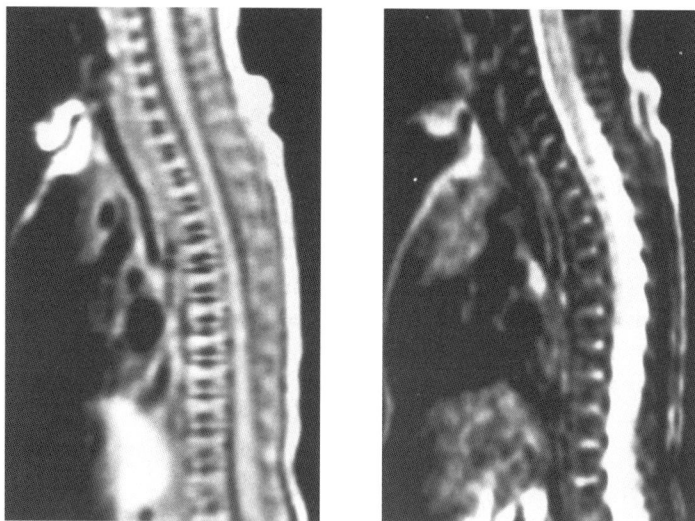

Fig. 11.1. *(Left)* Sagittal T$_1$-weighted image in an infant demonstrates relatively small hypointense vertebral bodies, with large intervening spaces of higher signal intensity which represent disk and adjacent unossified endplate cartilages. Prominent flow void of basivertebral plexus is seen at mid-posterior margin of each vertebral centrum (TR 500, TE 16, 30 mm). *(Right)* Vertebral bodies remain hypointense on T$_2$-weighted image due to predominance of hematopoietic bone marrow at this age (TR 3000, TE 96 effective, 3.0 mm).

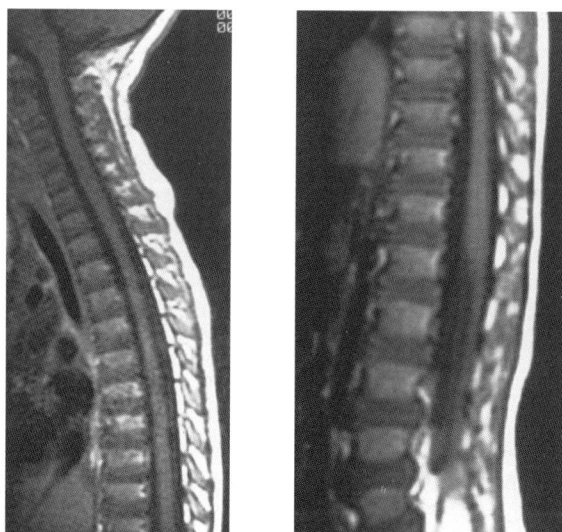

Fig. 11.2. By about age 2 years, increased vertebral body ossification results in better demarcation of vertebra from disk space. Although vertebral bone marrow signal intensity has increased compared to that of infancy, it is similar in intensity to muscle or soft tissue. This reflects continued predominance of red or hematopoietic bone marrow which persists until early adulthood (*Left*—TR 600, TE 11, 3.0 mm; *right*—TR 650, TE 11, 4.0 mm).

238

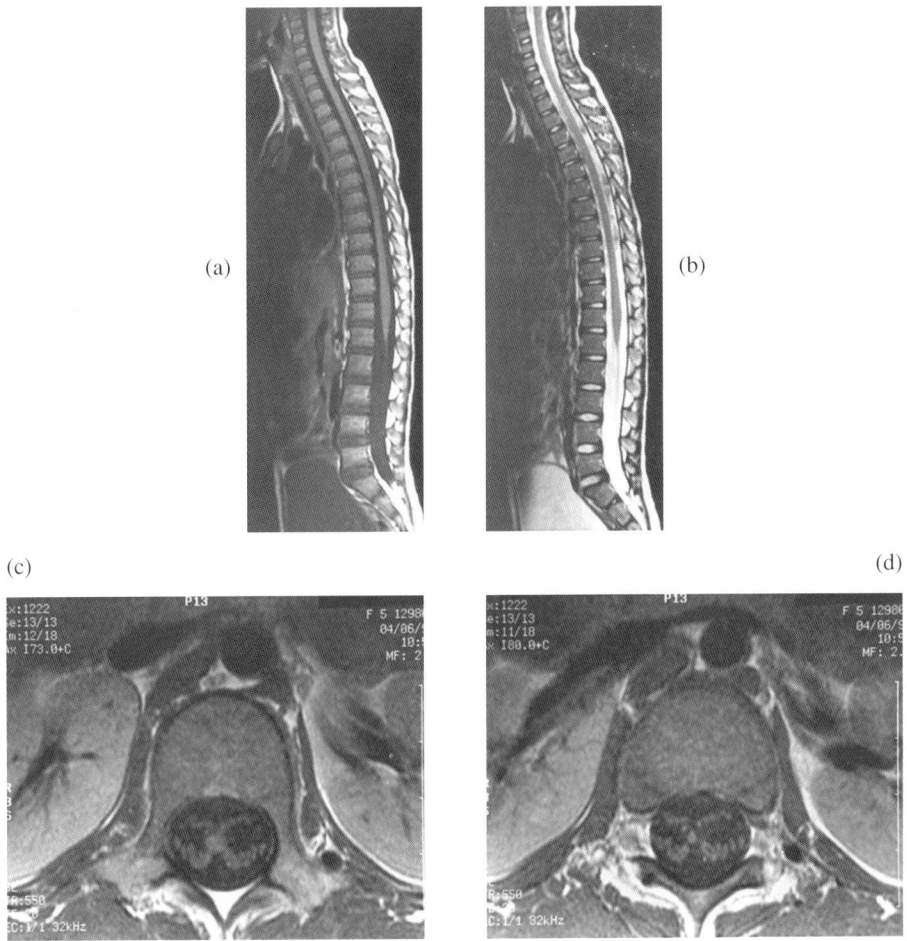

Fig. 11.3. Normal conus medullaris is located at L2–3 disk space or higher, and has smoothly tapered appearance (*a*—TR 500, TE 16, 3.0 mm; *b*—TR 3000, TE 96 effective, 3.0 mm). Axial images demonstrate nerve roots of cauda equina distributed around conus (*c*—TR 550, TE 20, 5.0 mm) and confirm transition from spinal cord to filum terminale (*d*—TR 550, TE 20, 5.0 mm).

conversion to hematopoietic marrow may be relatively rapid in response to physiologic stress; the reverse pattern of conversion from red to fatty marrow has been described with inactivity or immobilization (Minaire *et al.* 1974, Kricun 1985).

The normal conus terminates at or above the L2–3 disk space in infancy and childhood. A conus which terminates at the mid L3 vertebral body is indeterminate, and requires careful clinical evaluation and follow-up (Wilson and Prince 1989). Averaging of the conus with the cauda equina may obscure the level of conus termination if sagittal images alone are utilized; additional coronal or axial images aid in conus localization (Fig. 11.3). The normal filum is visible only on MRI images with sufficient resolution that the individual nerve roots of the cauda equina are detectable (Davis *et al.* 1988). The normal filum termin-ale has a maximum diameter of 2 mm and terminates at the coccyx (Byrd *et al.* 1991).

Other normal findings on pediatric spinal MRI include vertebral body enhancement following paramagnetic contrast in children less than 7 years old; enhancement of the vertebrae and the adjacent endplate cartilage is common in children less than 18 months old (Sze *et al.* 1991*b*). Remnants of the ossification centers, clefts due to notochord remnants, and a prominent basivertebral venous plexus are also common incidental findings. Focal fat deposition occurs when the normal hematopoietic bone marrow is replaced with fatty tissue; the MRI intensities of these foci follow those expected for fat on all pulse sequences. Hajek *et al.* (1987) found a 13 per cent incidence of focal fat deposition in children less than 10 years old; the incidence of focal fat deposition increases with age and pathologic changes such as spondylitis, kyphoscoliosis and spon-dylosis. Vertebral hemangiomas are occasionally encountered in children; they accounted for incidental findings in 11 per cent of the autopsy series of Ross *et al.* (1987). They show as focal areas of high signal intensity in a vertebral body on T_1-weighted images, and are iso- to slightly hyperintense on T_2-weighted images.

Scoliosis

MRI aids detection and localization of many spinal diseases which result in pediatric scoliosis; and scoliosis frequently results in referral for MRI evaluation (Nokes *et al.* 1987). Numerous etiologies account for pediatric onset of scoliosis, including neoplastic, congenital, metabolic, familial, idiopathic, and neuromuscular diseases (in particular, cerebral palsy); scoliosis may also result from surgery, radiation therapy, or infection. A tailored patient history permits choice of appropriate MRI sequences for these children. Imaging of the entire spinal column is necessary, so these examinations are lengthy and require careful planning. MRI scan planes are optimized to align with the child's curvature; oblique or angled images are often required.

An MRI algorithm based on patient history, used to direct and tailor the MRI evalua-tion of scoliosis, is presented opposite (Table 11.1).

Congenital pediatric spinal diseases
Chiari I malformation

Although Chiari I malformation is often thought of as an adult disease, its occurrence in children is well known (Hoffman *et al.* 1987). Presenting symptoms include lower cranial nerve palsies, hydrocephalus, scoliosis, nystagmus, or a dissociation in level of sensory and motor neurologic findings. Bony anomalies of the craniocervical junction or cervical spine associated with Chiari I include partial or complete assimilation of the ring of C1 to the clivus, a short or dysplastic clivus, or Klippel–Feil anomaly. Characteristic MRI findings include downward displacement of the cerebellar tonsils below the foramen magnum. Preliminary studies suggest that the distal cerebellar tonsils normally show progressive ascent with age: Mikulis *et al.* (1992) found them to be located as much as 6 mm below the foramen magnum during the first decade, decreasing to 5 mm in the second decade, in children without evidence of hydromyelia or CNS pathology. In Chiari

TABLE 11.1
MRI algorithm for the evaluation of scoliosis

A. Fatty mass, hairy patch, dermal sinus or surgical repair at several months/years of age = *occult dysraphism protocol*
   1. Sagittal and coronal T_1WI^* and sagittal fast spin echo (FSE) T_2WI^* of lumbosacral spine
   2. Axial T_1WI of sites of tether, hydromyelia, or axial T_2WI of clefts in cord
   3. Sagittal T_1WI, rest of spine

B. Frank myelomeningocele repaired at birth, usually with hydrocephalus = *Arnold–Chiari protocol*
   1. Rule out retether: sagittal and coronal T_1WI and sagittal FSE T_2WI of lumbosacral spine; axial T_1WI of tether site, axial T_2WI of inclusion masses or small clefts *vs* hydromyelia of cord; then sagittal T_1WI of rest of spine to include foramen magnum
   2. Infant with apnea/respiratory compromise: sagittal and coronal T_1WI of foramen magnum/brainstem/upper cord, sagittal T_2WI upper cervical spine and cord, then rest of spine with sagittal T_1WI

C. Congenital vertebral anomalies = *rule out diastematomyelia*
   1. Check level of conus (sagittal and coronal T_1WI lumbosacral spine)
   2. Sagittal and coronal T_1WI of thoracic cord
   3. Axial sequences (T_2WI or T_{2*}) through clefts or anomalies (diastematomyelia)
   4. Sagittal T_1WI of foramen magnum and cervical cord

D. Café-au-lait spots, neurofibromas, positive family history = *rule out neurofibromatosis*
   1. Sagittal FSE T_2WI and coronal T_1WI of area of interest; axial T_1WI or T_2WI and post-contrast T_1WI to define lesions identified
   2. Screen entire spine (coronal T_1WI, sagittal T_2WI)

E. None of above
   1. Check conus position (sagittal and coronal T_1WI lower sacral spine); if abnormal go to occult dysraphism protocol above
   2. If conus position is at L2–3 disc space or higher: coronal T_1WI of thoracic cord (rule out neurofibromatosis); sagittal T_2WI of thoracic cord (rule out cord tumor); sagittal T_1WI of cervical cord and foramen magnum (rule out Chiari I)

*$T1WI$, $T2WI$ = T1-, T2-weighted imaging.

I, the inferior cerebellar tonsils tend to have a peg-like or pointed configuration, with associated crowding of the cervicomedullary junction at the foramen magnum (Fig. 11.4). In some cases, the lack of certainty in differentiation between Chiari I malformation and tonsillar ectopia necessitates follow-up clinical and MRI examination.

Hydromyelia is a common accompaniment of Chiari I and is most prominent in the cervical spinal cord. Inferior extension into the thoracic cord or conus is variable. The spinal cord may be enlarged, normal or atrophic. The cystic contents of a hydromyelic cavity should match the intensity of normal CSF, and the cavity often has a multiseptated 'string of pearls' or 'stack of coins' appearance. Although there are reports of hydromyelic cavities with intensities which do not match those of CSF attributed to stasis or perhaps protein accumulation within the cavity, this finding should raise concern that another process is present such as neoplasia or infection (Davis *et al.* 1988).

After surgical posterior fossa and upper cervical decompression or cord myelotomy and shunting for Chiari I malformation, MRI demonstrates reduction in the size of the

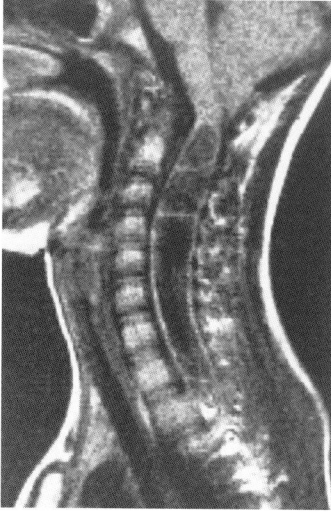

Fig. 11.4. MRI of child who presented at age 4 years with unexplained myelopathy. T_1-weighted image demonstrates characteristic 'stack of coins' appearance of hydromyelia with enlargement of spinal cord and pointed, inferiorly displaced cerebellar tonsils (TR 500, TE 50, 10mm). After surgical decompression, a follow-up examination confirmed decompression of hydromyelia.

hydromyelic cavity, cessation of pulsatile flow within the cavity, and diminished cervicomedullary compression at the foramen magnum (Enzmann *et al.* 1987, Slasky *et al.* 1987) (Fig. 11.4). T_2-weighted images without flow compensatory gradients or gating enhance MRI visualization of pulsatile flow within cavities of hydrosyringomyelia. Persistent enlargement of the hydrosyringomyelia cavity and/or demonstration of persistent pulsatile CSF flow suggest incomplete or unsuccessful decompression (Enzmann *et al.* 1987, Slasky *et al.* 1987). In a prospective study of children with Chiari I and scoliosis, Muhonen *et al.* (1992) found that craniocervical decompression in younger children (*i.e.* under 10 years) often resulted in stabilization or improvement of spinal curvature. Most children also had improvement in myelopathic findings of short preoperative duration or stabilization of long-standing myelopathy.

Chiari II malformation
Arnold–Chiari or Chiari II malformation is overwhelmingly associated with frank myelomeningocele which requires surgical repair within a few days of birth to prevent infection. The neural tube fails to close distally to form the central canal, resulting in an exposed neural placode. The overlying posterior spinal bone, dura and subcutaneous tissues are secondarily deficient. Most children born with Chiari II have or soon develop significant hydrocephalus and require shunting early in infancy. Intracranial findings include: fusion or dysplasia of the colliculi; downward displacement of the fourth ventricle, medulla, and cerebellum below the foramen magnum; a large massa intermedia; partial or complete agenesis of the corpus callosum; a hypoplastic cerebellar tentorium; absent or fenestrated falx; and gray matter heterotopias (Naidich *et al.* 1980*a,b,c*).

Spinal MRI examinations of children with Chiari II malformation are indicated for evaluation of symptomatology referable either to the foramen magnum or to the site of

242

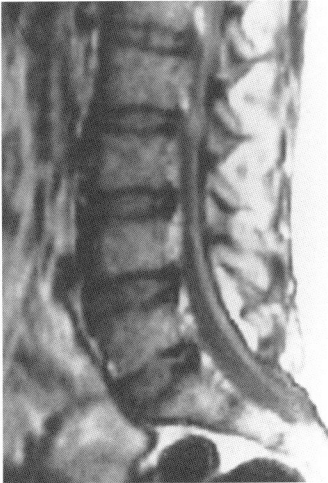

Fig. 11.5. Sagittal T$_1$-weighted image of lumbosacral spine demonstrates small dorsal defect in vertebral canal at S1 and S2. This is site of myelomeningocele repair in child with Chiari II malformation. Neural placode extends caudally to repair site and is usually scarred or retethered at site of closure (TR 516, TE 20, 4.0mm).

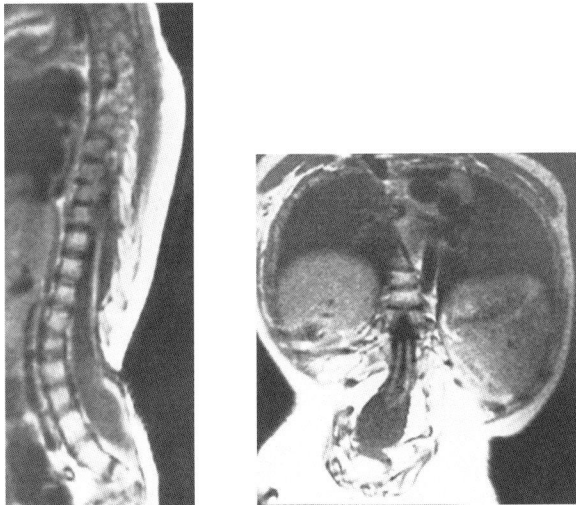

Fig. 11.6. MRI for symptoms suggesting retether in child with Chiari II. *(Left)* Scarring of neural placode at myelomeningocele repair site is apparent on sagittal T$_1$-weighted image (TR 700, TE 30, 5.0mm). *(Right)* Coexisting hydromyelia was confidently diagnosed only on coronal image (TR 700, TE 30, 5.0mm). (Reprinted by permission from Davis *et al.* 1988.)

the previously repaired myelomeningocele (*i.e.* retether). Sequences are described in the algorithm above. Children referred for foramen magnum symptoms have apnea or dysfunction of the medulla in association with dysplasia of brainstem nuclei, brainstem compression at the foramen magnum, arachnoid cyst, ventricular shunt malfunction, and/or syringobulbia. The spectrum of posterior fossa and foramen magnum anomalies in

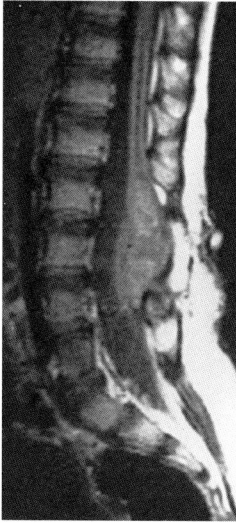

Fig. 11.7. Child with Chiari II and closure of myelomeningocele in infancy presented with progressive symptoms clinically related to retether. T_1-weighted image demonstrates focal expansion of distal neural placode by slightly hyperintense mass relative to adjacent spinal cord, surgically confirmed as epidermoid. Note also hydromyelia with slight cord enlargement and retether at myelomeningocele repair site (TR 720, TE 30, 4.0mm).

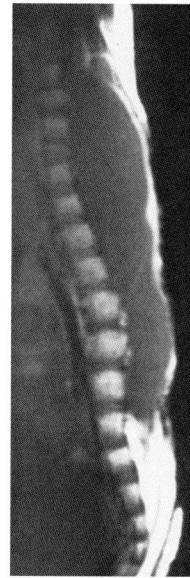

Fig. 11.8. Extensive hydromyelia is occasionally present in Chiari II, as demonstrated on T_1-weighted coronal image. Note 'stack of coins' appearance of upper thoracic spinal cord and secondary enlargement of vertebral canal (TR 700, TE 30, 5.0mm). (Reprinted by permission from Davis *et al.* 1988.)

Chiari II is variable in severity, and the role and appropriate timing of craniocervical surgical decompression is a subject of ongoing discussion (Park *et al.* 1985). Indeed, respiratory dysfunction attributed either to compression of the cervicomedullary junction within a relatively small bony foramen or to dysgenesis of the medullary nuclei is one of the leading causes of morbidity and mortality in Chiari II children.

More frequent presenting symptoms, particularly in older children, are related to the myelomeningocele repair site and thoracolumbar spine. These include loss of lower extremity function or continence, pain, scoliosis, or myelopathy. The initial operative closure of a myelomeningocele is complex, and may require skin or dural grafts to cover the deficient posterior spinal soft tissues. After closure, the distal spinal cord or neural placode is characteristically scarred ('retethered') to the dorsal spinal canal at the myelomeningocele repair site whether or not retether is apparent clinically (Tamaki *et al.* 1988) (Figs. 11.5, 11.6). Symptomatic tethering due to scarring of the neural placode includes progressive motor and sensory changes, incontinence, scoliosis, and back or leg pain (Yamada *et al.* 1981*b*). Postulated etiologies include continuous or intermittent traction on the spinal cord due to distal cord fixation with resultant spinal cord ischemia (Yamada *et al.* 1981*b*). Progressive deficits in Chiari II children may also result from hydromyelia,

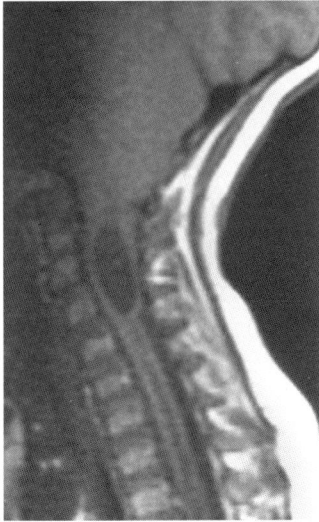

Fig. 11.9. Child with Chiari II and prior closure of myelomeningo-cele underwent MRI for evaluation of progressive apnea and lower cranial neuropathies. Sagittal T_1-weighted image demonstrates hydrobulbia at level of medulla and hydromyelia in cervical spinal cord (TR 450, TE 11, 3.0mm).

inclusion masses related to the primary surgical closure (*i.e.* lipoma, dermoid or epidermoid), bony subluxation, scoliosis, acquired arachnoid cysts or, infrequently, diastematomyelia (Scott *et al.* 1986, Rabb *et al.* 1992) (Figs. 11.7, 11.8). Evaluation of the entire spinal canal in the symptomatic child is essential in order to exclude these potential sources of disability.

Hydromyelia is present in 30 to 70 per cent of Chiari II children, and when severe, may produce vertebral canal expansion (Fig. 11.8). Hydrobulbia, although less frequent than hydromyelia, results in significant brainstem dysfunction (Fig. 11.9). Ventricular decompression, foramen magnum decompression and direct myelotomy are surgical techniques used to decompress symptomatic hydromyelia. Children with Chiari II often have localized or more severe hydromyelia in the lumbar and thoracic spinal cord than the cervical cord (Samuelsson *et al.* 1987). T_1-weighted MRI is useful to demonstrate the size and location of hydromyelic cavities, localize levels for surgical decompression, and assess adequacy of decompression postoperatively. In Chiari II as well as Chiari I, T_2-weighted imaging without flow compensatory techniques has a role in judging adequacy of decompression of these cavities and defining cord gliosis. MRI evaluation of cord motion or pulsatility has been studied for differentiation of symptomatic from asympto-matic retether, although demonstration of cord pulsatility with spinal ultrasonography has not correlated precisely with clinical evidence of tether (Levy *et al.* 1988, Curless *et al.* 1992).

Chiari III malformation
Chiari III malformation is described as a cervical myelomeningocele and/or occipital en-cephalocele with caudal displacement of the fourth ventricle. Hydromyelia and anomalies of the brainstem are associated findings. Chiari III is less common than the other Chiari

245

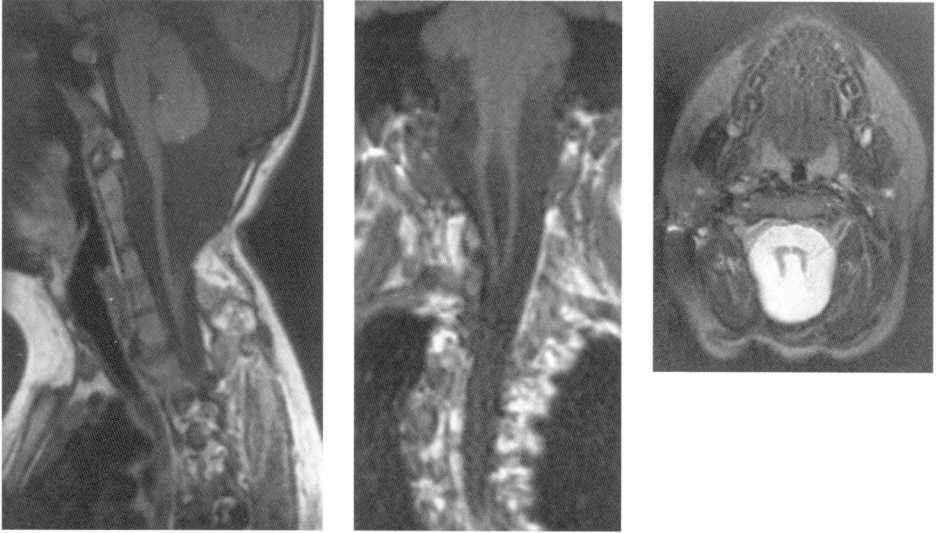

Fig. 11.10. Child who had postnatal surgical repair for occipital–cervical encephalocele/myelomeningocele (Chiari III). *(Left)* Cervicomedullary posterior meningocele is demonstrated on T_1-weighted image (TR 612, TE 20, 4.0mm). *(Centre)* Coronal image additionally reveals vertebral anomalies and hydromyelia (TR 415, TE 20, 4.0mm). *(Right)* Axial T_2-weighted image suggests dorsal expansion of hydromyelia into exophytic hydromyelia and/or myelocystocele (TR 2500, TE 90, 7.0mm).

malformations, and has a poorer prognosis for survival (Chapman *et al.* 1989, Castillo *et al.* 1992) (Fig. 11.10). The entire spinal cord should be assessed with MRI, primarily to exclude hydromyelia or myelocystocele.

Chiari IV malformation
This formerly used term refers to aplasia of the cerebellum, which is now classified with other cerebellar anomalies rather than with the Chiari malformations.

Occult dysraphism
The category of occult dysraphism includes skin-covered dorsal dysraphism (lipomyelo-meningocele, lipomyelocele, diastematomyelia, thickened filum, filum lipoma, dermal sinus, sacral dysgenesis, myelocystocele, meningocele), inclusion masses (dermoid, epidermoid, teratoma), caudal regression anomalies, and dysraphic lesions associated with congenital vertebral anomalies (neurenteric cysts, diastematomyelia). Children with occult forms of dysraphism have no overt myelomeningocele or other stigmata of Chiari II malformation; instead they have neurological or urogenital dysfunction and/or cutaneous stigmata such as a hairy patch (hypertrichosis), palpable lipoma, hemangioma, telangiectasia, nevus, asymmetric gluteal cleft, or dermal sinus. The cutaneous findings may be subtle or overlooked into late childhood or even adulthood. A focal failure of separation of neuroectodermal from mesodermal tissue during closure of the neural tube

246

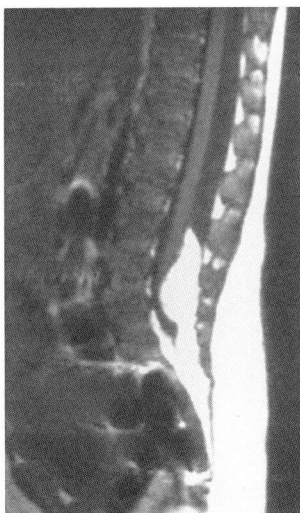

Fig. 11.11. Young child, referred because of sacral fatty mass, has lipomyelocele. Note that lipoma within paraspinal soft tissues is inseparable from normal subcutaneous fat. Lipoma is demonstrated in lower vertebral canal with cephalad extension to the dorsal conus. Conus is abnormally low, terminating at L4 or lower (TR 333, TE 20, 3.0mm).

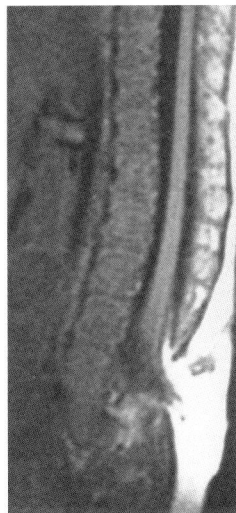

Fig. 11.12. Infant with lipomyelodysplasia has small intradural lipoma extending to dorsal conus, focal spina bifida at lumbosacral junction, and prominent sacral lipoma (TR 469, TE 30, 5.0mm).

is postulated as the etiology for many of these lesions; the result is development of dorsal inclusion masses, such as epidermoids, dermoids, lipomas and teratomas, which are inseparable from the dorsal spinal cord. Surgical untethering in infancy is advocated in order to prevent or halt progression of neurologic deficits (James and Walsh 1981).

In lipomyelomeningocele or lipomyelodysplasia, lipomatous tissue extends cephalad from the unfused bony lamina at the site of occult dysraphism to interface with the dorsal conus and/or filum terminale. The conus terminates caudal to the L2–3 disk space and is tethered primarily by the lipoma; symptoms result from tether rather than mass effect of the lipomatous tissue itself. Occasionally lipomyelodysplasia is associated with diastemato-myelia or hydromyelia; vertebral lesions including segmentation anomalies, butterfly vertebra, and partial sacral aplasia are common. The lipoma may be primarily intra- or extradural, or both intra- and extradural in location; those without enlargement of the spinal canal and thecal sac are referred to as lipomyelocele (Figs. 11.11–11.13). Since neural elements are often intermingled with the intraspinal components of the lipoma, careful surgical monitoring is required in order to untether the distal spinal cord without damaging the neural elements intermingled with it. Extensive resection of the intrathecal component of the lipoma itself may not be possible or desirable. Although the cutaneous and extradural lipoma is recognizable on MRI due to its mass effect, the extradural lipoma is inseparable from the normal subcutaneous tissues by signal intensity (Davis *et al.* 1988) (Fig. 11.11).

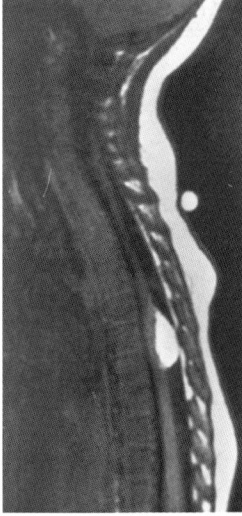

Fig. 11.13. Focal intraspinal lipoma, surgically confirmed, in child with intraspinal high signal intensity mass inseparable from dorsal aspect of thoracic spinal cord. Cutaneous stigmata of occult dysraphism are apparent overlying lesion (TR 612, TE 20, 3.0mm).

Although lipoma is the most common intraspinal neoplasia associated with dysraphism, other congenital spinal masses include dermoids, epidermoids and teratomas. Dermoid and epidermoid tumors arise from rests of dermal or epidermal tissues in association with incomplete developmental separation of the mesoderm (*i.e.* closed dysraphism or Chiari II malformation) or iatrogenic implantation (surgery, spinal puncture) (Scott *et al.* 1986). Dermoid tumors or cysts include tissues of dermal and epidermal origin, such as sebaceous glands, hair follicles, and keratinizing debris. Epidermoids contain keratinizing debris and epithelial cells. Although intracranial dermoids have a high signal intensity due to their associated fat content, spinal dermoids and epidermoids are variable in signal intensity and may be similar to CSF or neural tissue on all sequences. Intraspinal epidermoids may have signal intensities on MRI which mimic CSF on all sequences, rendering them difficult to diagnose and to differentiate from arachnoid cyst preoperatively (Barkovich *et al.* 1991). Epidermoids are frequently identified following closure of a myelomeningocele, perhaps related to inclusion of epidermal elements in the closure site (Fig. 11.7). Dermoids may have a slightly to definitely high signal intensity on T_1-weighted images, rendering differentiation from lipoma difficult. Spinal teratomas in association with dysraphism are uncommon; sacrococcygeal teratomas without dysraphism are discussed below. Teratomas contain tissues of all three germinal layers resulting in a complex and heterogeneous MRI pattern on all sequences. Lipoma, dermoid or teratoma are suspected when an intraspinal mass has a high signal intensity on T_1-weighted images; reliable criteria for differentiation between these entities on MRI have not been established. Those associated with occult dysraphism usually occur in the lumbar canal, with rare examples occurring in the thoracic or cervical regions (Figs. 11.13, 11.14).

Diastematomyelia refers to a division of the spinal cord (not a duplication), either partially or completely into two distinct hemicords. Diplomyelia refers to a duplication of

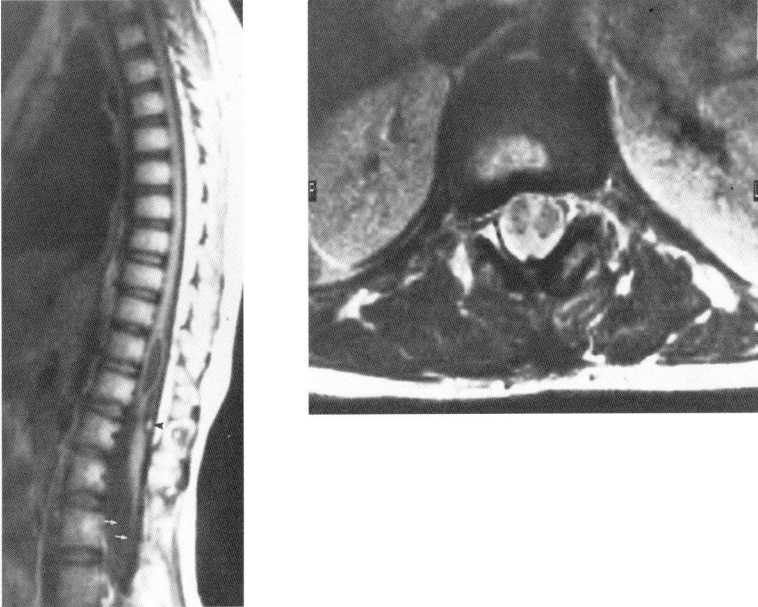

Fig. 11.14. Female child referred for suspected occult tether has abnormally low conus at L3–4 and two thickened fila *(arrows)*. *(Left)* Upper spinal cord contains small hydromyelic cavity, and small high signal intensity mass, surgically proven as teratoma, is present behind spinal cord *(arrowhead)* (TR 860, TE 30, 5.0 mm). A transverse image through upper CSF intensity lesion confirmed hydromyelia, while an axial image through distal conus at L3 demonstrated division of spine into two hemicords. *(Right)* T$_2$-weighted image reveals incomplete small posterior septum, indicating that hemicords are contained within one thecal sac (TR 1934, TE 100, 10 mm). (Reproduced by permission from Davis *et al.* 1988.)

the spinal canal or contents; this is very rare to non-existent in humans. Diastematomyelia has a female predominance and is associated with cutaneous stigmata in 50–75 per cent of cases. Vertebral anomalies include hemivertebra, butterfly vertebra, laminar anomalies, and intersegmental fusion. Diastematomyelia occurs in isolation, associated with other occult or skin covered dysraphism, or rarely with Chiari II malformation.

MRI demonstrates that the spinal cord division in diastematomyelia may be asymmetric, incomplete, or with one hemicord positioned more ventrally within the thecal sac than the other. The two hemicords often reunite into one cord distal to the diastematomyelia, and the distal cord is usually tethered by a thickened filum (Naidich and Harwood-Nash 1983). About half have associated splitting of the thecal sac into two separate sacs; the remainder have a divided spinal cord which is contained within one arachnoid–dural sheath (Schlesinger *et al.* 1986). A bony, cartilaginous or fibrous septum which results in tethering of the distal cord may be interposed between the hemicords; localization of this septum is important for surgical resection. Only about 40 per cent of diastematomyelic cords have this tethering band or septum between the hemicords; the remainder are tethered by other entities such as a thickened filum or a lipoma. Other

249

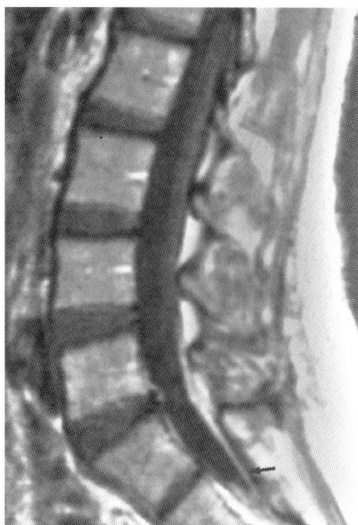

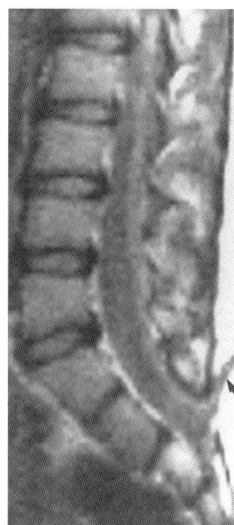

Fig. 11.15. Incidental fibrolipoma of filum is present in dorsal thecal sac on T_1-weighted image in patient studied with MRI for symptoms related to disk disease *(arrows)* (TR 498, TE 20, 4.0mm). Conus had normal position and configuration.

Fig. 11.16. Dermal sinus is visible posteriorly in sacral soft tissues *(arrow)* with intraspinal extension to tethered spinal cord (TR 550, TE 30, 5.0mm).

fibrous tethering bands may be additional sources of cord tether; CT with water soluble intrathecal contrast may be required to demonstrate these bands. Hydromyelia and/or congenital midline tumors may accompany diastematomyelia; one or both hemicords may contain hydromyelic cavities (Hilal *et al.* 1974, Schlesinger *et al.* 1986) (Fig. 11.14).

Children suspected of diastematomyelia or occult dysraphism, and those who harbor vertebral anomalies, should have MRI evaluation of the conus termination, distal spinal canal and focal vertebral anomalies. Confident differentiation between diastematomyelia and a small or localized hydromyelic cavity on T_1-weighted images may be difficult. Axial T_2-weighted imaging of the area of concern is helpful for exclusion of a tethering band or septum in diastematomyelia and identification of focal hydromyelia (Davis *et al.* 1988).

A thickened filum terminale may accompany other forms of occult or overt dysraphism or infrequently occur as an isolated anomaly. The normal filum is approximately the size of a spinal nerve root (2mm or less in diameter); a thickened filum is associated with fibrous, fatty or cystic enlargement of the filum and an abnormally low conus termination. Fatty or lipomatous infiltration of the filum without an abnormally low conus termination in adults may be asymptomatic and incidental; in children this finding warrants careful clinical and follow-up imaging studies (Fig. 11.15).

A dorsal dermal sinus may terminate in the spinal subcutaneous soft tissues or be associated with a dermal tract which extends to the spinal canal, the dura, or intrathecally to the filum (Barkovich *et al.* 1991, Byrd *et al.* 1991). The tract may be a source of spinal

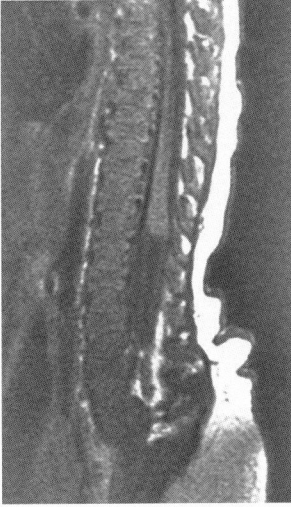

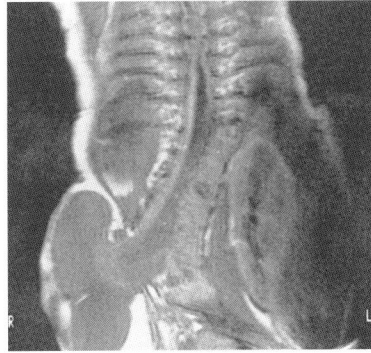

Fig. 11.18. Infant with large skin-covered dorsal mass related to lumbosacral dysraphism has distal cord expansion around CSF intensity cyst, or myelocystocele. Note associated vertebral anomalies (TR 500, TE 30, 4.0 mm).

Fig. 11.17. Child with caudal regression, with narrow pelvis, wide symphysis pubis, sacral hypoplasia and hip dislocation demonstrated on plain films. MRI demonstrates truncated appearance of distal conus associated with aplasia of sacral components of cord (TR 516, TE 20, 3.0 mm).

infection or CSF leakage, and may extend to an intrathecal thick filum, dermoid cyst, epidermoid or lipoma. MRI offers a noninvasive method for screening of intraspinal pathology associated with a dermal sinus; careful scrutiny of the extraspinal soft tissues may reveal the dermal tract itself in the overlying subcutaneous tissues (Fig. 11.16).

The caudal regression anomalies are associated with occult dysraphism and tether. Included in this category are children with the VATER syndrome (*v*ertebral anomalies, *a*nal atresia, *t*racheo-*e*sophageal fistula, and *r*adial and *r*enal anomalies), caudal regression syndrome and other anorectal anomalies (Barnes 1992). Spinal MRI can be combined with pelvic MRI for diagnosis of both pelvic and spinal anomalies (Carson *et al.* 1984, Sato *et al.* 1988). Renshaw (1978) suggested a classification of sacral agenesis; four types are recognized based on increasing incidence and severity of associated anomalies. The caudal regression syndromes may result in a truncated appearance of the distal conus on MRI which is thought to result from hypoplasia of the sacral neural elements (Barkovich *et al.* 1989) (Fig. 11.17).

Myelocystocele is characterized by expansion of the distal central canal at the neural placode into a large dorsal ependyma-lined cyst; the large cyst is enclosed within a meningocele but does not communicate with the subarachnoid space. This rare anomaly is often skin-covered, possibly a variant of myelomeningocele, and is associated with caudal regression syndromes and cloacal exstrophy (McLone and Naidich 1985, Vade and Kennard 1987) (Fig. 11.18).

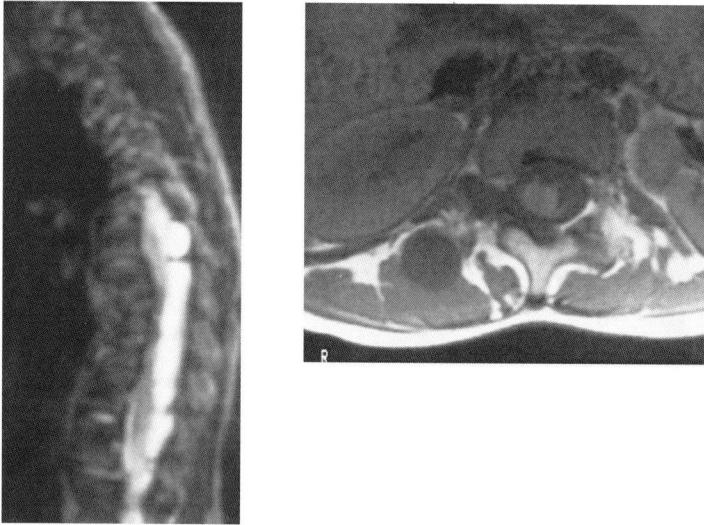

Fig. 11.19. *(Left)* Sagittal T$_2$-weighted image demonstrates several dorsal arachnoid cysts with ventral displacement of spinal cord in child with congenital vertebral anomalies and scoliosis (TR 2015, TE 90, 4.0mm). *(Right)* Lateral meningocele was confirmed on axial image (TR 685, TE 20, 5.0mm).

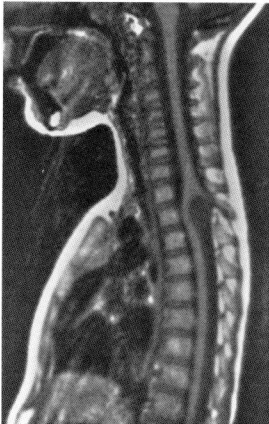

Fig. 11.20. Sagittal T$_1$-weighted image demonstrates small dorsal glial tract with small skin covered meningocele at T1–2 (TR 500, TE 15, 4.0mm).

Simple meningocele is a CSF-filled enlargement of the thecal sac which freely communicates with the subarachnoid space and has no associated abnormal neural elements. It may be enclosed by an enlarged but intact spinal canal (*i.e.* sacral meningocele) or herniated through unfused lamina into the dorsal spinal canal and soft tissues. Lateral meningocele is associated with neurofibromatosis and may be single or at multiple spinal levels. Anterior meningoceles are considered in the spectrum of neurenteric canal defects. MRI is useful to identify these anomalies, although CT following intrathecal contrast injection may be necessary to identify sites of communication with the thecal sac (Fig. 11.19). Other uncommon cystic lesions include congenital or acquired arachnoid cyst, enterogenous cysts and neurenteric cysts.

The upper thoracic and cervical spine is an infrequent primary site for dysraphic lesions. Upper spinal column disorders include myelomeningocele with or without Chiari III malformation, dermal sinus and tract, anterior or lateral meningocele, arachnoid cyst, neurenteric and duplication cysts, and rarely diastematomyelia (Beyerl *et al.* 1985) (Fig. 11.20).

Osteodystrophies and skeletal dysplasias

A variety of systemic diseases affect the spinal column, including biochemical disorders (calcium or phosphorus metabolism, glycogen storage diseases), hematopoietic disorders, chromosomal abnormalities, primary disorders of bone (osteogenesis imperfecta), connective tissue disorders, and phakomatoses (see below). Many types of osteochondro-dysplasias have been described; these often heritable disorders associated with short stature are characterized by intrinsic abnormalities in growth and remodeling of cartilaginous and osseous tissues. These entities may be associated with primary vertebral body abnormalities (platyspondyly, gibbus), kyphoscoliosis, structural instability (*i.e.* C1–2 ligamentous laxity or subluxation), spinal stenosis, pathologic fractures (osteomalacia, osteoporosis) and/or basilar impression.

Multiplanar MRI is useful for noninvasive demonstration of spinal canal or foramen magnum stenosis in children with varied craniocervical pathology or unexplained torticollis (Hawkes *et al.* 1983). Achondroplasia is the most common category of short limb dwarfism, and is transmitted as an autosomal dominant disorder with an 80 to 90 per cent incidence of new mutations. Standard growth curves for achondroplasia have been established (Horton *et al.* 1978, Hecht *et al.* 1985). In achondroplasia, enchondral bone formation is abnormal, and the spine and skull base are primarily affected. The subarachnoid spaces at the foramen magnum and the cisterna magna are very small, and dilated ventricles and subarachnoid spaces are common (Fig. 11.21). Macrocephaly and/or hydrocephalus have been documented in achondroplasia; reference to standard growth curves is helpful in evaluation of macrocephaly (Horton *et al.* 1978). Elevated venous sinus pressure, fourth ventricular outflow obstruction or obstruction in the subarachnoid space may contribute to macrocephaly or hydrocephalus in these children (Kao *et al.* 1989). Symptomatic spinal stenosis of the cervical spine presents early in childhood, while symptoms from thoracolumbar kyphosis and/or spinal stenosis develop later, from the late teens to early adulthood. A progressive lumbar decrease in interpediculate distance is characteristic; 40 to 50 per cent of persons with achondroplasia are affected (Yamada *et al.* 1981*a*). A variety of other short stature dysplasias are associated with spinal stenosis, craniovertebral instability and kyphoscoliosis (Hecht *et al.* 1985).

Children with mucopolysaccharidosis may have spinal canal compression due to ligamentous laxity, enlarged pedicles and lamina, or dural thickening and infiltration. Osseous dysplasia such as metatropic and diastrophic dysplasia are associated with kyphoscoliosis which may result in neurologic deficits. Spondyloepiphyseal dysplasia is

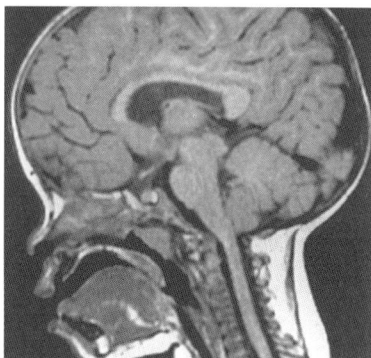

Fig. 11.21. Child with apnea and achondroplasia evaluated with MRI for foramen magnum stenosis. Sagittal T$_1$-weighted image (TR 50, TE 19, 4.0mm) reveals small foramen magnum; this was confirmed on axial T$_2$-weighted image.

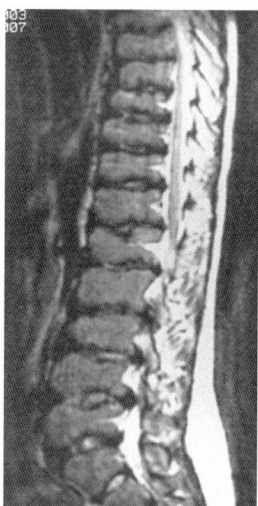

Fig. 11.22. This child with spondyloepiphyseal dysplasia underwent MRI because of myelopathy. T$_2$-weighted image demonstrates vertebral end-plate abnormalities and platyspondyly at many levels, and confirms multilevel spinal stenosis (TR 4000, TE 112 effective, 4.0mm).

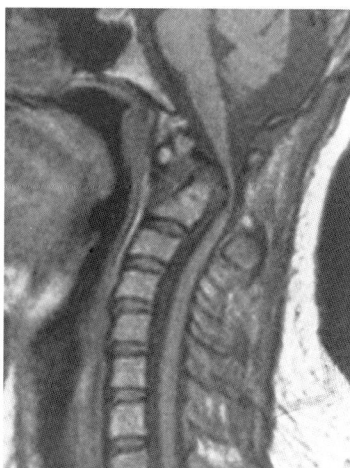

Fig. 11.23. MRI confirms spinal canal comprom-ise and cord compression associated with os odontoideum and C1–2 alignment abnormality in adolescent with Down syndrome (TR 700, TE 30, 5.0mm).

associated with progressive shortening of the trunk related to platyspondyly and spinal stenosis (Fig. 11.22). Atlantoaxial instability also contributes to neurologic symptoms.

Children with Down syndrome may have instability and subluxation or stenosis of the craniocervical junction due to a variety of anomalies of C1–2. Although ligamentous laxity is frequent, other craniocervical abnormalities include a hypoplastic odontoid, odontoid dysplasia, os odontoidium, and hypoplasia of the posterior arch of C1 (Martel and Tishler 1966, Martich *et al.* 1992) (Fig. 11.23). Pueschel and Scola (1987) identified an incidence of atlanto-axial instability in 14.6 per cent of individuals with Down syndrome. Multiplanar MRI allows noninvasive visualization of the foramen magnum and upper cervical spine for spinal cord compression; plain films or rapid sequence MRI in flexion and extension are used to confirm severity and level of subluxation and adequacy of the subarachnoid spaces (Pueschel and Scola 1987, White *et al.* 1993). The neural canal diameter measured on lateral radiographs from the posterior margin of the odontoid process to the posterior spinolaminar line of C1 correlates better with MRI-demonstrable cord compression and spinal canal compromise than measurement of the atlantodental interval (White *et al.* 1993).

Disorders of bone formation or maintenance which result in bone softening may result in basilar invagination and foramen magnum compromise, platyspondyly or pathologic fractures. Entities in this category include Cushing's disease, osteomalacia, osteoporosis and osteogenesis imperfecta. Standards for the range of normal neural canal diameter measurements in children at C1–2 have been reported by Hinck *et al.* (1962).

After plain films, MRI is best for demonstration of canal compromise, vertebral canal stenosis, and/or cord compression. A suggested approach to spinal MRI in these diseases is a combination of sagittal and coronal thin T_1- and T_2-weighted sequences followed by axial images of levels of pathology. Since these diseases are typically generalized, evaluation of the entire spinal column is appropriate. Bone marrow abnormalities may be demonstrated based on abnormal or inhomogeneous vertebral body signal intensity of T_1- and T_2-weighted images. Correlation with plain films, flexion and extension views or CT may be needed to document spinal column integrity or stability.

Spinal vascular malformations

Spinal arteriovenous malformations (AVMs) are commonly categorized as Type 1 (long dorsal or dural spinal AVMs), Type II (compact or glomus), Type III (large juvenile), and Type IV (direct arteriovenous fistula) (Di Chiro *et al.* 1971, Heros *et al.* 1986). Other vascular lesions of the spinal cord include cavernous malformation, venous malformation and angioma.

Intramedullary AVMs have characteristic signal abnormalities on MRI due to high flow, cord ischemia and/or associated hematomyelia, although angiography remains necessary to localize and plan operative resection of these lesions (Dormont *et al.* 1988) (Fig. 11.24). Rare Type III malformations are encountered in juveniles and young adults and have high flow, large size, and often involve adjacent tissues including the vertebrae (Spetzler *et al.* 1989) (Fig. 11.25). Dural fistulae usually occur in adults and are easily overlooked on MRI. Sequelae of spinal vascular malformations include clinical signs of myelopathy, myelomalacia, syringohydromyelia and hemorrhage.

MRI of vascular malformations includes multiplanar T_1- and T_2-weighted imaging, with additional flow sensitive gradient echo and MR angiography (MRA) sequences. Even with very detailed MR techniques, a significant percentage of spinal vascular malformations are not detected on MRI or MRA perhaps due to small size, slow vascular flow, or obscuration by motion related respiratory or CSF artifacts. Definitive surgical mapping of spinal vascular malformations requires selective spinal angiography.

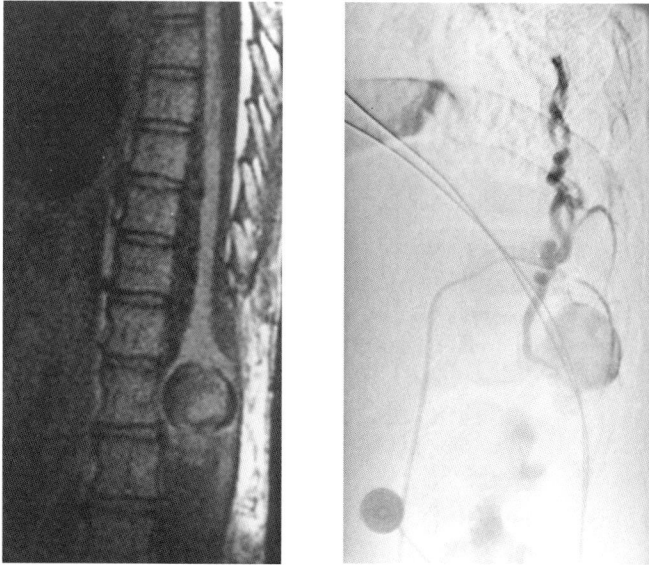

Fig. 11.24. *(Left)* Sagittal MRI of thoracolumbar junction (TR 650, TE 30, 3.0 mm) reveals large vascular lesion with aneurysmal flow void in 9-year-old child with conus arteriovenous malformation. *(Right)* Vascular malformation with focal aneurysm formation confirmed by spinal angiography.

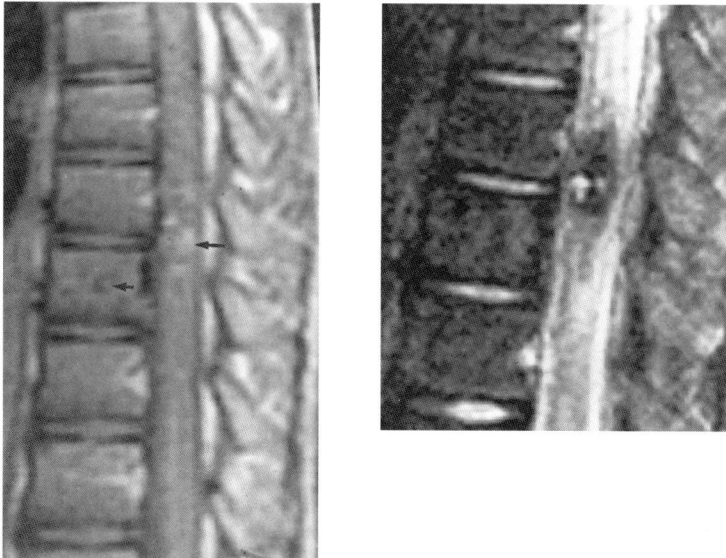

Fig. 11.25. *(Left)* Juvenile or type III arteriovenous malformation (AVM) resulted in subtle intramedullary high signal intensity *(arrow)* and minor inhomogeneity of the adjacent involved vertebra *(arrows;* TR 750, TE 30, 3.0 mm). *(Right)* Intramedullary component is better localized on T_2-weighted image (TR 1800, TE 90, 4.0 mm).

256

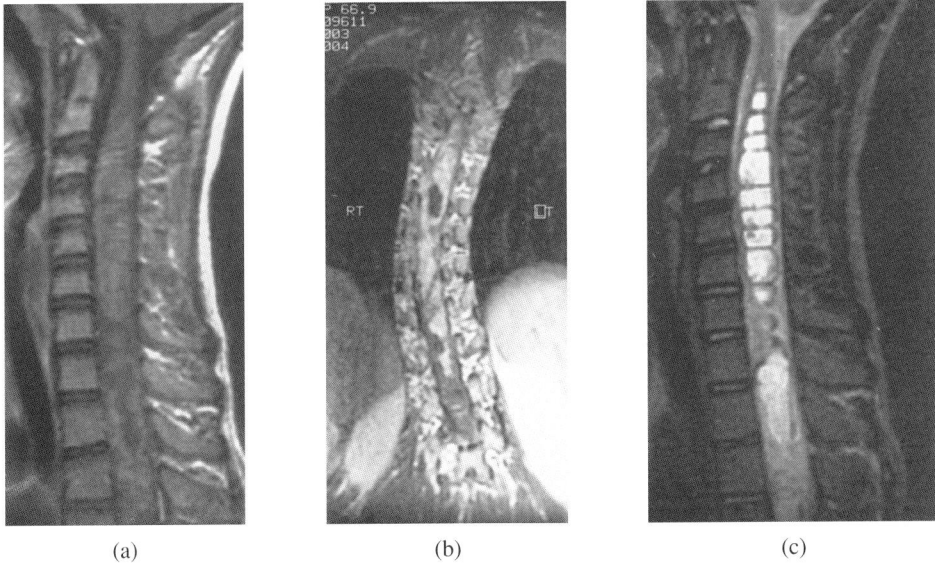

(a)   (b)   (c)

Fig. 11.26. Diffuse astrocytoma of spinal cord was confirmed surgically in 12-year-old child with scoliosis and mild foot drop. *(a,b)* Contrast-enhanced T_1-weighted images demonstrate diffuse inhomogeneous enlargement of spinal cord with several foci of cyst formation and syringomyelia (*a*—TR 600, TE 20, 4.0mm; *b*—TR 800, TE 20, 4.0mm). *(c)* T_2-weighted image confirms heterogeneous nature of this cystic and solid neoplasm (TR 1980, TE 100, 4.0mm).

Spinal neoplasia

Intramedullary tumors

MRI has replaced other imaging technologies for initial evaluation of suspected spinal cord disease. Intramedullary diseases of childhood include neoplasia (astrocytoma, ependymoma, rarely neurofibroma, metastases, lipoma or hemangioblastoma), AVMs, hydrosyringomyelia, transverse myelitis, demyelinating disease, traumatic contusion or hematomyelia, and infarction. The clinical presentation, MRI appearance, and pattern of contrast enhancement allow localization and characterization of these abnormalities for therapeutic planning. Initial sagittal T_1- and T_2-weighted images are used to identify intramedullary pathology. Other imaging planes and contrast-enhanced T_1-weighted sequences are useful to localize biopsy sites and to aid differentiation of cystic/necrotic from solid masses (Sze *et al.* 1988*b*, 1990; Parizel *et al.* 1989; Brunberg *et al.* 1991).

In children, about 60 per cent of intramedullary tumors are astrocytomas, and about 28 per cent are intramedullary ependymomas (Reimer and Onofrio 1985). Diffuse spinal cord tumors with or without cystic components tend to be grade I or II astrocytic tumors; included are an occasional malignant astrocytoma or glioblastoma multiforme (Fig. 11.26). Spinal cord astrocytomas are slightly more frequent in males and tend to involve the cervical or cervicothoracic cord. Average symptom duration before diagnosis can be quite long (Reimer and Onofrio 1985). Symptoms include pain, gait disturbance, sensory

257

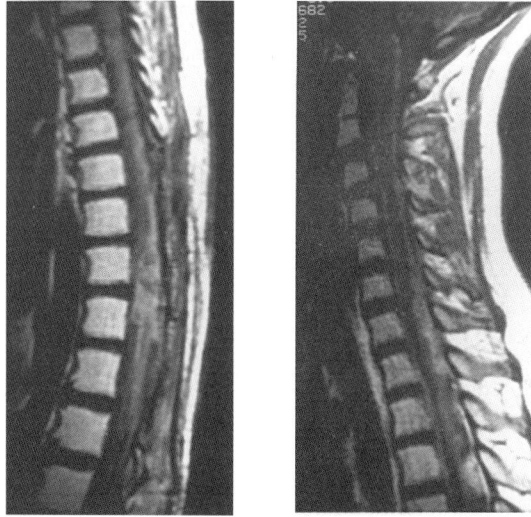

Fig. 11.27. MRI of child who underwent partial resection of thoracic spinal cord malignant astrocytoma followed by radiation therapy. Contrast enhanced T_1-weighted images reveal extensive recurrence in thoracic spinal canal (*left*—TR 550, TE 11, 3.0mm) and dissemination in cranial and spinal leptomeninges (*right*—TR 550, TE 11, 3.0mm.). Note hyperintense thoracic vertebral bone marrow related to radiation therapy.

deficits and sphincter dysfunction. Up to 12 per cent have symptoms of increased intracranial pressure or hydrocephalus; this has been attributed to seeding from malignant tumors or to elevated CSF protein (Ammerman and Smith 1975) (Fig. 11.27). Spinal cord astrocytoma may be eccentric, focal, or have exophytic extension into the subarachnoid space. The benefits of surgical resection, decompression and radiation therapy are controversial since there are reports of long-term survivors without resection or radiation (Epstein and Epstein 1981, Reimer and Onofrio 1985). Survival correlates with tumor grade; long-term survivors with low grade astrocytomas frequently develop postoperative kyphoscoliosis or subluxation requiring operative intervention.

Spinal cord ependymoma tends to be more focal and well demarcated than astrocytoma and is associated with spontaneous subarachnoid hemorrhage (Nemoto *et al.* 1992). Ependymoma tends to involve the conus and filum, and may be intramedullary or present partially or completely as an intradural extramedullary mass associated with the filum terminale. Spinal ependymoma may result in leptomeningeal spread caudal to the primary lesion. Focal or localized ependymoma has a good prognosis for survival following complete surgical excision.

Hemangioblastoma is unusual in pediatric patients unless they are being closely evaluated due to a family history of von Hippel–Lindau syndrome. Usual age at diagnosis is young adulthood, and about one-third of those with proven hemangioblastoma have a family history of von Hippel–Lindau syndrome (Dorwart *et al.* 1983). This is an autosomal dominant disorder associated with cerebellar hemangioblastoma, retinal angioma, renal carcinoma and pheochromocytoma. Spinal hemangioblastoma is a highly vascular lesion which may be solitary or multiple and result in syringomyelia.

Spinal cord tumors result in enlargement of the spinal cord on T_1-weighted images. The intramedullary lesions are better localized on T_2-weighted images, although differentiation among myelomalacia, syringomyelia, cyst, solid tumor and edema is imprecise. Although essentially all spinal cord tumors are recognizable on T_2-weighted images, contrast enhanced T_1-weighted images aid tumor characterization and localization for biopsy or resection. Both astrocytoma and ependymoma often enhance following paramagnetic contrast administration; enhancement aids separation of more solid portions of tumor apart from adjacent cysts or edema. Cysts occurring within solid cord tumors may be tumor lined; those rostral or caudal to the primary tumor may represent syringomyelia without direct involvement by tumor. Overlap between the MRI appearance of spinal cord tumors is common. As a result, confident differentiation between ependymoma and astrocytoma requires histologic examination (Parizel *et al.* 1989).

Extramedullary intradural neoplasia
Intradural extramedullary tumors of childhood include congenital tumors associated with occult dysraphism (see above), neurofibroma and schwannoma, leptomeningeal neoplastic seeding from a central nervous system (CNS) or hematologic malignancy, and rarely meningioma.

Nerve sheath tumors may occur in isolation or in association with neurofibromatosis. Two genetically distinct forms of neurofibromatosis have been designated neurofibromatosis type 1 (NF-1) and neurofibromatosis type 2 (NF-2) (Martuza and Eldridge 1988, National Institutes of Health Consensus Development Conference 1988). Other forms are not yet classified as distinct genetic disorders. NF-1 is associated with an abnormality of chromosome 17 and is often manifested by optic pathway glioma. NF-2 is associated with chromosome 22, and affected children have acoustic neuroma (unilateral or bilateral), meningioma, other dural or nerve sheath neoplasia, and a positive family history for this disorder. NF-1 is strongly associated with spinal neurofibroma, while NF-2 is more often associated with schwannoma (Halliday *et al.* 1991) (Fig. 11.28). Sporadic spinal nerve sheath tumors without stigmata of neurofibromatosis are usually schwannomas. Other spinal abnormalities described with neurofibromatosis include kyphoscoliosis, enlargement of the neural foramina due to schwannoma erosion or lateral meningocele, and dural ectasia (Figs. 11.29, 11.30). Malignant degeneration is suggested based on invasiveness and bone destruction (Fig. 11.30). Spinal meningioma, although quite uncommon in children, tends to arise in children with evidence of neurofibromatosis.

Leptomeningeal dissemination of malignancy may accompany a variety of primary brain tumors including ependymoma, glioblastoma multiforme, germinoma, primitive neuroectodermal tumors (PNETs) (*i.e.* medulloblastoma, pineoblastoma, neuroblastoma, medulloepithelioma, ependymoblastoma), and systemic hematologic malignancies such as leukemia or lymphoma. Spinal seeding may be subtle or inapparent on non-contrast MRI; detection is substantially improved following contrast enhancement (Krol *et al.*

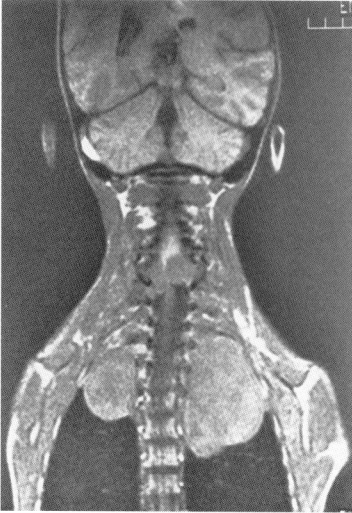

Fig. 11.28. Child with known neurofibromatosis complained of progressive dyspnea. Multiple dumb-bell neurofibromas are noted on sagittal T₁-weighted image with compression of the trachea and spinal cord (*a*—TR 575, TE 30, 5.0 mm).

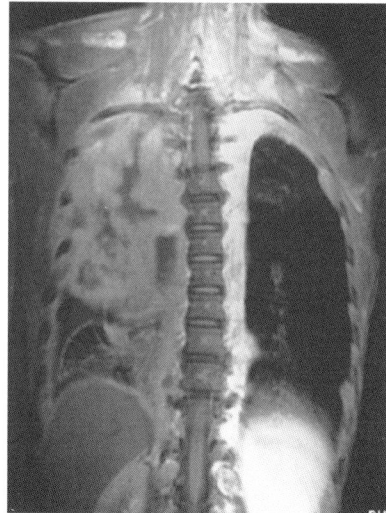

Fig. 11.29. Child with known neurofibromatosis developed aggressive chest wall neurofibrosarcoma shown following contrast enhancement to invade spinal canal (TR 1045, TE 20, 8.0 mm). (Courtesy Dr Turner I. Ball, Egleston Children's Hospital at Emory University, Atlanta, GA.)

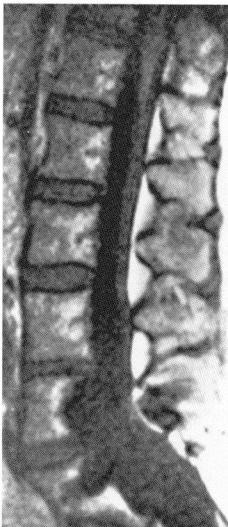

Fig. 11.30. Dural ectasia demonstrated on MRI in patient with neurofibromatosis (TR 500, TE 30, 5.0 mm).

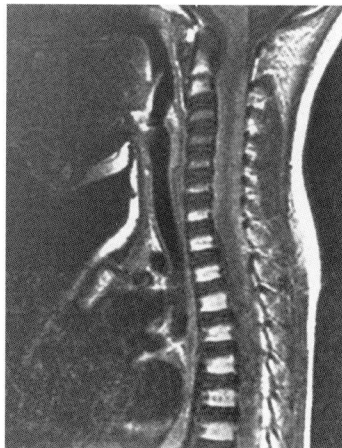

Fig. 11 31. Child with pineoblastoma, who developed cranial and spinal metastases. Diffuse enhancement of surface of spinal cord and entire cervical spinal canal noted on T₁-weighted image following contrast administration (TR 500, TE 30, 5.0 mm).

260

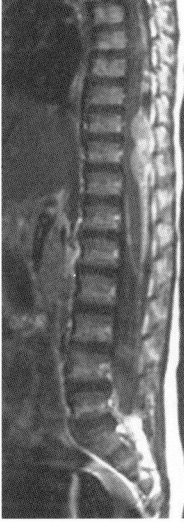

Fig. 11.32. Multiple enhancing nodules within thecal sac and on surface of spinal cord resulting from leptomeningeal dissemination of medulloblastoma (TR 500, TE 20, 4.0 mm).

1988, Sze *et al.* 1988*a*) (Figs. 11.31, 11.32). Contrast-enhanced MRI examination of the spinal column aids staging of the child who is newly diagnosed with a primary CNS malignancy; leptomeningeal dissemination is present at the time of diagnosis in up to 30 per cent of children with medulloblastoma. Leptomeningeal tumor produces a diffuse linear enhancement on the surface of the spinal cord, a coated appearance of enhancement of the spinal nerve roots, or multiple focal nodules of enhancement; larger masses result in spinal cord compression. A normal contrast-enhanced spinal MRI examination does not exclude spinal seeding; small foci of neoplasia may be present which can only be detected by repeated CSF cytological testing.

Extradural neoplasia

Extradural spinal tumors of childhood include diffuse or metastatic diseases of the vertebral column, paraspinal masses with intraspinal extension, and primary osseous tumors. Neoplastic bone marrow infiltration results in hypointense vertebral foci on T_1-weighted images and variable hyperintensity on T_2-weighted images; lesion heterogeneity and multiplicity aid recognition in children who have not received prior radiation or chemotherapy. After these therapies, it is difficult to distinguish between regenerating hematopoietic marrow, bone marrow changes in response to therapy, and recurrent or residual marrow neoplasia.

Vertebral metastatic disease in children results from primary neuroblastoma, rhabdomyosarcoma, leukemia, lymphoma, hepatoblastoma, Ewing's sarcoma, histiocytosis X, and other hematopoietic and neoplastic disorders. Leukemia is the most common malignancy of childhood; the most common type is acute lymphoblastic leukemia. Spinal findings in leukemia include diffuse bone marrow infiltration, osteoporosis with pathologic fracture, epidural soft tissue masses, and leptomeningeal dissemination.

261

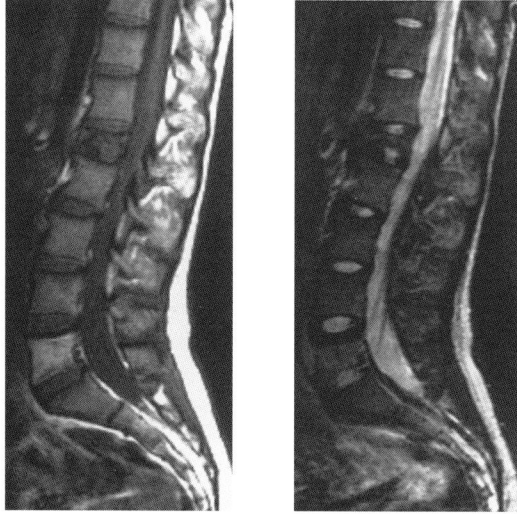

Fig. 11.33. Compression fracture of L1 and several focal areas of abnormal bone marrow signal in child who had undergone chemotherapy for lymphoma (*left*—TR 500, TE 20, 4.0mm; *right*—TR 1800, TE 90, 4.0mm). These bone marrow changes may reflect persistent tumor or regenerating hematopoietic tissue.

Measurement of T_1 relaxation times has a role in differentiation between regenerating bone marrow following therapy and recurrent leukemic bone marrow disease. Moore *et al.* (1986) found a longer T_1 in primary and relapsing leukemia compared to regenerating or normal marrow. Lymphoma, like leukemia, may involve the vertebrae or affect the epidural and paraspinous spaces with sparing of the vertebral bodies themselves (Fig. 11.33). Non-Hodgkin's lymphoma, often a disease of adulthood, results in primary osseous disease of long bones and metastases to spinal bone marrow. Hodgkin's disease is most prevalent in young adults but may occur in children or adolescents. Eventual involvement of spinal bone marrow may develop as the disease progresses.

Paraspinal neoplasia may extend into the spinal canal and compress the spinal cord; this pattern has been described in sarcoma, ganglioneuroma, ganglioneuroblastoma and neuroblastoma. Neuroblastoma is the most common solid tumor of childhood; children under 5 years of age are most often affected. Neuroblastoma originates from neural crest tissues, with the adrenal gland being the most frequent primary tumor site. Other primary tumor sites arise anywhere along the parasympathetic chain, thus paravertebral lesions in the abdomen, chest or neck are not uncommon. Children with neuroblastoma frequently have spinal metastases at the time of diagnosis, and intraspinal extension from adjacent paraspinal or abdominal neuroblastoma is well known (Siegel *et al.* 1986, Brodeur 1991) (Figs. 11.34, 11.35). Ganglioneuroblastomas and ganglioneuromas are more differentiated, more mature tumors which, like neuroblastomas, originate from neural crest cells. These may extend into the extradural or intradural extramedullary spinal canal with resultant nerve root or spinal cord compression.

262

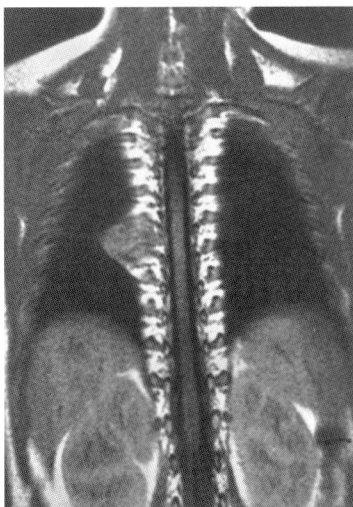

Fig. 11.34. Paraspinal mass with extension into adjacent neural foramina identified on MRI (TR 700, TE 30, 5.0 mm); no cord compression was present. Surgical excision confirmed ganglioneuroblastoma.

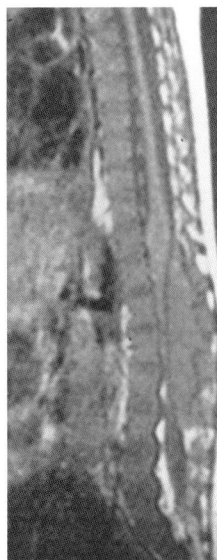

Fig. 11.35. Extensive intraspinal extension with spinal canal and cord compromise in child with abdominal neuroblastoma (TR 450, TE 20, 4.0 mm).

A combination of T_1-, T_2- and contrast enhanced T_1-weighted images can be helpful in defining extradural neoplasia. Focal lesions confined to the vertebral bone marrow are typically hypointense relative to normal marrow on non-contrast T_1-weighted images in older children and adults. Bone marrow infiltration is more difficult to recognize in younger children due to a predominance of hematopoietic marrow. Diffuse marrow replacement by metastasis may result in a reversal of normal bone marrow intensities such that the marrow is hypointense on T_1-weighted and hyperintense on T_2-weighted images (Ruzal-Shapiro *et al.* 1991). In predominantly fatty marrow, contrast enhancement may render vertebral metastases less visible on T_1-weighted images unless a fat-suppression technique is applied (Sze *et al.* 1988*b*).

Ongoing investigations address the role of MRI in staging of bone marrow abnormalities including those associated with tumor, storage diseases (Gaucher's disease) and hematologic disorders (sickle cell disease, thalassemia). Bone marrow undergoing repopulation following radiation or chemotherapy is difficult to distinguish from recurrent neoplasia. Radiation therapy results in fatty infiltration and secondary high signal intensity bone marrow on T_1-weighted images (Ramsey and Zacharias 1985). MRI signal changes may be recognized as early as two to three weeks after radiation therapy; later sequelae in skeletally immature children include secondary scoliosis or growth abnormalities with doses of more than 1000 rad (Stevens *et al.* 1990). CT may still be required for detailed bone anatomy in diseases which destroy or infiltrate bone, or for surgical planning of spinal decompression, tumor resection or stabilization.

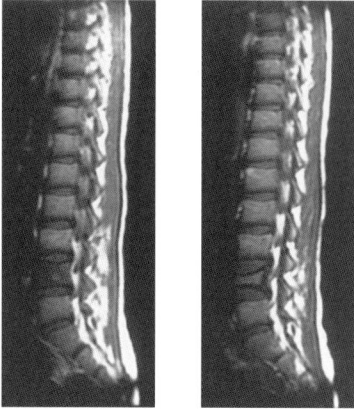

Fig. 11.36. Young girl with back pain due to pathologic fracture of L4. T$_1$-weighted images confirmed this as solitary vertebral lesion without spinal canal compression (TR 650, TE 23, 4.0mm). A CT-guided biopsy of this focal destructive lesion confirmed eosinophilic granuloma.

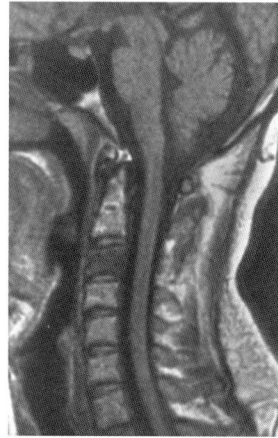

Fig. 11.37. Adolescent with neck pain due to sclerotic process involving C3 vertebral body. MRI indicated diffuse involvement of vertebra without cord compression (TR 700, TE 30, 5.0mm); this was surgically confirmed as osteoblastoma.

With few exceptions (*i.e.* histiocytosis X, aneurysmal bone cyst, and rare giant cell tumors), primary osseous vertebral neoplasms of childhood rarely extend across disk spaces or levels to involve adjacent vertebrae. Benign vertebral neoplasias of childhood include eosinophilic granuloma, osteochondroma, osteoid osteoma, osteoblastoma, aneurysmal bone cyst and hemangioma. Eosinophilic granuloma should be considered in a child who presents with a solitary marked vertebral compression fracture (vertebra plana). Age of incidence is typically 2 to 6 years, and the wedged vertebra occurs with little or no preceding trauma (Fig. 11.36). These benign lesions heal spontaneously, although systemic or progressive disease requires intervention. Histiocytosis X results in multifocal disease, so the entire spine may require MRI evaluation. Osteoid osteoma is a painful lesion of children and young adults (second decade predominance); a central lucency with a sclerotic border and increased activity on a radionuclide bone scan are typical. These small lesions are subtle and readily overlooked on MRI. Osteoblastomas are over 2cm in size, occur predominately in males under age 30, and have a good prognosis if completely resected. They tend to present as mixed sclerotic and lytic lesions of the lamina or pedicle, with occasional cases limited to the vertebral body (Figs. 11.37, 11.38).

About 80 per cent of aneurysmal bone cysts are identified in adolescents. These vascular lesions are large at presentation and tend to involve the posterior elements. Sediment levels on MRI reflect the vascular and complex cystic matrix of these lesions, and extension to involve adjacent vertebral levels is not uncommon. Spinal canal compromise and cord compression are well demonstrated on MRI, although associated pathologic fractures may require CT for demonstration.

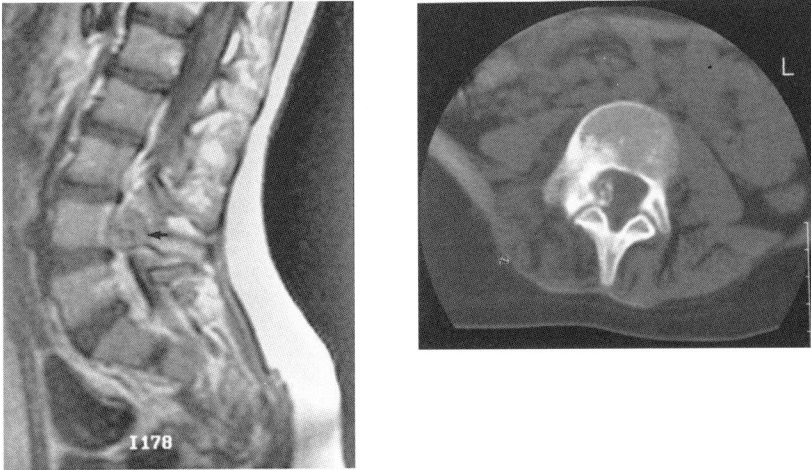

Fig. 11.38. T$_1$-weighted image *(left)* shows eccentric lesion *(arrow)* in 12-year-old boy with painful scoliosis (TR 700, TE16, 4.0mm). Focal sclerotic lesion involving right L4 pedicle is more apparent on CT *(right)*; this was surgically confirmed as osteoblastoma.

Vertebral hemangioma is a common incidental finding which is recognized with increased frequency with advancing age. These tend to be hyperintense on both T$_1$- and T$_2$-weighted images, and have characteristic coarsened trabeculae surrounded by a non-calcified matrix on CT. Infrequently hemangioma is expansile with cord or foraminal compression, or is associated with pathologic fracture requiring surgical or interventional therapy.

More aggressive or variably aggressive lesions include giant cell tumor, sacro-coccygeal teratoma and chordoma. Giant cell tumor is less common in children than aneurysmal bone cyst, tends to occur in the sacrum, and may present in late adolescent years (Fig. 11.39).

Teratoma occurs in association with occult dysraphism (see above) or as a primary sacral, coccygeal, or pelvic tumor of infancy. Those without associated dysraphism are predominantly posterior and external, presacral and pelvic, or both (Figs. 11.40, 11.41). Teratoma is more likely to be benign if identified before 4 months or after 5 years of age; those diagnosed in the interval between these ages have a 50–60 per cent chance of malignancy (Dorwart *et al.* 1983). Spinal teratoma remote from the sacrococcygeal region is unusual and tends to be benign. The inhomogeneous MRI intensities on all pulse sequences reflect the complex nature of these masses.

Ewing's sarcoma involves the long bones, scapula, ribs and pelvis, affecting the spine in only about 5 per cent of cases. Presenting features include localized pain, fever, and leukocytosis suggestive of diskitis or osteomyelitis. Sites of metastasis include the lungs, other bones, and lymph nodes. MRI is used to demonstrate the extent of marrow involvement of the primary lesion, and to demonstrate spinal metastases. Osteosarcoma

265

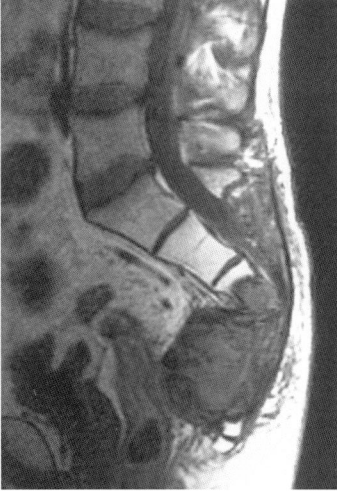

Fig. 11.39. Complex sacral and presacral mass in adolescent male (TR 500, TE 20, 4.0mm), histologically confirmed as giant cell tumor.

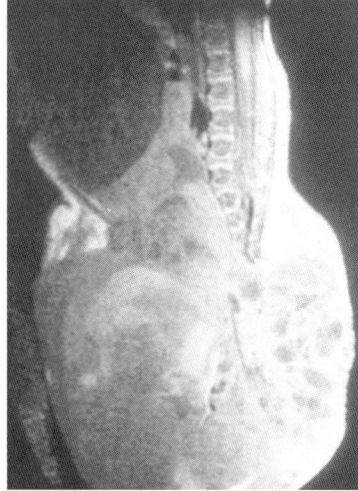

Fig. 11.40. Complex pelvic and sacral teratoma is inhomogeneous on T_1-weighted image in this infant (TR 500, TE 30, 10mm). (Courtesy of Dr Turner I. Ball, Egleston Children's Hospital at Emory University, Atlanta, GA.)

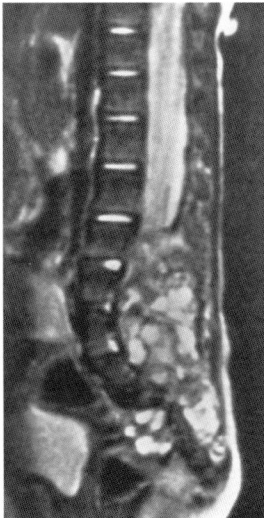

Fig. 11.41. Intraspinal and presacral complex mass, later confirmed as teratoma, in toddler with lower extremity spasticity and delayed walking (TR 2000, TE 90, 4.0mm).

rarely originates in the vertebral column, although metastases to the spinal column are not unusual. As for Ewing's sarcoma, MRI is used to assess spinal involvement, cord compression, and paraspinal extension. Chondrosarcoma is infrequent in children and uncommonly originates in the spine. CT is complementary to MRI for these osseous lesions, and may better demonstrate the tumor matrix.

MRI and CT are complementary for assessment of spinal osseous tumors. Sequences include multiplanar T_1- and T_2-weighted imaging with selective use of gradient echo, fat suppressed T_1-weighted imaging, and inversion recovery sequences. Although paramagnetic contrast aids differentiation of cystic/necrotic tumor from solid masses and definition of tumor margins, a non-contrast T_1-weighted or fat suppression sequence is required in order to avoid masking of bone marrow disease. MRI advantages include depiction of internal lesion morphology (fluid levels, hemorrhage), and demonstration of spinal cord, canal, or foraminal compromise. CT is preferable for characterization of calcified tumor matrix, pathologic fracture, and in individuals with MRI artifact from surgery or instrumentation. MRI has generally supplanted myelography for localization or staging of these diseases.

Spinal infections
A high index of suspicion is necessary for diagnosis of spinal infection in a timely fashion. Few or no systemic signs may be apparent. Risk factors in children, as in adults, include any cause for bacteremia (endocarditis, surgical manipulation, congenital heart disease) or immune compromise, although disk space infection may occur with no recognizable predisposing illness. Children have a greater vascular supply to the disk and/or its adjacent endplate; therefore, infections in childhood may begin primarily in the disk rather than in the vertebral endplates. Simple diskitis of childhood is commonly due to staphylococcal infection and occurs mainly in females under 5 years of age. Spontaneous resolution without antibiotic therapy and negative cultures from disk space aspiration are common.

Diskitis with osteomyelitis may result from *Staphylococcus* or other pyogenic organisms (Figs. 11.42, 11.43). Tuberculous spondylitis may soon be encountered with increased frequency coincident with the increased incidence of tuberculous infections of recent years (Snider and Roper 1992) (Fig. 11.44). Children acquire tuberculous spondylitis from close contact with an infectious host adult, and present with an insidious onset of a localized painful kyphosis. Sequelae of tuberculous spondylitis include kyphosis with secondary respiratory or neurologic problems from cord compression (Hsu and Yau 1985). Other infectious agents are uncommon in developed countries, although actinomycosis or blastomycosis could result in a similar presentation.

Both T_1- and T_2-weighted images are essential for recognition of inflammatory spinal disease (Modic *et al.* 1985, de Roos *et al.* 1986, Post *et al.* 1988). On T_1-weighted images, the vertebral endplate destruction which is the hallmark of a disk space infection may be subtle, incomplete or not apparent. On T_2-weighted images, the involved disk often has an abnormally high signal intensity with associated increased intensity of the adjacent involved vertebral bodies. A narrowed disk space as a sequela of trauma or herniated nucleus pulposus should be desiccated and have a less intense signal than adjacent normal disk. Thrush and Enzmann (1990) described the highly variable spectrum of disk and vertebral signal intensities on MRI in infectious spondylitis; atypical MRI findings are not unusual in proven diskitis/osteomyelitis. A narrow disk space with an intensity which is as bright as a normal disc on T_2-weighted imaging should be viewed

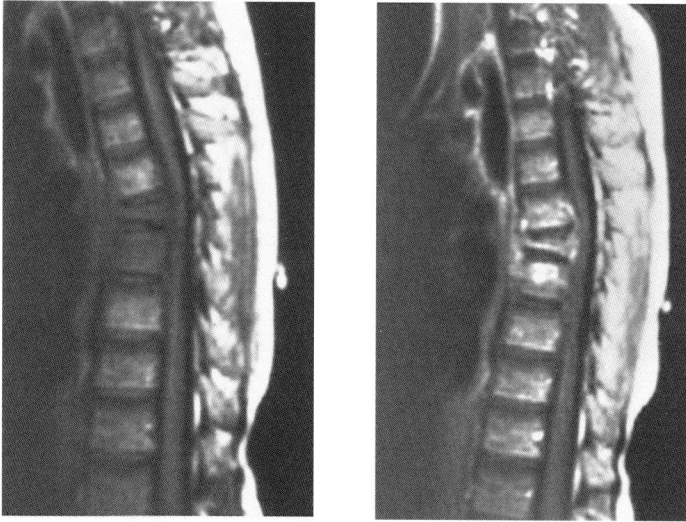

Fig. 11.42. Child with recurrent thoracic back pain, partially treated with various antibiotics. *(Left)* MRI reveals compression fracture with abnormal signal intensity in adjacent vertebral body and abnormal soft tissues along anterior spinal ligament and prevertebral fascia (TR 726, TE 20, 4.0mm). These findings are typical of diskitis and osteomyelitis. A T_2-weighted image confirmed vertebral body abnormalities. *(Right)* After administration of paramagnetic contrast, prespinal and epidural inflammatory enhancement is apparent (TR 726, TE 20, 4.0mm). Biopsy and aspiration revealed inflammatory material; cultures were sterile and no cytological evidence of malignancy was noted.

with suspicion for infection; diskitis may result in little or no abnormal disk space signal intensity. Few neoplastic lesions of childhood cross a disk space to involve adjacent regions of the vertebrae; occasionally this occurs with aneurysmal bone cyst, giant cell tumor or aggressive sarcoma. Degenerative disk disease may result in abnormal endplate intensities, but this is unusual in the pediatric population. Subligamentous spread, more than two adjacent involved vertebrae, paraspinal abscess, sparing of the posterior elements, and skip lesions are typical of infection with tuberculosis (Smith *et al.* 1989). Paramagnetic contrast may be helpful for demonstration of epidural abscess, paraspinal abscess or meningitis.

Spinal trauma
Spinal fractures without neurologic findings in children tend to heal well with little secondary kyphoscoliosis. However, significant neurologic injury is well documented in children without bony injury. Children aged under 10 years are more prone to injuries of the upper cervical spine or craniocervical junction than older juveniles and adolescents (Pang and Wilberger 1982, Hill *et al.* 1984). Children may have significant spinal cord injury which is remote from levels of bone injury or unassociated with a bony abnormality; this has been termed SCIWORA (*s*pinal *c*ord *i*njury *w*ithout *r*adiographic *a*bnormality) (Pang and Wilberger 1982). These age-related differences in spinal injury

268

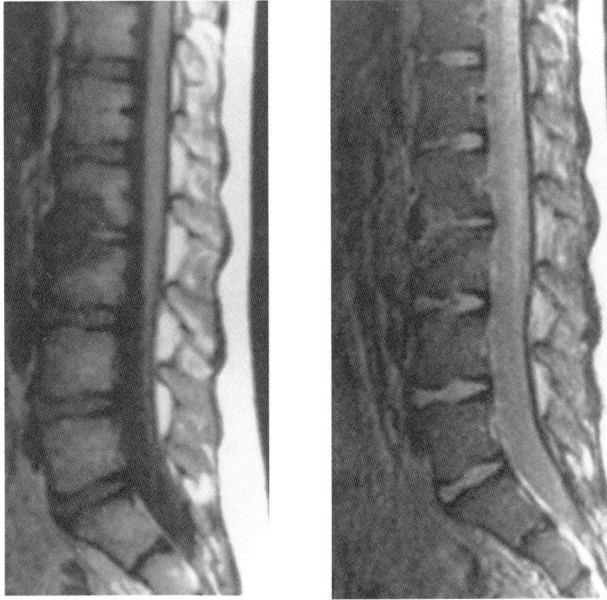

Fig. 11.43. Child with history of thyroid malignancy, referred for MRI due to low back pain. T_1-weighted (*left*—TR 500, TE 30, 4.0mm) and T_2-weighted (*right*—TR 1800, TE 50, 5.0mm) images demonstrate abnormal vertebral marrow signal in adjacent regions of L2 and L3 vertebrae. Anterior disk space margins are blurred, and signal intensity of narrow L2–3 disk is similar to that of adjacent normal disks. Aspirate and culture confirmed pyogenic infection with *Staphylococcus*.

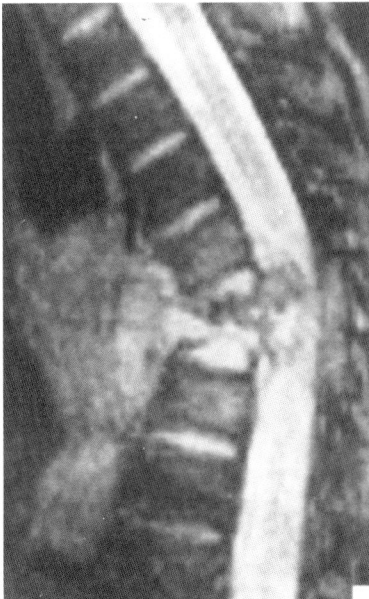

Fig. 11.44. Child with painful kyphosis, initially thought to have aggressive malignancy based on plain films. T_2-weighted gradient echo scan demonstrates abnormal vertebral signal in at least three adjacent levels, marked compression fracture and prominent subligamentous spread anteriorly. Spinal cord is significantly compressed by extensive associated epidural abscess in this child with proven tuberculous spondylitis (TR 500, TE 17, 7° flip angle, 3.0mm).

269

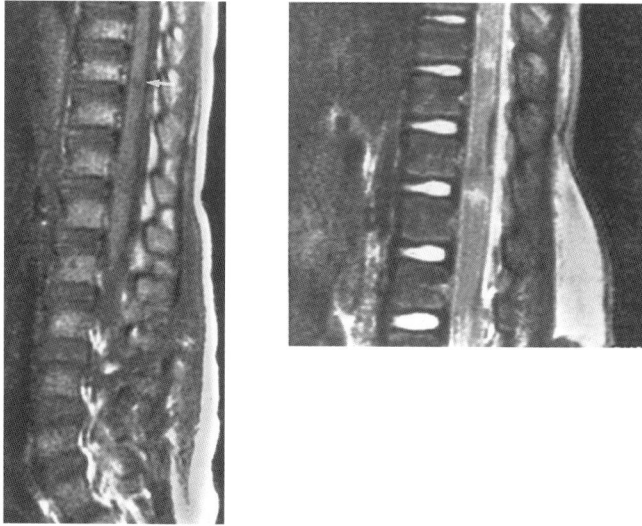

Fig. 11.45. Child with unexplained paraplegia following seat-belt type motor vehicle injury. T_1-weighted image (*left*—TR 498, TE 20, 4.0mm) shows area of abnormal signal *(arrow)*, confirmed as hemorrhagic cord contusion on localized T_2-weighted image *(right*—TR 2000, TE 90, 4.0mm*)* of the lower thoracic spinal canal.

have been attributed to the increased flexibility of the pediatric spine, lesser mineralization, incomplete fusion of ossification centers, relatively greater cranial weight by proportion, and more horizontally oriented cervical facet joints of preteen children (Hill *et al.* 1984, Matsumura *et al.* 1990). Infants also experience birth injuries of the spinal cord or craniocervical junction associated with difficult delivery, forceps delivery and breech delivery (Byers 1975, Stanley *et al.* 1985).

Lap belt injuries in children also differ from those of adults (Taylor and Eggli 1988, Sivit *et al.* 1991). Lap belt injuries in children are caudal in location compared to those of adults, and associated abdominal injuries may overshadow spinal injury. Reasons for these differences include the difficulty in properly positioning a lap belt at the pelvis rather than the abdomen of younger children, and the greater spinal flexibility resulting in a lower fulcrum of maximum flexion. In some cases remote cord/conus contusions explain paraplegia following a Chance-type fracture (Chance 1948). Spinal injuries in children with otherwise unexplained lower extremity paresis, kyphosis, or wedge fracture have been described as sequelae of the battered child syndrome (Swischuk 1969, Cullen 1975).

Plain radiographs with supervised flexion and extension views and/or CT are the initial imaging modalities for fracture localization or confirmation of spinal column stability. The wider range of normal soft tissue measurements in children must be considered. The atlantodental interval in children ranges up to 4mm, the prevertebral soft tissues up to 7mm, and the retrotracheal space up to 14mm in normal children (Wholey *et al.* 1958, Locke *et al.* 1966). Soft tissue swelling is a helpful localizing sign in trauma, but may be absent in spite of significant spinal injury.

MRI has a role in evaluation of the traumatized child with suspected spinal cord or ligament injury after clinical stabilization and radiographic evaluation of bony integrity (Davis *et al.* 1993) (Fig. 11.45). T_1- and T_2-weighted imaging provides localization of sites of traumatic cord contusion and cord infarction, and gradient echo images improve detection of intramedullary hemorrhage (Hackney *et al.* 1986, Mirvis *et al.* 1988). Extra-dural spinal cord compression or canal impingement by hematoma is well demonstrated; traumatic disk herniation is unusual in childhood. Since MRI noninvasively depicts abnormalities of the spinal cord, the extent of cord injury and hematomyelia, these images may have significance for recovery prognosis of neurologic function (Kulkarni *et al.* 1987, 1988; Bondurant *et al.* 1990; Davis *et al.* 1993). Myelography and post-myelographic CT have a role in confirmation of dural tears, penetrating injury and nerve root avulsion. Late sequelae of spinal cord injury, including myelomalacia, post-traumatic syrinx and incomplete spinal canal decompression, are well demonstrated on MRI, which should be considered if late deterioration occurs in a spinal injured individual (Quencer *et al.* 1986).

Miscellaneous spinal disorders
Disk herniation and avulsed ring apophysis
Although disk herniation sometimes occurs with physical activity or mild trauma in juveniles, strains, sprains and contusions associated with sports activities are far more common. Disk herniation in association with major trauma is unusual in childhood and early adolescence although it is described in older adolescence and early adulthood. In the younger population, a slipped vertebral ring apophysis may be retropulsed into the spinal canal and mimic disk herniation (Techakapuch 1981). The ring apophysis appears at about age 6, and fusion is complete by about age 18. The fibers of the annulus are strongly imbedded in the ring apophysis; thus the weak point in juveniles is at the junction of the vertebral body with the ring apophysis (Banerian *et al.* 1990). A fracture occurs at the ring apophysis and the intact disk is retropulsed along with the apophysis into the spinal canal. These injuries tend to occur at the L4 level, may occur at several levels, and may not respond to conservative therapy as readily as a conventional disk herniation. Visualization of the avulsed calcified ring apophysis posteriorly displaced into the ventral spinal canal is key to this diagnosis, hence plain films or CT may be preferable to MRI for this entity.

Spondylolysis and spondylolisthesis
Abnormalities of the pars interarticularis associated with spondylolisthesis or pain include stress or fatigue fractures, acute pars fracture, dysplastic or deficient facet joint development, or elongated intact pars. Five types have been described by Wiltse *et al.* (1976); included are degenerative and pathologic fractures which are uncommon in children. By far the most common pars abnormality is the fatigue fracture which is estimated to occur in 5 per cent of the adult population. Since this entity is unknown in

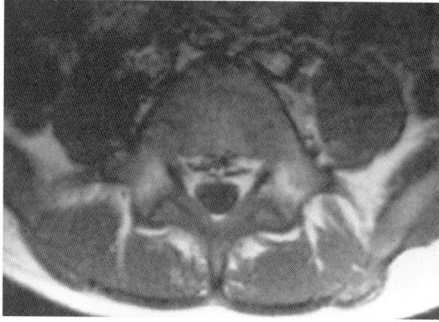

(a)

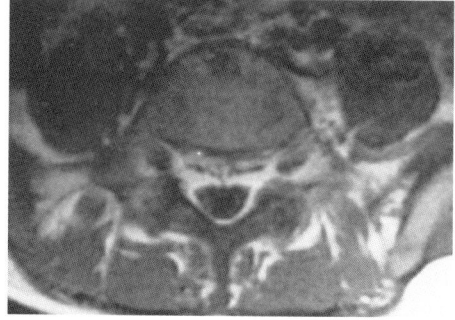

(b)

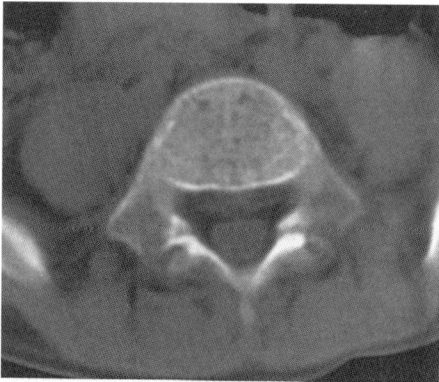

(c)

Fig. 11.46. *(a)* T_1 weighted image at L5–S1 demonstrates intact facet joints (TR 500, TE 30, 5.0 mm). *(b)* Adjacent image reveals hypointensity and loss of discrete bone contours in posterior elements at level of pars interarticularis (TR 500, TE 30, 5.0 mm). *(c)* CT better demonstrates this bilateral spondylolysis. (Reproduced by permission from Davis and Rao 1993.)

animals and has not been described in non-weight-bearing humans, upright posture seems to increase the likelihood of this occurrence. Secondary vertebral body subluxation associated with pars interarticularis abnormalities is graded from I to IV based on the quartile of subluxation of the vertebral body anteriorly. Spondylolysis most commonly occurs at L5 with secondary subluxation at L5–S1. MRI findings of spondylolysis include signal hypointensity across the pars on T_1-weighted images (Grenier *et al.* 1989) (Fig. 11.46). A developmentally small pars, a sclerotic pars, or one which contains little bone marrow or abnormal bone marrow could have a similar appearance on MRI. Recognition of pars defects is facilitated in the axial plane based on absence of the normal facet joint space, departure from the expected oblique angle of the facet joints, and a pseudo disk herniation appearance due to subluxation (Teplick *et al.* 1986). CT or upright weight-bearing plain films facilitate diagnosis of spondylolysis and grading of severity of spondylolisthesis (Teplick *et al.* 1986).

Disk calcification
Symptomatic disk space calcification is of uncertain etiology, although associations with trauma (30 per cent), recent upper respiratory tract infection (15 per cent), and fever (23

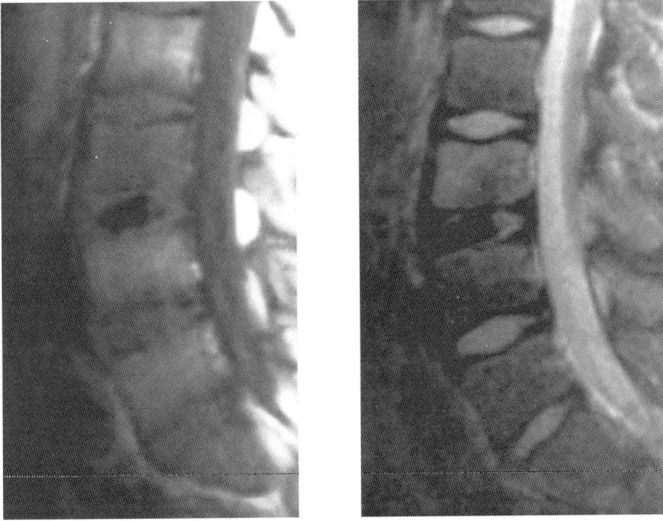

Fig. 11.47. Adolescent with back pain, in whom plain films had revealed focal disk space calcification. No spinal canal compromise was demonstrated on MRI (*left*—TR 500, TE 15, 4.0 mm; *right*—TR 1800, TE 80, 4.0 mm). (Reproduced by permission from Davis and Rao 1993.)

per cent) have been noted (Sonnabend *et al.* 1982). An infectious etiology has not been confirmed, although there is speculation that this is a nonspecific inflammatory reaction. Disk calcification predominates in males by a two to one ratio, and is not often encountered in association with metabolic disorders. Disk space calcification may be incidental and asymptomatic, although detectable disk protrusions have been described in symptomatic patients which later resorb with no resultant disk space narrowing (Urso *et al.* 1987) (Fig. 11.47).

Scheuermann's disease

Scheuermann's disease is a disorder of unknown etiology which presents in adolescence with a thoracic kyphosis. Early interpretations speculated that this painful kyphosis was due to aseptic necrosis of the ring apophysis; however, this has not been supported by later investigations. Associations include heavy mechanical stress, family history, and hormonal or calcium disorders, but a direct result from spinal trauma has not been confirmed (Ascani and Montanaro 1985). According to Sorenson (1964), radiographic criteria for this diagnosis include three or more wedged adjacent vertebrae, vertebral wedging by five degrees or more, and endplate irregularities. Schmorl's nodes may accompany this entity, and the associated disk spaces may be narrow (Hensinger 1985).

Summary

MRI plays an increasingly essential role in diagnosis and management of a wide variety of spinal disorders in children. It is now the study of choice for investigation of scoliosis and dysraphism. Invasive procedures such as myelography which were commonplace a mere 10 years ago are now rarely required, and technical advances continue to enhance image resolution and reduce scan times. Newer MRI sequences offer a demonstration of CSF and vascular flow not previously achieved noninvasively, and development of MR spectroscopy holds out the promise of insights into functional disturbances which are unavailable based on anatomical abnormalities. With such rapid technological advancements, MRI has an increasingly broad and practical application for pediatric spinal imaging of all children regardless of age or severity of illness.

ACKNOWLEDGEMENTS

The author gratefully acknowledges the efforts of Carol Ann Padgett for editorial assistance and manuscript preparation, and Jack Kearse for medical photography.

REFERENCES

Ammerman, B.J., Smith, D.R. (1975) 'Papilledema and spinal cord tumors.' *Surgical Neurology*, **3**, 55–57.

Ascani, E., Montanaro, A. (1985) 'Scheuermann's disease.' *In:* Bradford, D.S., Hensinger, R.M. (Eds.) *The Pediatric Spine.* New York: Thieme, pp. 307–324.

Banerian, K.G., Wang, A.M., Samberg, L.C., Kerr, H.H., Wesolowski, D.P. (1990) 'Association of vertebral end plate fracture with pediatric lumbar intervertebral disk herniation: value of CT and MR imaging.' *Radiology*, **177**, 763–765.

Barkovich, A.J., Wippold, F.J., Sherman, J.L., Citrin, C.M. (1986) 'Significance of cerebellar tonsillar position on MR.' *American Journal of Neuroradiology*, **7**, 795–799.

—— Raghavan, N., Chuang, S., Peck, W.W. (1989) 'The wedge-shaped cord terminus: a radiographic sign of caudal regression.' *American Journal of Neuroradiology*, **10**, 1223–1231.

—— Edwards, M.S.B., Cogen, P.H. (1991) 'MR evaluation of spinal dermal sinus tracts in children.' *American Journal of Neuroradiology*, **12**, 123–129.

Barnes, P.D. (1992*a*) 'Developmental abnormalities of the spine and spinal neuraxis.' *In:* Wolpert, S.M., Barnes, P.D. (Eds.) *MRI in Pediatric Neuroradiology.* St. Louis: Mosby Year Book, pp. 331–411.

—— (1992*b*) 'Acquired abnormalities of the spine and spinal neuraxis.' *In:* Wolpert, S.M., Barnes, P.D. (Eds.) *MRI in Pediatric Neuroradiology.* St. Louis: Mosby Year Book, pp. 412–464.

—— Lester, P.D., Yamanashi, W.S., Prince, J.R. (1986) 'Magnetic resonance imaging in infants and children with spinal dysraphism.' *American Journal of Neuroradiology*, **7**, 465–472.

Beyerl, B.D., Ojemann, R.G., Davis, K.R., Hedley-Whyte, E.T., Mayberg, M.R. (1985) 'Cervical diastematomyelia presenting in adulthood. Case report.' *Journal of Neurosurgery*, **62**, 449–453.

Bondurant, F.J., Cotler, H.B., Kulkarni, M.V., McArdle, C.B., Harris, J.H. (1990) 'Acute spinal cord injury. A study using physical examination and magnetic resonance imaging.' *Spine*, **15**, 161–168.

Brodeur, G. M. (1991) 'Neuroblastoma and other peripheral neuroectodermal tumors.' *In:* Fernbach, D.J., Vietti, T.J. (Eds.) *Clinical Pediatric Oncology.* St. Louis: C.V. Mosby, pp. 437–464.

Brunberg, J.A., DiPietro, M.A.,Venes, J.L., Dauser, R.C., Muraszko, K.M., Berkey, G.S., D'Amato, C.J., Rubin, J.M. (1991) 'Intramedullary lesions of the pediatric spinal cord: correlation of findings from MR imaging, intraoperative sonography, surgery, and histologic study.' *Radiology*, **181**, 573–579.

Byers, R.K. (1975) 'Spinal-cord injuries during birth.' *Developmental Medicine and Child Neurology*, **17**, 103–110.

Byrd, S.E., Darling, C.F., McLone, D.G. (1991) 'Developmental disorders of the pediatric spine.' *Radiologic Clinics of North America*, **29**, 711–752.

Carson, J.A., Barnes, P.D., Tunell, W.P., Smith, E.I., Jolley, S.G. (1984) 'Imperforate anus: the neurologic implication of sacral abnormalities.' *Journal of Pediatric Surgery*, **19**, 838–842.

Castillo, M., Quencer, R.M., Dominguez, R. (1992) 'Chiari III malformation: imaging features.' *American Journal of Neuroradiology*, **13**, 107–113.

Chance, G.Q. (1948) 'Note on a type of flexion fracture of the spine.' *British Journal of Radiology*, **21**, 452–453.

Chapman, P.H., Swearingen, B., Caviness, V.S. (1989) 'Subtorcular occipital encephaloceles: anatomical considerations relevant to operative management.' *Journal of Neurosurgery*, **71**, 375–381.

Cullen, J. (1975) 'Spinal lesions in battered babies.' *Journal of Bone and Joint Surgery*, **57B**, 364–366.

Curless, R.G., Quencer, R.M., Katz, D.A., Campanioni, M. (1992) 'Magnetic resonance demonstration of intracranial CSF flow in children.' *Neurology*, **42**, 377–381.

Davis, P.C., Rao, K.C.V.G. (1993) 'Trauma.' *In:* Rao, K.C.V.G, Williams, J.P., Lee, B.C.P., Sherman, J.L. (Eds.) *MRI and CT of the Spine.* Baltimore: Williams & Wilkins, pp. 277–346.

—— Hoffman, J.C., Ball,T.I., Wyly, J.B., Braun, I.F., Fry, S.M., Drvaric, D.M. (1988) 'Spinal abnormalities in pediatric patients: MR imaging findings compared with clinical, myelographic, and surgical findings.' *Radiology*, **166**, 679–685.

—— Reisner, A., Hudgins, P.A., Davis, W.E., O'Brien, M.S. (1993) 'Spinal injuries in children: role of MR.' *American Journal of Neuroradiology*, **14**, 607–617.

De Roos, A., Van Persijn Van Meerten, E.L., Bloem, J.L., Bluemm, R.G. (1986) 'MRI of tuberculous spondylitis.' *American Journal of Roentgenology*, **147**, 79–82.

Di Chiro, G., Doppman, J.L., Ommaya, A.K. (1971) 'Radiology of spinal cord arteriovenous malformations.' *Progress in Neurological Surgery*, **4**, 329–354.

Dooms, G.C., Fisher, M.R., Hricak, H., Richardson, M., Crooks, L.E., Genant, H.K. (1985) 'Bone marrow imaging: magnetic resonance studies related to age and sex.' *Radiology*, **155**, 429–432.

Dormont, D., Gelbert , F., Assouline, E., Reizine, D., Helias, A., Riche, M.C., Chiras, J., Bories, J., Merland, J.J. (1988) 'MR imaging of spinal cord arteriovenous malformations at 0.5 T: a study of 34 cases.' *American Journal of Neuroradiology*, **9**, 833–838.

Dorwart, R.H., Lamasters, D.L., Watanabe, T.J. (1983) 'Tumor.' *In:* Newton, T.H., Potts, D.G. (Eds.) *Modern Neuroradiology. Vol.1. Computed Tomography Of The Spine And Spinal Cord.* San Anselmo, CA: Clavadel Press, pp. 115–147.

Enzmann, D.R., O'Donohue, J., Rubin, J.B., Shuer, L., Cogen, P., Silverberg, G. (1987) 'CSF pulsations within nonneoplastic spinal cord cysts.' *American Journal of Neuroradiology*, **8**, 517–525.

Epstein, F., Epstein, N. (1981) 'Surgical management of holocord intramedullary spinal cord astrocytomas in children. Report of three cases.' *Journal of Neurosurgery*, **54**, 829–832.

Grenier, N., Kressel, H.Y., Schiebler, M.L., Grossman, R.I. (1989) 'Isthmic spondylolysis of the lumbar spine: MR imaging at 1.5T.' *Radiology*, **170**, 489–493.

Hackney, D.B., Asato, R., Joseph, P.M., Carvlin, M.J., McGrath, J.T., Grossman, R.I., Kassab, E.A., DeSimone, D. (1986) 'Hemorrhage and edema in acute spinal cord compression: demonstration by MR imaging.' *Radiology*, **161**, 387–390.

Hajek, P.C., Baker, L.L., Goobar, J.E., Sartoris, D.J., Hesselink, J.R., Haghighi, P., Resnick, D. (1987) 'Focal fat deposition in axial bone marrow: MR characteristics.' *Radiology*, **162**, 245–249.

Halliday, A.L., Sobel, R.A., Martuza, R.L. (1991) 'Benign spinal nerve sheath tumors: their occurrence sporadically and in neurofibromatosis types 1 and 2.' *Journal of Neurosurgery*, **74**, 248–253.

Hawkes, R.C., Holland, G.N., Moore, W.S., Corston, R., Kean, D.M., Worthington, B.S. (1983) 'Craniovertebral junction pathology: assessment by NMR.' *American Journal of Neuroradiology*, **4**, 232–233.

Hecht, J.T., Nelson, F.W., Butler, I.J., Horton, W.A., Scott, C.I., Wassman, E.R., Mehringer, C.M., Rimoin, D.L., Pauli, R.M. (1985) 'Computerized tomography of the foramen magnum: achondroplastic values compared to normal standards.' *American Journal of Medical Genetics*, **20**, 355–360.

Hensinger, R.M. (1985) 'Back pain in children.' *In:* Bradford, D.S., Hensinger, R.M. (Eds.) *The Pediatric Spine.* New York: Thieme, pp. 41–60.

Heros, R.C., Debrun, G.M., Ojemann, R.G., Lasjaunias, P.L., Naessens, P.J. (1986) 'Direct spinal arteriovenous fistula: a new type of spinal AVM.' *Journal of Neurosurgery*, **64**, 134–139.

Hilal, S.K., Marton, D., Pollack, E. (1974) 'Diastematomyelia in children. Radiographic study of 34 cases.' *Radiology*, **112**, 609–621.

Hill, S.A., Miller, C.A., Kosnik, E.J., Hunt, W.E. (1984) 'Pediatric neck injuries. A clinical study.' *Journal of Neurosurgery*, **60**, 700–706.

Hinck, V.C., Hopkins, C.E., Savara, B.S. (1962) 'Sagittal diameter of the cervical spinal canal in children.' *Radiology*, **79**, 97–108.

Ho, P.S.P, Yu, S., Sether, L.A., Wagner, M., Ho, K-C., Haughton, V.M. (1988) 'Progressive and regressive changes in the nucleus pulposus. Part I. The neonate.' *Radiology*, **169**, 87–91.

Hoffman, H.J., Neill, J., Crone, K.R., Hendrick, E.B., Humphreys R.P. (1987) '(1990) Hydrosyringomyelia and its management in childhood.' *Neurosurgery*, **21**, 347–351.

Horton, W.A., Rotter, J.I., Rimoin, D.L., Scott, C.I., Hall, J.G. (1978) 'Standard growth curves for achondroplasia.' *Journal of Pediatrics*, **93**, 435–438.

Hsu, L.C.S., Yau, A.C.M.C. (1985) 'Tuberculosis of the spine.' *In:* Bradford, D.S., Hensinger, R.M. (Eds.) *The Pediatric Spine*. New York: Thieme, pp. 68–79.

Hudgins, P.A., Davis, P.C., Hoffman, J.C. (1991) 'Gadopentetate dimeglumine-enhanced MR imaging in children following surgery for brain tumor: spectrum of meningeal findings.' *American Journal of Neuroradiology*, **12**, 301–307.

James, H.E., Walsh, J.W. (1981) 'Spinal dysraphism' *Current Problems in Pediatrics*, **11**, 1–25.

Kao, S.C.S., Waziri, M.H., Smith, W.L., Sato, Y., Yuh, W.T.C., Franken, E.A. (1989) 'MR imaging of the craniovertebral junction, cranium, and brain in children with achondroplasia.' *American Journal of Roentgenology*, **153**, 565–569.

Kricun, M.R. (1985) 'Red–yellow marrow conversion: its effect on the location of some solitary bone lesions.' *Skeletal Radiology*, **14**, 10–19.

Krol, G., Sze, G., Malkin, M., Walker, R. (1988) 'MR of cranial and spinal meningeal carcinomatosis: comparison with CT and myelography.' *American Journal of Neuroradiology*, **9**, 709–714.

Kulkarni, M.V., McArdle, C.B., Kopanicky, D., Miner, M., Cotler, H.B., Lee, K.F., Harris, J.H. (1987) 'Acute spinal cord injury: MR imaging at 1.5 T.' *Radiology*, **164**, 837–843.

—— Bondurant, F.J., Rose, S.L., Narayana, P.A. (1988) '1.5 Tesla magnetic resonance imaging of acute spinal trauma.' *Radiographics*, **8**, 1059–1082.

Levy, L.M., Di Chiro, G., McCullough, D.C., Dwyer, A.J., Johnson, D.L., Yang, S.S.L. (1988) 'Fixed spinal cord: diagnosis with MR imaging.' *Radiology*, **169**, 773–778.

Locke, G.R., Gardner, J.I., Van Epps, E.F. (1966) 'Atlas–dens interval (ADI) in children. A survey based on 200 normal cervical spines.' *American Journal of Roentgenology*, **97**, 135–140.

Martel, W., Tishler, J.M. (1966) 'Observations on the spine in mongoloidism.' *American Journal of Roentgenology*, **97**, 630–638.

Martich, V., Ben-Ami, T., Yousefzadeh, D.K., Roizen, N.J. (1992) 'Hypoplastic posterior arch of C-1 in children with Down syndrome: a double jeopardy.' *Radiology*, **183**, 125–128.

Martuza, R.L., Eldridge, R. (1988) 'Neurofibromatosis 2. (Bilateral acoustic neurofibromatosis.)' *New England Journal of Medicine*, **318**, 684–688.

Matsumura, A., Meguro, K., Tsurushima, H., Kikuchi, Y., Wada, M., Nakata, Y. 'Magnetic resonance imaging of spinal cord injury without radiologic abnormality.' *Surgical Neurology*, **33**, 281–283.

McLone, D.G., Naidich, T.P. (1985) 'Terminal myelocystocele.' *Neurosurgery*, **16**, 36–43.

Mikulis, D.J., Diaz, O., Egglin, T.K., Sanchez, R. (1992) 'Variance of the position of the cerebellar tonsils with age: preliminary report.' *Radiology*, **183**, 725–728.

Minaire, P., Meunier, P., Edouard, C., Bernard, J., Courpron, P., Bourret, J. (1974) 'Quantitative histological data on disuse osteoporosis: comparison with biological data.' *Calcified Tissue Research*, **17**, 57–73.

Mirvis, S.E., Geisler, F.H., Jelinek, J.J., Joslyn, J.N., Gellad, F. (1988) 'Acute cervical spine trauma: evaluation with 1.5-T MR imaging.' *Radiology*, **166**, 807–816.

Modic, M.T., Feiglin, D.H., Piraino, D.W., Boumphrey, F., Weinstein, M.A., Duchesneau, P., Rehm, S. (1985) 'Vertebral osteomyelitis: assessment using MR.' *Radiology*, **157**, 157–166.

Moore, S.G., Gooding, C.A., Brasch, R.C., Ehman, R.L., Ringertz, H.G., Ablin, A.R., Matthay, K.K., Zoger, S. (1986) 'Bone marrow in children with acute lymphocytic leukemia: MR relaxation times.' *Radiology*, **160**, 237–240.

Muhonen, M.G., Menezes, A.H., Sawin, P.D., Seinstein, S.L. (1992) 'Scoliosis in pediatric Chiari malformations without myelodysplasia.' *Journal of Neurosurgery*, **77**, 69–77.

Naidich, T.P., Harwood-Nash, D.C. (1983) 'Diastematomyelia: hemicord and meningeal sheaths; single and double arachnoid and dural tubes.' *American Journal of Neuroradiology*, **4**, 633–636.

—— Pudlowski, R.M., Naidich, J.B. (1980*a*) 'Computed tomographic signs of Chiari II malformation. II. Midbrain and cerebellum.' *Radiology*, **134**, 391–398.

—— —— —— (1980*b*) 'Computed tomographic signs of the Chiari II malformation. III. Ventricles and cisterns.' *Radiology*, **134**, 657–663.

—— —— —— Gornish, M., Rodriguez, F.J. (1980*c*) 'Computed tomographic signs of the Chiari II malformation. I. Skull and dural partitions.' *Radiology*, **134**, 65–71.

National Institutes Of Health Consensus Development Conference (1988) 'Neurofibromatosis conference statement.' *Archives of Neurology*, **45**, 575–578.

Nemoto, Y., Inoue, Y., Tashiro, T., Mochizuki, K., Oda, J., Kogame, S., Katsuyama, J., Hakuba, A., Onoyama,

Y. (1992) 'Intramedullary spinal cord tumors: significance of associated hemorrhage at MR imaging.' *Radiology*, **182**, 793–796.

Nokes, S.R., Murtagh, F.R., Jones, J.D., Downing, M., Arrington, J.A., Turetsky, D., Silbiger, M.L. (1987) 'Childhood scoliosis: MR imaging.' *Radiology*, **164**, 791–797.

Pang, D., Wilberger, J.E. (1982) 'Spinal cord injury without radiographic abnormalities in children.' *Journal of Neurosurgery*, **57**, 114–129.

Parizel, P.M., Baleriaux, D., Rodesch, G., Segebarth, C., Lalmand, B., Christophe, C., Lemort, M., Haesendonck, P., Niendorf, H.P., *et al.* (1989) 'Gd-DTPA-enhanced MR imaging of spinal tumors.' *American Journal of Roentgenology*, **152**, 1087–1096.

Park, T.S., Cail, W.S., Maggio, W.M., Mitchell, D.C. (1985) 'Progressive spasticity and scoliosis in children with myelomeningocele. Radiological investigation and surgical treatment.' *Journal of Neurosurgery*, **62**, 367–375.

Post, M.J.D., Quencer, R.M., Montalvo, B.M., Katz, B.H., Eismont, F.J., Green, B.A. (1988) 'Spinal infection: evaluation with MR imaging and intraoperative US.' *Radiology*, **169**, 765–771.

Pueschel, S.M.F., Scola, F.H. (1987) 'Atlantoaxial instability in individuals with Down syndrome: epidemiologic, radiographic, and clinical studies.' *Pediatrics*, **80**, 555–560.

Quencer, R.M., Sheldon, J.J., Post, M.J.D., Diaz, R.D., Montalvo, B.M., Green, B.A., Eismont, F.J. (1986) 'Magnetic resonance imaging of the chronically injured cervical spinal cord.' *American Journal of Neuroradiology*, **7**, 457–464.

Rabb, C.H., McComb, J.G., Raffel, C., Kennedy, J.G. (1992) 'Spinal arachnoid cysts in the pediatric age group: an association with neural tube defects.' *Journal of Neurosurgery*, **77**, 369–372.

Ramsey, R.G., Zacharias, C.E. (1985) 'MR imaging of the spine after radiation therapy: easily recognizable effects.' *American Journal of Roentgenology*, **144**, 1131–1135.

Reimer, R., Onofrio, B.M. (1985) 'Astrocytomas of the spinal cord in children and adolescents.' *Journal of Neurosurgery*, **63**, 669–675.

Renshaw, T.S. (1978) 'Sacral agenesis. A classification and review of twenty-three cases.' *Journal of Bone and Joint Surgery*, **60A**, 373–383.

Ross, J.S., Masaryk, T.J., Modic, M.T., Carter, J.R., Mapstone, T., Dengel, F.H. (1987) 'Vertebral hemangiomas: MR imaging.' *Radiology*, **165**, 165–169.

Ruzal-Shapiro, C., Berdon, W.E., Cohen, M.D., Abramson, S.J. (1991) 'MR imaging of diffuse bone marrow replacement in pediatric patients with cancer.' *Radiology*, **181**, 587–589.

Samuelsson, L., Bergström, K., Thuomas, K-Å., Hemmingsson, A., Wallensten, R. (1987) 'MR imaging of syringohydromyelia and Chiari malformations in myelomeningocele patients with scoliosis.' *American Journal of Neuroradiology*, **8**, 539–546.

Sato, Y., Pringle, K.C., Bergman, R.A., Yuh, W.T.C., Smith, W.L., Soper, R.T., Franken, E.D. (1988) 'Congenital anorectal anomalies: MR imaging.' *Radiology*, **168**, 157–162.

Schlesinger, A.E., Naidich, T.P., Quencer, R.M. (1986) 'Concurrent hydromyelia and diastematomyelia.' *American Journal of Neuroradiology*, **7**, 473–477.

Scott, R.M., Wolpert, S.M., Bartoshesky, L.E., Zimbler, S., Klauber, G.T. (1986) 'Dermoid tumors occurring at the site of previous myelomeningocele repair.' *Journal of Neurosurgery*, **65**, 779–783.

Siegel, M.J., Jamroz, G.A., Glazer, H.S., Abramson, C.L. (1986) 'MR imaging of intraspinal extension of neuroblastoma.' *Journal of Computer Assisted Tomography*, **10**, 593–595.

Sivit, C.J., Taylor, G.A., Newman, K.D., Bulas, D.I., Gotschall, C.S., Wright, C.J., Eichelberger, M.R. (1991) 'Safety-belt injuries in children with lap-belt ecchymosis: CT findings in 61 patients.' *American Journal of Roentgenology*, **157**, 111–114.

Slasky, B.S., Bydder, G.M., Niendorf, H.P., Young, I.R. (1987) 'MR imaging with gadolinium-DTPA in the differentiation of tumor, syrinx, and cyst of the spinal cord.' *Journal of Computer Assisted Tomography*, **11**, 845–850.

Smith, A.S., Weinstein, M.A., Mizushima, A., Coughlin, B., Hayden, S.P., Lakin, M.M., Lanzieri, C.F. (1989) 'MR imaging characteristics of tuberculous spondylitis vs vertebral osteomyelitis.' *American Journal of Neuroradiology*, **10**, 619–625.

Snider, D.E., Roper, W.L. (1992) 'The new tuberculosis.' *New England Journal of Medicine*, **326**, 703–705.

Sonnabend, D.H., Taylor, T.K.F., Chapman, G.K. (1982) 'Intervertebral disc calcification syndromes in children.' *Journal of Bone and Joint Surgery*, **64B**, 25–30.

Sorenson, H.K. (1964) *Scheuermann's Kyphosis: Clinical Appearances, Radiography, Aetiology, and Prognosis.* Copenhagen: Munksgaard.

277

Spetzler, R.F., Zabramski, J.M., Flom, R.A. (1989) 'Management of juvenile spinal AVM's by embolization and operative excision. Case report.' *Journal of Neurosurgery*, **70**, 628–632.

Stanley, P., Duncan, A.W., Isaacson, J., Isaacson, A.S. (1985) 'Radiology of fracture–dislocation of the cervical spine during delivery.' *American Journal of Roentgenology*, **145**, 621–625.

Stevens, S.K., Moore, S.G., Kaplan, I.D. (1990) 'Early and late bone-marrow changes after irradiation: MR evaluation.' *American Journal of Roentgenology*, **154**, 745–750.

Swischuk, L.E. (1969) 'Spine and spinal cord trauma in the battered child syndrome.' *Radiology*, **92**, 733–738.

Sze, G., Abramson, A., Krol, G., Liu, D., Amster, J., Zimmerman, R.D., Deck, M.D.F. (1988a) 'Gadolinium-DTPA in the evaluation of intradural extramedullary spinal disease.' *American Journal of Roentgenology*, **150**, 911–921.

—— Krol, G., Zimmerman, R.D., Deck, M.D.F. (1988b) 'Intramedullary disease of the spine: diagnosis using gadolinium-DTPA-enhanced MR imaging.' *American Journal of Neuroradiology*, **9**, 847–858.

—— —— —— —— (1988) 'Malignant extradural spinal tumors: MR imaging with Gd-DTPA.' *Radiology*, **167**, 217–231.

—— Stimac, G.K., Bartlett, C., Dillon, W.P., Haughton, V.M., Orrison, W., Kashanian, F., Goldstein, H. (1990) 'Multicenter study of gadopentetate dimeglumine as an MR contrast agent: evaluation in patients with spinal tumors.' *American Journal of Neuroradiology*, **11**, 967–974.

—— Baierl, P., Bravo, S. (1991) 'Evolution of the infant spinal column: evaluation with MR imaging.' *Radiology*, **181**, 819–827.

—— Bravo, S., Baierl, P., Shimkin, P.M. (1991) 'Developing spinal column: gadolinium-enhanced MR imaging.' *Radiology*, **180**, 497–502.

Tamaki, N., Shirataki, K., Kojima, N., Shouse, Y., Matsumoto, S. (1988) 'Tethered cord syndrome of delayed onset following repair of myelomeningocele.' *Journal of Neurosurgery*, **69**, 393–398.

Taylor, G.A., Eggli, K.D. (1988) 'Lap-belt injuries of the lumbar spine in children: a pitfall in CT diagnosis.' *American Journal of Roentgenology*, **150**, 1355–1358.

Techakapuch, S. (1981) 'Rupture of the lumbar cartilage plate into the spinal canal in an adolescent. A case report.' *Journal of Bone and Joint Surgery*, **63A**, 481–482.

Teplick, J.G., Laffey, P.A., Berman, A., Haskin, M.E. (1986) 'Diagnosis and evaluation of spondylolisthesis and/or spondylolysis on axial CT.' *American Journal of Neuroradiology*, **7**, 479–491.

Thrush, A., Enzmann, D. (1990) 'MR imaging of infectious spondylitis.' *American Journal of Neuroradiology*, **11**, 1171–1180.

Urso, S., Colajacomo, M., Migliorini, A., Fassari, F.M. (1987) 'Calcifying discopathy in infancy in the cervical spine: evaluation of vertebral alterations over a period of time.' *Pediatric Radiology*, **17**, 387–391.

Vade, A., Kennard, D. (1987) 'Lipomeningomyelocystocele.' *American Journal of Neuroradiology*, **8**, 375–377.

White, K.S., Ball, W.S., Prenger, E.C., Patterson, B.J., Kirks, D.R. (1993) 'Evaluation of the craniocervical junction in Down syndrome: correlation of measurements obtained with radiography and MR imaging.' *Radiology*, **186**, 377–382.

Wholey, M.H., Bruwer, A.J., Baker, H.L. (1958) 'The lateral roentgenogram of the neck. (With comments on atlanto-odontoid-basion relationship.)' *Radiology*, **71**, 350–356.

Wilson, D.A., Prince, J.R. (1989) 'MR imaging determination of the location of the normal conus medullaris throughout childhood.' *American Journal of Roentgenology*, **152**, 1029–1032.

Wiltse, L.L., Newman, P.H., Macnab, I. (1976) 'Classification of spondylolysis and spondylolisthesis.' *Clinical Orthopaedics and Related Research*, **117**, 23–29.

Yamada, H. Nakamura, S., Tajima, M., Kageyama, N. (1981a) 'Neurological manifestations of pediatric achondroplasia.' *Journal of Neurosurgery*, **54**, 49–57.

—— Zinke, D.E., Sanders, D. (1981b) 'Pathophysiology of "tethered cord syndrome".' *Journal of Neurosurgery*, **54**, 494–503.

Yousem, D.M., Schnall, M.D. (1991) 'MR examination for spinal cord compression: impact of a multicoil system on length of study.' *Journal of Computer Assisted Tomography*, **15**, 598–604.

12
PROTON MAGNETIC RESONANCE SPECTROSCOPY IN HYPOXIC–ISCHEMIC DISORDERS

Brian D. Ross, Thomas Ernst and Roland Kreis

Historical introduction

The experimental pathobiochemistry of hypoxic–ischemic injury to the brain is discussed in detail (Volpe 1987) and has now been confirmed in studies in neonates and infants. Figure 12.1 is a summary of some of the events of hypoxia–ischemia cascade, as defined by the work of Lowry (summarized in Volpe 1987). Thus, after the alterations in membrane function, the effects of oxygen deprivation, including the failure of electron transport and of oxidative phosphorylation, are all 'metabolic'. While the order of these events is still unclear, free radical damage, lipid release, dissolution of cell membranes and cell swelling all contribute to edema. Edema is probably the first event that would be obvious to an imaging examination such as MRI. Indeed, this may be related more to recovery from hypoxia and the immediate post-hypoxia events (which include cell swelling and obstruction of capillary blood-flow) described as the 'no-reflow phenomenon'. At the microscopic level, the effects of hypoxia on neocortex are fully documented, including the predilection of neurons in layer 2 of the hippocampal gyrus as the most sensitive, and hence the earliest targets of damage (Volpe 1987). A role for glutamate (Glu) as a neurotoxin capable of mediating such damage is also postulated. At the gross anatomic level, many decades of experience emphasize the heterogeneous distribution of hypoxic– ischemic brain injury, which can nevertheless be reduced to three or four major patterns (Volpe 1987).

Ultrasound, CT and MRI have contributed substantially to our understanding and management of these clinical emergencies. Positron emission tomography (PET) has been applied on rare occasions and helps to link the events throughout the brain with the experimental findings. An important finding in PET studies (also discussed by Volpe), which will be echoed in the MR spectra shown here, is the occurrence of abnormal metabolism distant from those areas most obviously affected by an ischemic or hypoxic lesion. The presence of PET changes even in the opposite hemisphere is now generally accepted to mean that the hypoxic damage in newborns is widespread. However, because PET is not widely available and requires an injection of a radioactive isotope, it is to magnetic resonance spectroscopy (MRS) that we must turn for any knowledge of the early biochemical events in a routine clinical setting.

[31]Phosphorus MRS was first used in this context in 1979, and showed decreased phosphocreatine (PCr) and ATP and intracellular pH after carotid artery ligation in the gerbil (Gadian 1982). By 1983, it had been conclusively shown that neonatal and pediatric

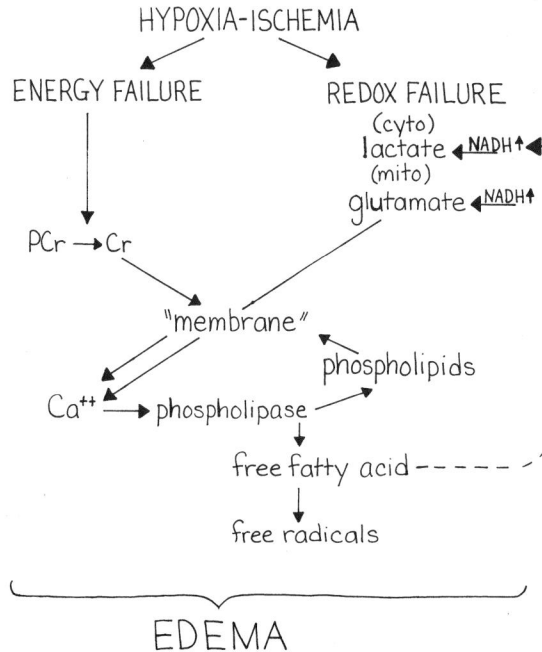

HYPOXIA-ISCHEMIA

ENERGY FAILURE   REDOX FAILURE
                                     (cyto)
                                   lactate ◂NADH↑◂
                                     (mito)
                                   glutamate ◂NADH↑
    PCr ➝ Cr

                    "membrane"
                                phospholipids

    Ca⁺⁺ ➝ phospholipase

                    free fatty acid ------
                              ↓
                    free radicals

EDEMA

Fig. 12.1. Hypoxia–ischemia cascade. A simplified schema of the metabolic events which follow ischemia and/or hypoxia in the intact brain. Some events, including free-radical formation and edema are more popularly associated with restoration of oxygen delivery after a period of ischemia.

hypoxic encephalopathy should be accompanied by decreases in intracerebral high energy phosphate (PCr and ATP) concentrations and increases in inorganic phosphate (Pi) and [H⁺] (Cady *et al.* 1983). The latter is detected as a change in pH, apparent from the chemical shift of inorganic phosphate by means of ^{31}P MRS. Despite severe technical constraints, including the absence of any serious attempt at anatomic localization for the brain spectra, and a magnet so small that follow-up beyond a few weeks of postnatal age was precluded by growth of the patient, the predictive power of the new technique was demonstrated.

At about this time, ^{1}H MRS was used to show the accumulation of lactate and loss of the putative neuronal marker *N*-acetylaspartate (NAA) in the ischemic rat and rabbit brain. There were also changes in lactate, creatine (Cr) and NAA content in the human infant, all of which are readily detected by means of long echo time (TE) ^{1}H MRS (Peden *et al.* 1990). More detailed evaluation of the effects of neonatal hypoxia has emerged with the introduction of routine methods using short TEs (Kreis *et al.* 1991*a*), and quantitative MRS (Ernst *et al.* 1993, Kreis *et al.* 1993*a,b*).

Neuropathology
Histopathologic studies show that neurons are selectively sensitive to hypoxia, astrocytes being relatively resistant. As we shall see, NAA, a prominent metabolite observed in the

280

NEUROPATHOLOGY

Edema (? newborn)

^{1}H
MRS $\left\{\begin{array}{l}\end{array}\right.$ **Selective neuronal necrosis (neuron > oligodendroglia > astrocyte)**

Parasaggital + posterior cortex

Periventricular leukomalacia

Focal ischemia → cysts

Fig. 12.2. Hypoxic encephalopathy: role of ^{1}H MRS in early diagnosis and neuropathology. By assaying NAA, MRS offers a first-line discriminator between neuronal and astrocyte damage due to hypoxia. Using a reliable localization technique (such as STEAM), MRS can readily distinguish parasagittal from periventricular metabolic changes. However, the inconvenient shape and location prevents the application to hippocampal gyrus, while relative insensitivity means that individual neuron 'layers' are at present not distinguishable from each other (*i.e.* minimum STEAM volume *ca.* 0.5–1cm^3).

^{1}H spectrum, is essentially a neuronal marker and a valuable new tool in neonatal medicine. Furthermore, the many studies of the blood flow to brain have emphasized the regional differences in oxygen distribution and the existence of particular areas of sensitivity to oxygen lack. Notably, 'watershed' areas are defined in the parasagittal and posterior cortical regions. Anatomically, children studied after 'recovery' from severe hypoxia show periventricular leukomalacia and focal cysts, both of which are presumed to be a reflection of the brain regions most susceptible to hypoxic damage. By reliably assaying NA*, image guided ^{1}H MRS is particularly sensitive to neuronal damage and can distinguish between parasagittal and parietal distribution of hypoxic damage (Ross *et al.* 1992) (Fig. 12.2). As expected, the former location is affected earlier, and more severely (see later, and Fig. 12.20). More sensitive areas defined by studies on brain slices and isolated neurons from the hippocampal gyrus or in the basal ganglia, or the more 'resistant' areas of the brainstem, are currently not routinely examined by MRS *in vivo*, but may offer yet more insights. These regional events will not be discussed further.

Temporal aspects
Despite the overwhelming experimental evidence that hypoxic–ischemic injury begins within minutes of the 'insult', histopathologic changes associated with neuron damage (pyknosis of nuclei) and demonstrable cell necrosis, take much longer to appear (24–36

*By now, NAA is a familiar abbreviation. However, for technical reasons, the precise proportion of the *N*-acetyl (NA) resonance attributable to NAA (and the neuronal dipeptide marker *N*-acetylaspartylglutamate, NAAG) is uncertain, so it is more appropriate to use the abbreviation NA to describe the MRS peak.

TEMPORAL ASPECTS

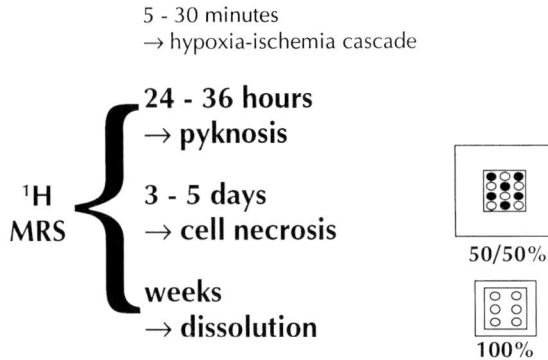

5 - 30 minutes
→ hypoxia-ischemia cascade

**24 - 36 hours
→ pyknosis**

¹H
MRS {

**3 - 5 days
→ cell necrosis**

50/50%

**weeks
→ dissolution**

100%

Fig. 12.3. Hypoxic encephalopathy: role of ¹H MRS in early diagnosis—temporal aspects. The second, slower cascade of events which follow those illustrated in Fig. 12.1, concern neuronal death. Inset are diagrammatic representations of voxels in the 'normal' volume of severely hypoxic cortex; viable neurons which still contain NA are shown as open circles. Half of the neuronal number are assumed to have undergone necrosis, with loss of NAA. NA/Cr may fall. A purely speculative model describes later cortical atrophy, represented by reduced brain volume *(lower inset)*. The voxel may now contain only viable neurons. NA/Cr may rise or even be normal. Absolute quantitation of Cr may reveal underlying loss of cells. However, with this simplified model, both [NA] and [Cr] could become 'normal', the neuronal loss being measured only by the anatomical extent of cortical atrophy in MRI.

hours, and 3–5 days, respectively) (Fig. 12.3). It is this model, rather than the more classical descriptions of Lowry and colleagues (see Volpe 1987), which is needed to describe the results of MRS examinations. In survivors of hypoxic injury, those early and medium term events are long passed. This is perhaps fortunate, because in clinical practice the opportunities to examine infants during the primary episode of hypoxia are very limited. On the other hand, the knowledge that 'delayed' effects are also amenable to detection with ¹H MRS, offers a very practical solution. As we have already briefly described elsewhere (Kreis *et al.* 1992*a*), the loss of NA from the brain spectrum occurs after some days. This is compatible with the hypothesis underlying Fig. 12.3. The upper box views the first events as resulting in loss of neurons (black circles) compared with surviving neurons (open circles). The next series of events concern dissolution, which refers to the reorganization of surviving neural tissues; 'dead' neurons are removed, leaving a thinned cortex in which largely intact neurons remain. The 'density' of open circles is seen to increase, though less than in normal brain. This process may take a number of weeks. Atrophy is notable after two weeks, and the dramatic MR images observed in the survivors of cerebral hypoxia are finally established after months. This sequence of events indicates that the pattern of changes observable in MR spectra is likely to be strongly time-dependent. This will be discussed below.

Despite earlier studies showing very abnormal ³¹P MRS in infants suffering from intracranial hemorrhage, 'normal' phosphorus spectra are occasionally recorded from brains which in MRI are clearly disorganized following ischemic birth injury (unpublished observations; and see Fig. 12.16). The histopathologic explanation for this may be summarized as in Figure 12.3. After an infarct, surviving brain tissue consolidates, while necrotic tissues are removed. Within the residual volume assayed with MRS, the metabolite profile, *i.e.* metabolite ratios, will 'recover' and be closer to that of normal brain tissue. With the advent of quantitative ^{1}H MRS, this paradox has been resolved. When the signal intensity is corrected, the MR spectrum may show lower absolute [NA] (and [Cr]), correctly identifying loss of neurons and the loss of tissue 'mass'.

Based on such models, we believe that from the pattern of changes in cerebral metabolites we may even be able to define the *time* of the hypoxic insult more accurately. There is already copious literature concerning the impact of prenatal *vs* perinatal hypoxia in preterm *vs* term infants on MR images of the brain. In future, ^{1}H MRS may also have an important part to play in this distinction.

Major clinical questions in hypoxic encephalopathy

At the cot-side, the questions that arise for which answers would affect management and outcome in hypoxic encephalopathy are:

1. Can MRS improve the sensitivity with which we detect hypoxic damage? Is there any neuronal damage in an at-risk baby in whom imaging, including ultrasound, is non-contributory or normal?
2. Can prognostic value be placed upon these MRS tests for hypoxic encephalopathy, especially those which are reported quantitatively? Does measurable biochemical change imply irrecoverable hypoxic damage? Can therapy be positively influenced by MRS findings?
3. Can the time of injury be more precisely identified? Is the hypoxic damage identified the result of intrauterine events, or was it sustained during or after the moment of birth? This question has copious legal implications for health professionals in neonatology and obstetrics.

If MRS can begin to address these issues, it will probably find a warm welcome in neonatal and pediatric intensive care units.

Methods of clinical MRS

MRS differs from MRI (which images the protons at the single frequency of water) in that it records the concentrations of protons at all their different frequencies. The frequency 'map' is the spectrum in which chemical shift is identified and peak area (or height) is proportional to concentration. In this chapter, we deal exclusively with one group of tests: qualitative, quantitative or semi-quantitative short TE ^{1}H MRS of single voxels (volumes of interest).

Early ^{1}H MR spectra which laid the groundwork for diagnosis in medicine used long TEs (TE 270, 135 ms). The use of 270 ms allows clear identification of three major peaks, and elimination of much of the unwanted lipid, which has a short T_2. A TE of 135 ms may be selected because specific inversion of lactate is achieved, which allows separation of that metabolite from lipid. Recently, short TE techniques (20, 30 ms) became available.

Shielded gradients, minimizing eddy currents, permitted even ultra-short TE acquisitions. This meant the visualization of a considerably larger number of metabolites; the protons of several neurometabolites have a short T_2 and have disappeared from spectra acquired with longer TE. Newly visualized metabolites are *myo*-inositol, *scyllo*-inositol (or taurine?), glutamate, glutamine, GABA, fatty acid chains, glucose and ketone bodies. The problem of short TE techniques is the baseline. However, the flatter baseline and greater simplicity of long TE techniques do not outweigh the loss of diagnostic information.

Localized MRS has superseded non-localized MRS for diagnostic purposes. It has become very uncommon to see MR spectra without a prior proton localizer image. This prevents acquisition of spectra from skull regions contaminated by fat, and from regions of magnetic field inhomogeneity which distort spectra detail. Three localization schemes are now in widespread use: STEAM (90–180–180), PRESS (90–90–90) and ISIS (180–180–180). Water suppression is usually achieved by either presaturation (with two or three pulses) or selective excitation (generally 1:3:3:1), centered on the water resonance. Other, less satisfactory schemes are slowly being superseded. Adequate water suppression is of great importance in proton MRS. Instability of water suppression during acquisition of a clinical MR spectrum is one of the most insidious sources of artifacts, and may result in unusual spectra, in this way compromising a most useful test. Recent improvements have been very successful in eradicating or greatly minimizing the proton signal of water at 4.7 parts per million (ppm). With these methods, resonances as close as 4.1 ppm can be reliably identified, including several peaks upfield of water, in the aromatic region.

Standardization and quantitation

The best means to interpret data obtained in ^{1}H MRS has also evolved considerably since the first clinical studies. As with MRI, if the acquisition parameters are accurately known and adhered to, a system of pattern recognition is an acceptable means of diagnosis. In earlier times, when only three resonances were defined, present or absent (for NAA and Cr) and higher or lower (for the choline/creatine [Cho/Cr] ratio) was a common *modus operandi*. For two reasons this is unacceptable. First, quite serious pathology is missed if 10–20 per cent changes in even these three metabolites cannot be defined; and second, in infants there are well defined modulations of cerebral metabolites with age. The two factors are compounded by the realization that no single metabolite peak can be assumed constant in either healthy or diseased brain so that no reliable internal reference is available. Interpretation of single ^{1}H MR spectra becomes problematic. Two new approaches have minimized, if not eliminated, this problem: standardization and quantitation.

Bottomley (1991, 1992) summarizes the faults in many clinical MRS studies. Several of these can be traced to a lack of critical attention to detail. In no other clinical area is it acceptable to vary the technique from one day to the next. Yet, spectra acquired from different total volumes, in different brain areas, with different acquisition parameters and under seemingly trivially different acquisition conditions are often compared. Correcting these basic faults can be termed 'standardization'. One such routine is described in this chapter. Adoption of this or a similar routine will greatly enhance the progress of MRS in neonatal hypoxia.

Until recently, the use of peak ratios to define metabolite ratios was common in the absence of other means of quantitation. But now, at least four independent methods of absolute quantitation have been proposed and tested clinically. It is premature to choose one among them, and the present authors believe an ideal method will incorporate some features from each. To date, the following components of the ^{1}H MRS examination have been successfully addressed (Ernst *et al.* 1993, Kreis *et al.* 1993*a*): (a) an external reference; (b) coil 'loading', recorded; (c) compartment correction for CSF and 'solid' brain material; (d) water referencing; (e) determined water content.

At present, different 'absolute' results are obtained. The largest source of these 'errors' is a failure to standardize the method of expressing the results (millimolar, millimolal, per volume or per wet weight). A second, unresolved problem is the baseline contribution to the spectrum. It is widely accepted that this baseline is composed of unassigned metabolites (Behar 1991), and therefore any attempt to 'correct' it may introduce a new error. A temporary solution is the use of 'institution units', since standardized acquisitions in one MR scanner result in reproducible baselines (Kreis *et al.* 1991*b*). On this basis, good longitudinal studies can be performed (Ross *et al.* 1992).

Finally, it should be noted that all efforts concerning absolute quantition have been devoted to ^{1}H MRS and that no such endeavor has been concluded for ^{31}P MRS. Without this, it is unlikely that current interpretations can be viewed as final.

Chemical shift imaging (CSI)

Phase encoding with gradients allows many spectra to be acquired at the same time. Chemical shift information is retained, so that each peak of the spectrum can be mapped to provide a spatial image or metabolite map. Even though spatial resolution is much more limited than water proton imaging, a great deal has been learned of the heterogeneity of metabolic changes in seemingly focal lesions, such as tumors, stroke and multiple sclerosis. It is likely that this method will throw some light on hypoxic–ischemic disease by allowing definition of the anatomic extent of a biochemical lesion and visualization of heterogeneity in metabolic derangements, for instance, distribution of NAA and of lactate. Much can also be learned from repeated CSI. In particular, as lesions enlarge or contract, biochemical events may precede histologic changes.

The major disadvantages at present include the necessity for long TEs (thus making imaging of several potentially useful metabolites including glutamine more difficult), and the lack of any quantitative information. The spatial resolution of ^{1}H metabolite images is reasonable.

In localized ^{31}P MRS, the advent of proton decoupling is the most important advance. With decoupling, phosphoethanolamine is separated from phosphocholine in the PME peak and glycerophosphocholine is separated from glycerophosphoethanolamine within the PDE peak. As the PDE peak and, to a lesser extent, the PME peak, changes in height in demyelinating disorders, it may be worthwhile to examine the contributions of phosphoethanolamine, phosphocholine, glycerophosphoethanolamine and glycerophosphocholine. However, the resolution of ^{31}P metabolite images, including CSI, is rather poor. Typically, eight to twelve pixels are available for each metabolite image in an entire brain slice.

^{13}C MRS of the brain is feasible and is becoming widely available. Detection of organic compounds and following their metabolism is highly interesting and may be the most direct approach to diagnosis. This technique generally necessitates the infusion of ^{13}C-enriched precursors.

Information content of short TE ^{1}H MR spectra
The proton spectrum, which is potentially rather richer in information than that of ^{31}P, has the enhanced sensitivity which allows us to examine smaller volumes of interest, and the enormous practical advantage that, at field strengths of around 1.5 T, existing hardware on clinical imagers can be used to perform the examination. Integration of MRI and ^{1}H MRS is thereby readily achieved, and MRS can be completed in between six and 30 minutes.

Interpretation of a brain spectrum: short TE proton MRS
Figure 12.4 is an adult human ^{1}H brain spectrum. At least 17 peaks are identified, including the residual water and lipid peaks. Simplification of the spectrum, by procedures generally described as 'editing', can be achieved. Metabolites not at present visualized in the spectrum shown might been seen if yet other editing procedures were to be applied during initial acquisition of the signal. Another form of simplification, the long TE acquisition which results in a proton spectrum of brain with only the most prominent three resonances, is a commonly encountered profile. By artificially subdividing the spectrum, the ensuing discussions of biochemical and clinical significance of ^{1}H MRS are straightforward.

Area I is the simplest grouping of major resonances [NAA], [Cr] and [Cho] observed in the brain. NA actually has two resonances, and creatine also has two, so that the simplest analysis nevertheless ascribes five peaks to three metabolites.

Area II is in fact not a spectrum but an area in which lactate (Lac), alanine (Ala) and a number of other 'methyl' protons, including ethanol, would resonate. Lactate and alanine are normal and important metabolites which existing techniques can demonstrate only at pathologically (or physiologically) elevated concentrations.

Area III selects from the remaining peaks those associated with three further metabolites: glutamate and glutamine (abbreviated as Glx) and *myo*-inositol (mI). The biochemistry of glutamate, glutamine and *myo*-inositol has been described by Ross (1991). The coincidence of the most prominent *myo*-inositol resonance with that of the alpha protons of the amino acid glycine, is to be noted.

This chapter deals exclusively with our experience with ^{1}H MRS. Most of the critical early work in this field was performed with ^{31}P MRS. The reader is referred to valuable papers by Cady *et al.* (1983), Hope *et al.* (1984), Boesch *et al.* (1989) and van der Knaap *et al.* (1992). In addition, important methodologic and conceptual advances in neonatal MRS were made by Peden *et al.* (1990), van der Knaap *et al.* (1990, 1992), Zimmerman and Wang (1991), and others.

The method evolved for use in neonatal and pediatric emergencies at Huntington Medical Research Institutes (HMRI) in Pasadena, California, is briefly described here and given in detail by Kreis *et al.* (1991*b*, 1992*b*, 1993*a*,*b*), Ernst *et al.* (1992, 1993) and Kreis and Ross (1992).

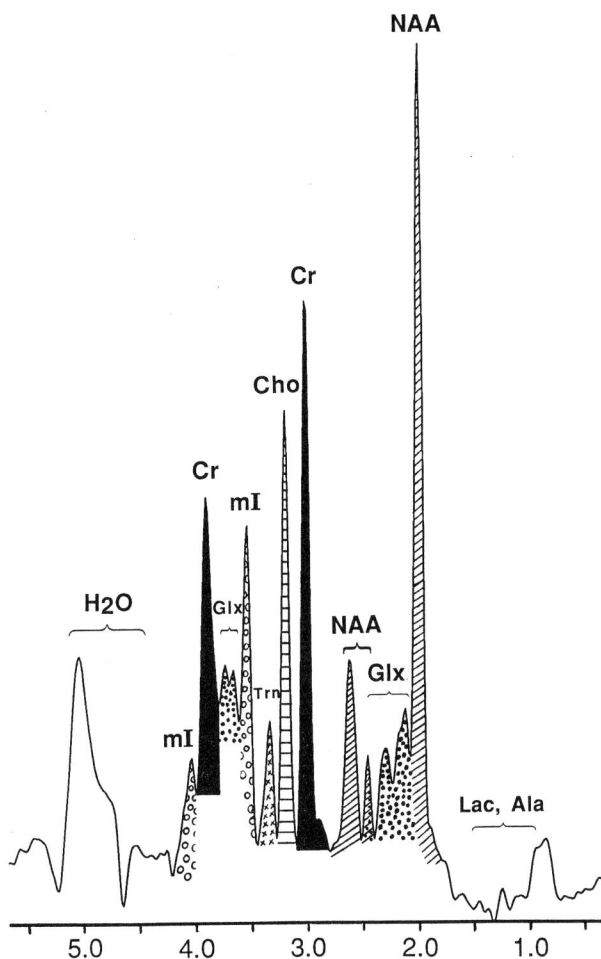

Fig. 12.4. Proton spectrum of human cerebral cortex. The central spectrum was obtained at 1.5 T after water suppression, and with a relatively short TE (30 ms). Detailed assignments are given elsewhere. The peaks correspond to the main metabolites discussed in this volume: N-acetylaspartate, creatine and choline (I). Lactate and alanine (barely perceptible at physiological concentration) (II), and glutamate, glutamine and *myo*-inositol (III). More detail concerning the brain spectrum and additional assignments are given by Kreis and Ross (1992).

Practical details

Over 100 children have been examined at HMRI, from 19 hours post-partum to 12 years old and from a gestational age of 31 weeks upwards (Kreis *et al.* 1993*b*). Many were transferred to the MRS unit in incubators and while on life-support, and were thereafter returned to the intensive care unit at Huntington Memorial Hospital (Pasadena, CA). No formal monitoring incubator was used during MRS (*cf.* Cady *et al.* 1983, Boesch *et al.* 1989), but pulse oximetry, manual ventilation (with extended gas tubing and T-piece to

287

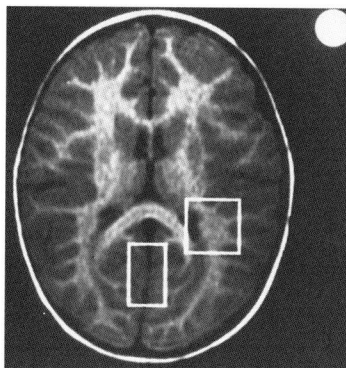

LOCATION

Hippocampus

Basal ganglia

^{1}H $\left\{\begin{array}{l}\text{Occipital cortex}\\[4pt] \text{Parietal cortex}\end{array}\right.$

MRS

Fig. 12.5. Hypoxic encephalopathy: role of ^{1}H MRS in diagnosis—location. Low resolution MRI is sufficient to place voxels for MRS examinations. The two locations described in this article are chosen for their robustness in clinical use, even though theoretical and experimental considerations might indicate improved sensitivity in other brain regions (see also legend to Fig. 12.2). Visible in this field of view is the calibration standard, an important modification for full quantitation in clinical ^{1}H MRS.

minimize respiratory dead-space), and a syringe infusion pump with 4–5 m of intravenous or intra-arterial tubing to maintain safe distances from the magnet, were used. A full-time specialist nurse and respiratory therapy nurse, but no anesthetist, were deemed necessary participants in the examination. Occasionally, the additional presence of the neonatologist was desirable.

MRS in hypoxia
A rigorous reproducible examination was the aim, since age differences and regional differences in the spectrum must be thoroughly understood. This in turn makes heavy demands on quality control. Without this rigorous approach, no clinical conclusions could be justified. One or both of only two brain regions of interest (voxels) were consistently examined (Fig. 12.5): the parietal cortex, as representative of white matter, and the occipital cortex, as representative of gray matter and watershed vascular supply. Exceptions were made in either of two special circumstances: (1) if the standard voxel included blood or obviously damaged tissue, then the voxel of interest was shifted to *exclude* this region; and (2) if location was crucial to diagnosis, *e.g.* middle cerebral infarct. For the interpretation and significance of deviations from 'normal', age-related curves were constructed (Fig. 12.6) based on metabolite ratios and dependent on the presumption that [Cr] (*i.e.* creatine conentration) is constant. Detailed information may be obtained from Kreis *et al.* (1993*b*).

Quantitation
Because of hypoxia-associated cerebral cortical atrophy, and because the metabolic response to hypoxia may include changes in all metabolites of an MR spectrum, increasingly we believe that quantitative MRS will become the preferred method in pediatric hypoxia. Accordingly, the reader is referred to a number of recent methods of quantition. The present

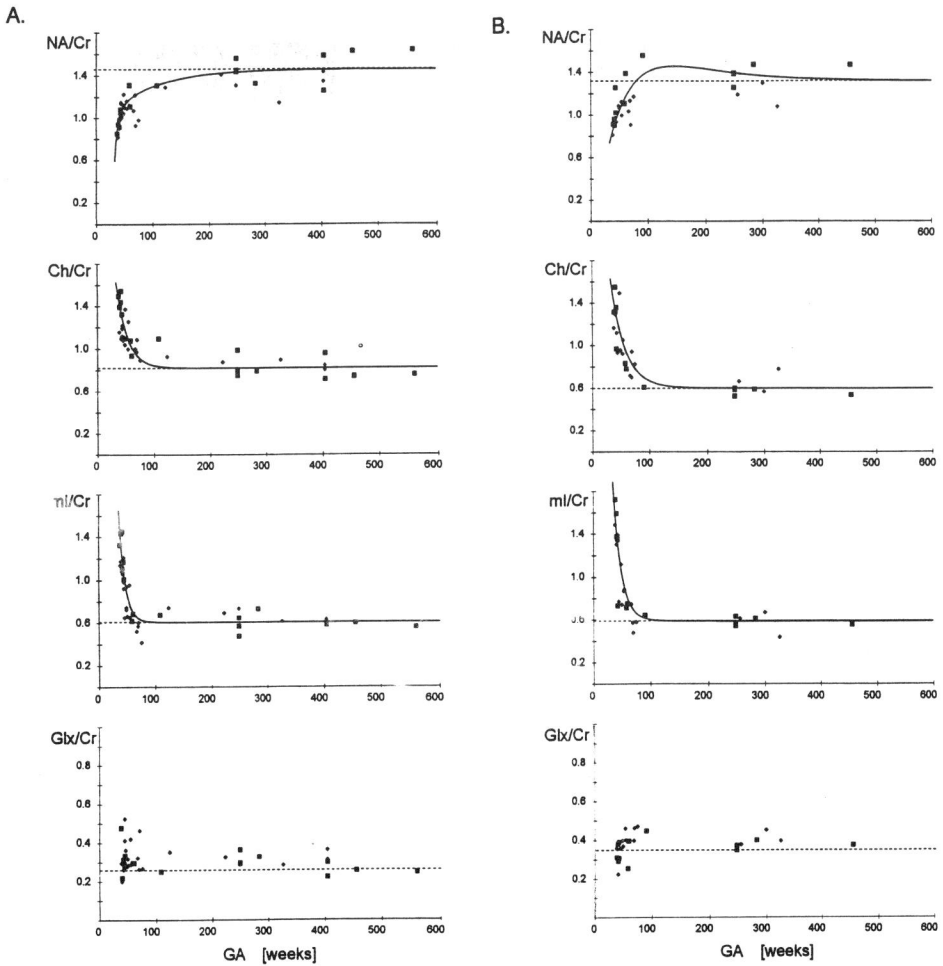

Fig. 12.6. Time courses of metabolite peak amplitude ratios *vs* gestational age of subject (modified by permission from Kreis *et al.* 1993*b*). *(A)* and *(B)* contain the normative curves for the parietal (mostly white matter) and occipital (predominantly gray matter) locations, respectively. The curves are well defined for the first year of life, where the most dramatic changes take place. The normative curves are specific for the acquisition parameters used.

results were largely acquired according to the methods of Ernst *et al.* (1993) and Kreis *et al.* (1993*a*). The method we employ in clinical practice is rapid and robust, but is not strictly quantitative since it makes no allowance for T_1 and T_2 variations in single patients. Results are expressed in Institutional Units, rather than mmol/kg wet weight of brain. Fortunately, this is an acceptable compromise. The alternative, the accurate determination of metabolite T_1 and T_2 saturation factors in each patient (Kreis *et al.* 1993*b*), requires an examination of ≥1 hour and is therefore probably impractical in emergency studies.

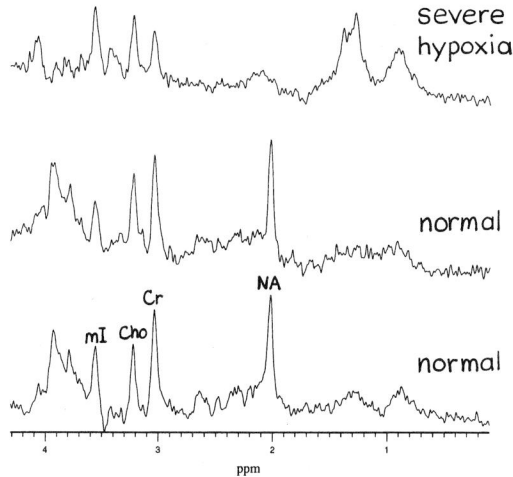

Fig. 12.7. Late MRS changes in severe hypoxia. This child, a term birth (gestational age 38 weeks), suffered an hypoxic insult at age 8 months and was re-examined after 'recovery' when severe cortical atrophy with ventricular dilatation was present on MRI, spastic paraplegia and cortical blindness on clinical examination. The upper spectrum was obtained from parietal cortex at age 11 months (13 weeks post-hypoxia). Lower two spectra are from age-matched normal infant and normal adult respectively.

MRS findings in hypoxia–ischemia: three types of injury

The patterns of hypoxic–ischemic damage in MRS appear to follow a pattern noted in the MR image. We can best illustrate this in a series of case studies. MRI and localized ^{1}H MRS were performed in each case. We point out that our experience is confined to two regions of the brain. A strong case could be made that increased sensitivity to hypoxia would be achieved by examinations of the basal ganglia or of the hippocampal gyrus, but this awaits rigorous testing to determine their clinical utility.

Pure hypoxic injury

Figure 12.7 illustrates a common pattern of cerebral metabolites after severe hypoxia. Whereas normal spectra show NA, Cr, Cho and mI, there is dramatically disorganized metabolism in the upper, hypoxic, spectrum. NA is absent, Cho 'exceeds' Cr, and two new broad resonances, assigned to intracerebral lipids or free fatty acids, dominate the spectrum. In this example, acquired from an 11-month-old infant several weeks after injury, it is not possible to unequivocally assign any resonances to lactate, although excess lactate is a frequent finding.

A specific case illustrates the MRI and ^{1}H MRS findings in this common clinical setting (Fig. 12.8). Changes in MRI are subtle and may indicate bilateral 'hypoxic' damage, slightly more obvious on the left. No obvious hemorrhage is seen on T$_2$-weighted images. Proton MRS is dramatically affected in both of the regions identified; in addition to lactate and lipid accumulation, NA is depleted. The changes on the MRS right are very obvious, despite the only modest changes in the MR image.

290

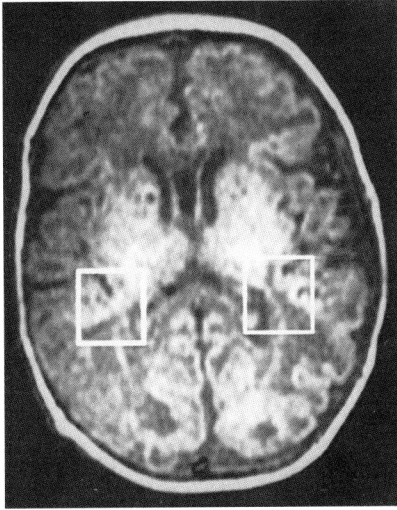

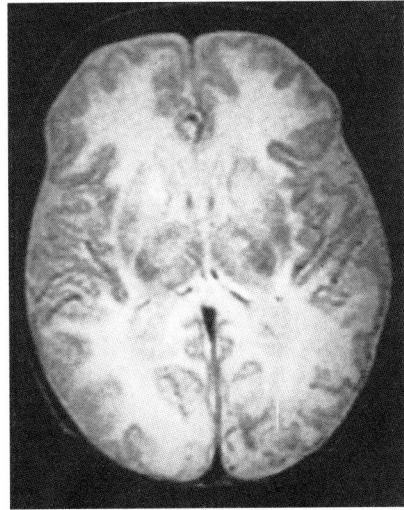

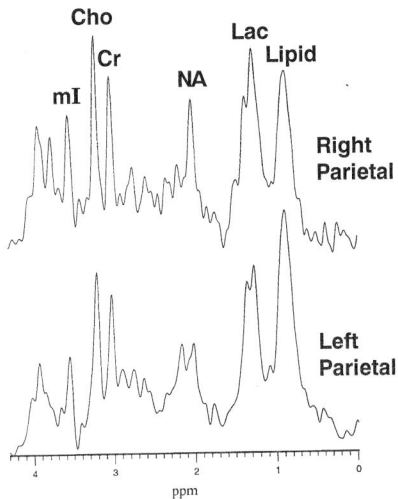

Fig. 12.8. Hypoxic encephalopathy. *(Above)* T_1- and T_2-weighted images of infant, postnatal age 2 weeks (42 weeks GA at birth). Hypoxic episode at birth; improving clinically. MRI reported as demonstrating left posteroparietal and occipital ischemic infarction and right occipital ischemia, with changes more marked on left. (CT showed only the left parieto-occipital lesion.) *(Left)* ^{1}H MR spectra. Severe hypoxic changes include reduced NA/Cr, excess lactate and intra-voxel lipid. Ischemic damage is considerably more severe on left, but lactate and lipid are prominent on both left and right parietal spectra.

Intracerebral hemorrhage

Spectra obtained from within obvious areas of intracerebral hemorrhage are severely disorganized (Fig. 12.9) and are of poor quality due to local magnetic field susceptibility problems. Indeed, it is a rather pointless exercise, adding nothing to the diagnosis. However, the extent of hypoxic damage exceeds that detectable in MRI (as predicted earlier by PET studies) (Volpe 1987), so that the spectrum from the right parietal region, which avoids the 'visible' hemorrhage, while also of rather poor quality, shows reduced NA/Cr, and possible presence of lactate.

291

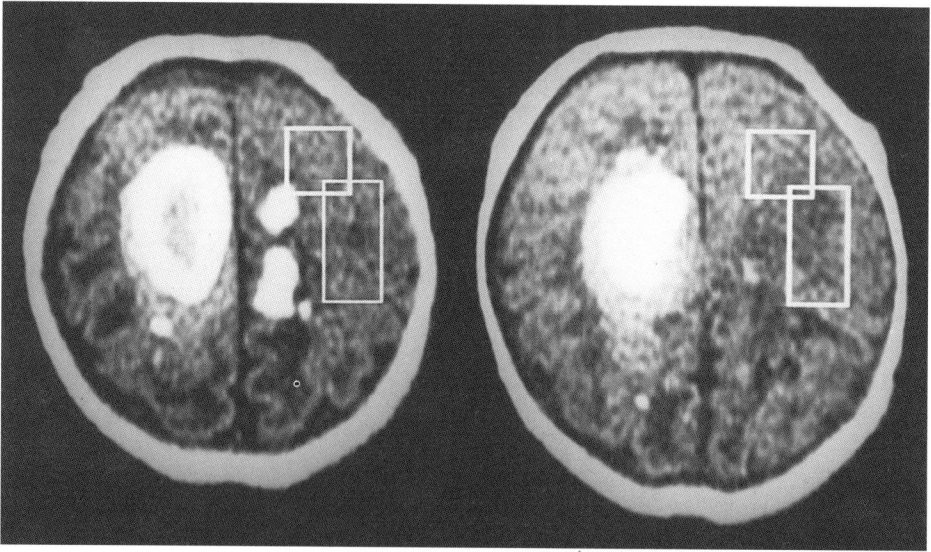

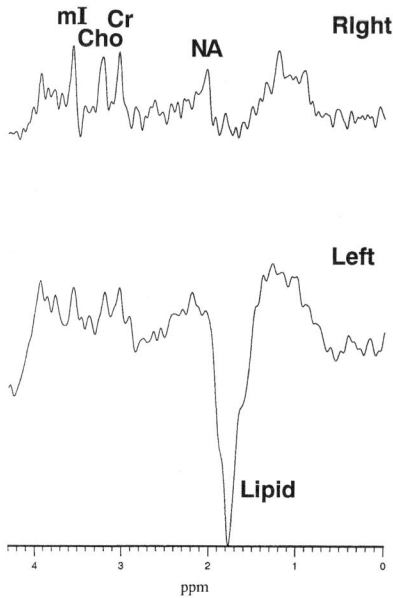

Fig. 12.9. Hemorrhagic infarction or primary brain hemorrhage. MRI and MRS of $3\frac{1}{2}$-week-old infant (GA at birth 38 weeks) showing extensive hemorrhage and severe frontal encephalomalacia. Lower spectrum (from left) is hardly interpretable due to susceptibility effects of local hemorrhage. Probably only Cr, Cho and mI are recognizably present, but no NA. Upper spectrum is acquired from the right hemisphere where little or no obvious hemorrhage is present on MRI. Again signal-to-noise is uncharacteristically poor. Nevertheless, NA/Cr is well below the age-related normal which should be close to 1.0 ppm (see Fig. 12.6). The presence of lactate (1.3 ppm), though suggestive, cannot be evaluated with certainty in this spectrum.

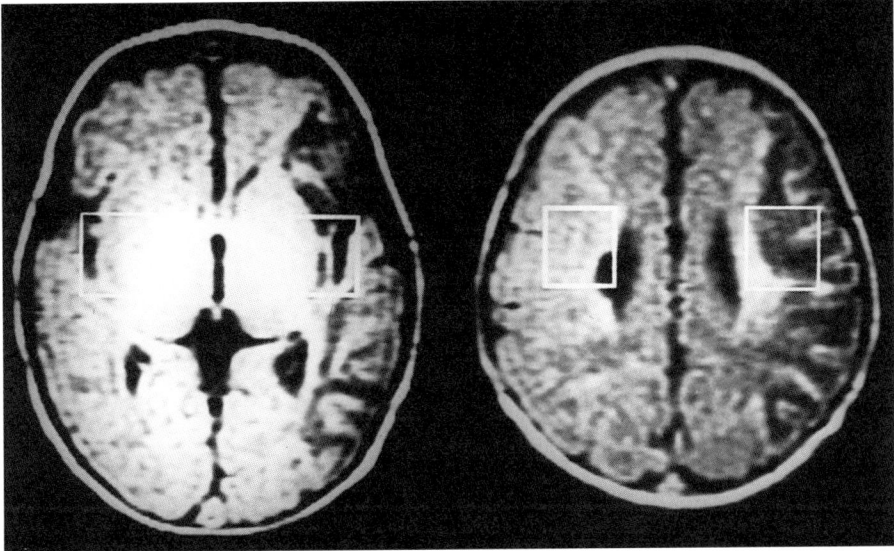

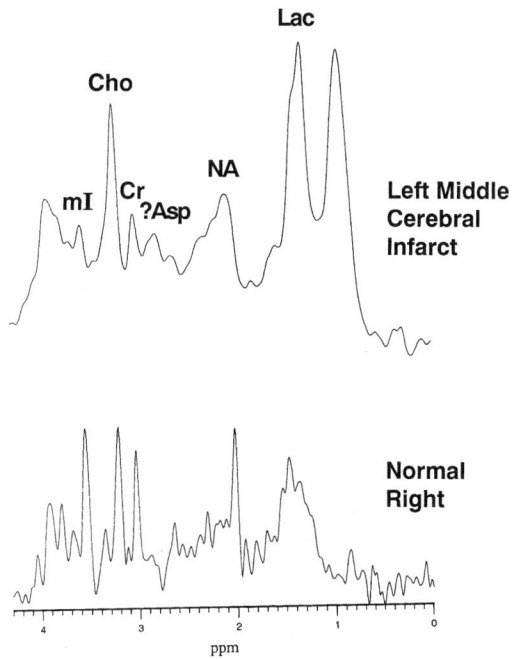

Fig. 12.10. Cerebral infarction at birth. MRI and MRS of 10-day-old infant (GA at birth 41 weeks). A left middle cerebral infarct was diagnosed with CT and readily confirmed by MRI. Sedation was inadequate so that the quality of the spectrum obtained from the (?normal) right hemisphere is poor. NA/Cr, Cho/Cr and mI/Cr are approximately correct for age. Within the infarct on the left, NA is virtually absent and Cr is much reduced. Lactate and intracerebral lipid, characteristic of chronic 'stroke', dominate the spectrum.

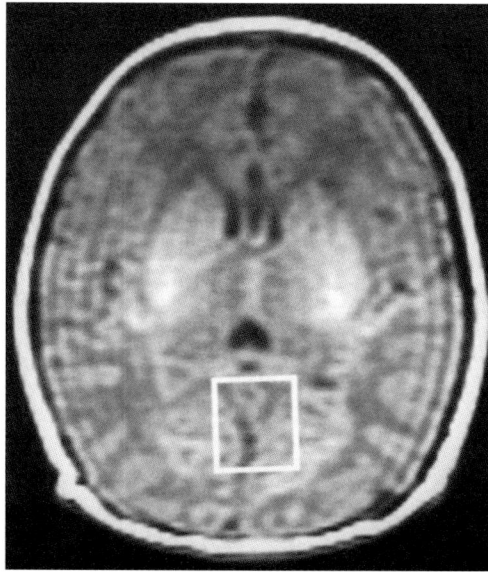

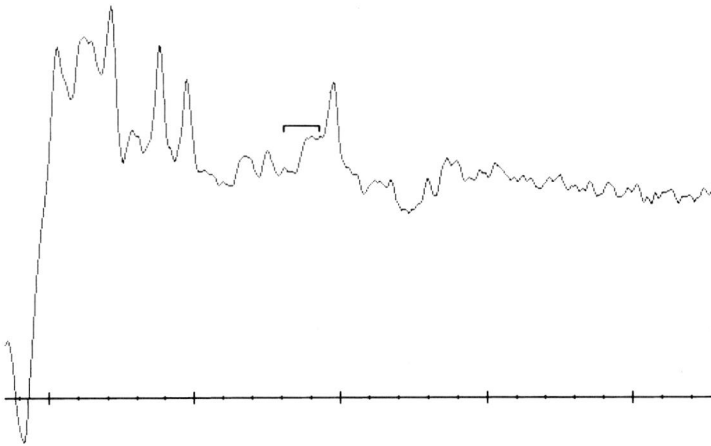

Fig. 12.11. PROBE reverses diagnosis in 'hypoxic' infant. A newborn infant 36 hours after a very difficult birth was thought to have suffered severe hypoxic brain damage. No spontaneous breathing or pulse for 20 minutes after delivery by caesarean section (mother had *abruptio placentae*). Respiratory assistance and external cardiac massage were continued. However, clinical progression was very poor, with apparently severe neurologic damage with fixed dilated pupils. The neonatologist's prognosis was, "severely guarded with virtually no chance of neurologically intact infant." MRS (including PROBE) was performed in the occipital location, normally highly diagnostic and predictive of outcome in hypoxic encephalopathy. MRI was also performed and appeared normal. The MRS showed no lactate; normal NA/Cr, Cho/Cr, mI/Cr ratios; matched to correct age-related curves. PROBE confirmed these findings in semi-quantitative form. based upon the MRS findings, the infant was maintained on ventilator and full support for a further 48 hours. The baby was subsequently weaned off the ventilator and commenced sucking. The baby was discharged neurologically *normal* on the 10th day, and was normal at follow-up at 5$\frac{1}{2}$ months.

294

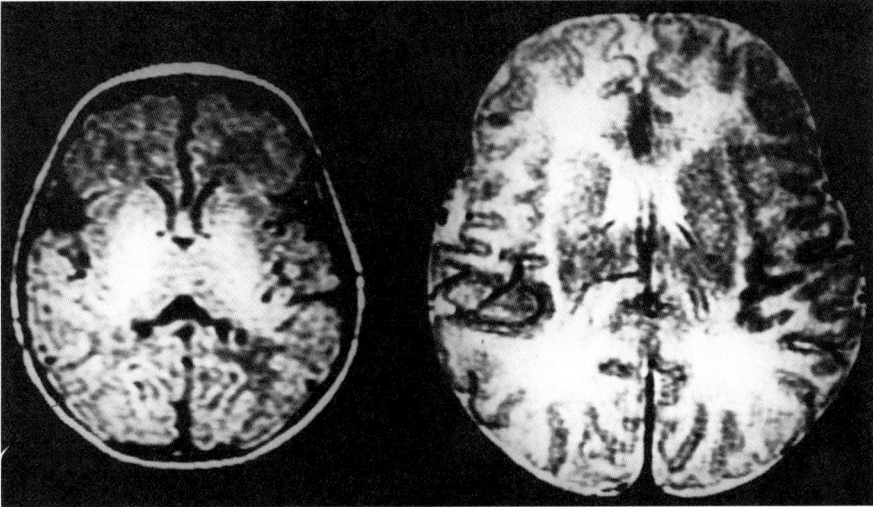

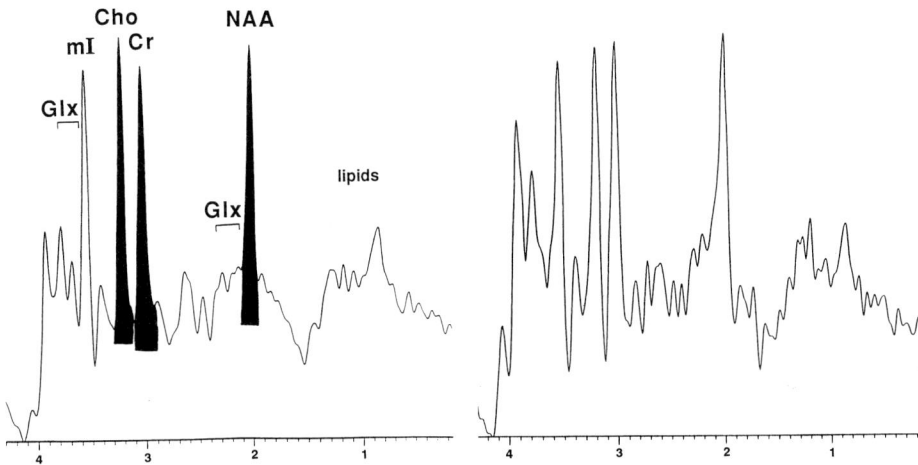

Fig. 12.12. MRI and MRS of left–right parietal hemispheres after arteriovenous ECMO. ^{1}H MRS showed normal spectrum in both parietal hemispheres. The patient was 26 days post-partum. No significant differences in principal metabolites.

Infarct

Occlusion of the middle cerebral artery with a sequential cerebral infarct is a readily recognized complication in neonates. The region of the infarct (Fig. 12.10) yields a spectrum with loss of NA and Cr, and accumulation of lactate and intracerebral lipid. The contralateral spectrum, although technically unsatisfactory due to motion, shows a much more normal pattern of metabolites with only the dubious resonance in the lipid/lactate area.

Recovery after prolonged birth apnea or after successful arteriovenous extracorporeal membrane oxygenation (ECMO) life support

By way of contrast with these dramatically abnormal ^1H spectra, we can state with some certainty that infants exposed to hypoxia but clinically recovered show essentially normal MR spectra. Two examples are presented.

The first patient, examined 36 hours after birth when flaccid and neurologically severely abnormal, showed a normal MRI, and a relatively normal MRS (Fig. 12.11). The spectra shown were obtained with PROBE (a fully automated MRS examination) in six minutes; quantitative results were also obtained with the routine ^1H MRS method, confirming the pattern of findings and providing the required information that actual metabolite amounts were appropriate.

The second (Fig. 12.12) was taken from a child after ECMO. In MR spectra obtained on day 20, cerebral metabolism is near-normal and is symmetrical. Spectra from the left and right hemispheres are so similar as to be superimposable, despite the fact that the right carotid artery was ligated as part of the ECMO procedure.

Evolution of MRS changes after cerebral hypoxia

While much can be inferred from infants studied once, it is most convincing to follow the progressive biochemical changes as they occur in a single infant at varying times after the hypoxic insult.

Early detection and progression of abnormality

Figures 12.13–12.15 show this progression with time, and at the same time, the varying degrees of severity of changes in different brain regions. Thus, although as yet we have no histologically verified cases, it is hard to escape the conclusion that progression in both severity and duration after hypoxia is an important piece of information inherent in the ^1H MR spectrum.

These figures illustrate that severe changes in the MR spectrum occurred where the hypoxic damage was greatest. Furthermore, the progressive loss of NA, Cr and mI with time must reflect evolution of hypoxic damage between days 5, 12 and 42 after birth. The frontoparietal cortex appears to be essentially spared (Fig. 12.15D) and provides a 'control' spectrum for this infant. In parentheses, we may note that MRI, equivocal on day 5, clearly reflects the changes in MRS by day 12 (Fig. 12.14). The final dissolution of the occipital lobes, by day 42, was undoubtedly predicted by the severity of MRS disturbances already present on day 5. From this we may anticipate an increasing frequency of MRS examinations which are positive for hypoxic brain damage, when MRI is equivocal or even normal.

A point of some technical interest is the demonstration in this subject that lipid seen in the MR spectrum is probably of intracerebral location. The peak intensity observed in voxels sited in the same brain location (Figs. 12.13, 12.15) increases with time. The signal is 'in phase' and is less likely to be an artifact of extracerebral lipid superimposed from poorly localized MR. This lipid is therefore one of the metabolic markers of hypoxia and must be further investigated.

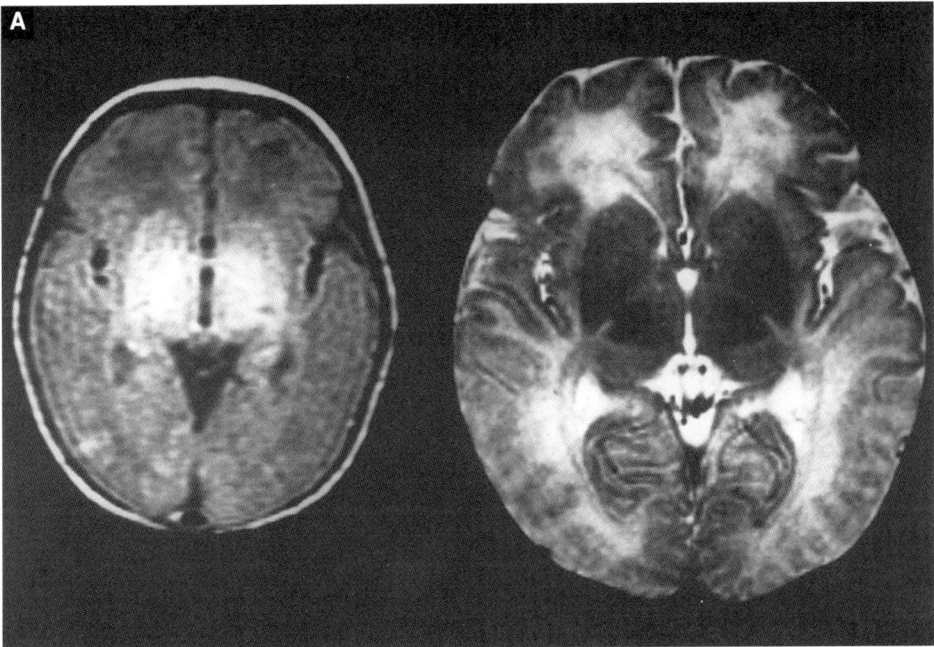

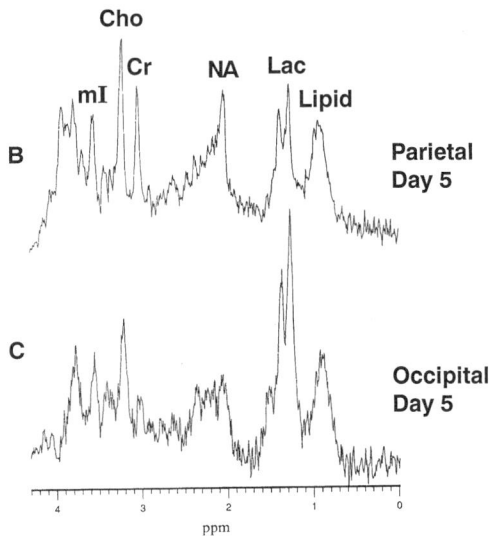

Fig. 12.13. This and Figs. 12.14 and 12.15 show the progression of hypoxic encephalopathy in a term infant, delivered by caesarean section, with severe bradycardia. Apgar scores 2, 8 and 9, and thereafter intermittent apnea. EEG was reported abnormal. On day 5, MRI is equivocal, showing normal or modest edema *(A)*, but MRS is dramatically abnormal *(B,C)*. The occipital cortex is marked by overall low signal with virtually absent NA and great excess of lactate and lipid. Even in the parietal cortex, lactate and lipid are prominent; mI is considerably below normal for age in both locations.

297

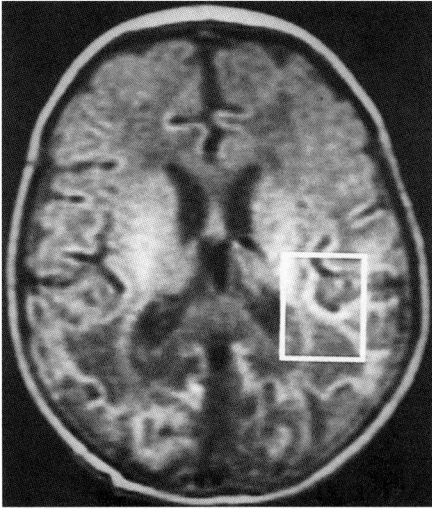

Fig. 12.14. Day 12. MRI in the occipital lobe shows encephalomalacia. A progressive change from normal or modest edema is evident. MRS on day 12 is shown as Fig. 12.15B.

Paradoxical regression: progression to apparent normality

As already mentioned, it has been a paradox of MRS that apparently 'normal' spectra might be observed even when hypoxia and tissue damage are severe and unequivocal (Fig. 12.16). The patient illustrated in Figures 12.17 and 12.18 emphasizes this point, and Figure 12.3 offers a reasonable explanation. The infant is a girl with hypoxic encephalopathy with a probable gestational age at caesarean delivery of 31–34 weeks. At this age, NA is normally very low indeed, so that as a clue to hypoxia further loss of NA is equivocal (Fig. 12.17B). From the parallel examination of a 'normal' infant of 35 weeks gestational age (Fig. 12.17A), we must conclude that absence of NA in the patient is truly abnormal, and a sign of severe intracerebral hypoxia. The presence of lactate and lipid are also pointers to severe hypoxic damage.

The lower spectrum (Fig. 12.17c) was obtained from the thinned occipital cortex after 12 weeks (GA now ~47 weeks) and appears to indicate 'recovery' of NA and apparent normalization of the spectrum. The presence of lipid in the spectrum may indicate the presence of extracerebral lipid signals, which can contaminate the voxel. MRS appears to suggest 'normalization' in an infant who was still severely abnormal to clinical and neurologic testing. The evidence to the contrary comes from the image and from the clinical course. Ventricular dilatation and thinning of the cortex (Fig. 12.18) means that the voxel contains only around 50 per cent brain. Using Figure 12.3 as a guide, we propose that the 50 per cent of brain remaining is that which survived the hypoxic insult with near-normal NAA content. The remainder has suffered necrosis and removal. What we see in the spectrum is a 'normal' metabolic profile, with low absolute metabolite content and less than half of the normal brain mass and is surely not evidence of recovery.

298

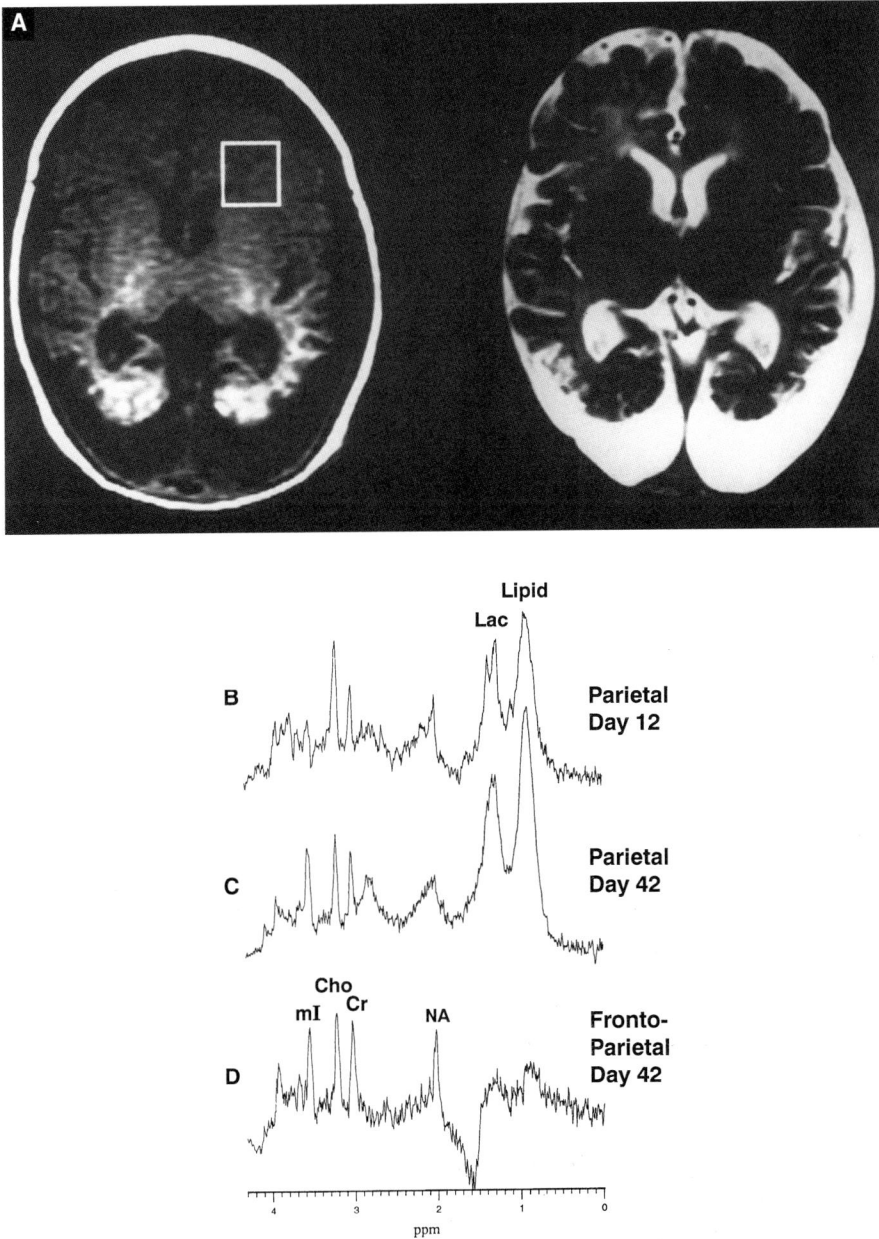

Fig. 12.15. MRI on day 42 *(A)* shows complete occipital lobe atrophy. Changes in parietal cortex on day 12 are reflected by the progressive loss of NA and Cr and apparent increasing lactate and lipid intensities *(B)*, which by 6 weeks *(C)* dominate the spectrum, as total signal falls. There is some increase in mI/Cr at this late stage of hypoxia. Even at this late stage, MRS of the frontoparietal cortex is virtually normal *(D)* (the inverted lipid peak is from outside the voxel of interest and probably outside the brain). MRI of the frontoparietal cortex was also normal.

299

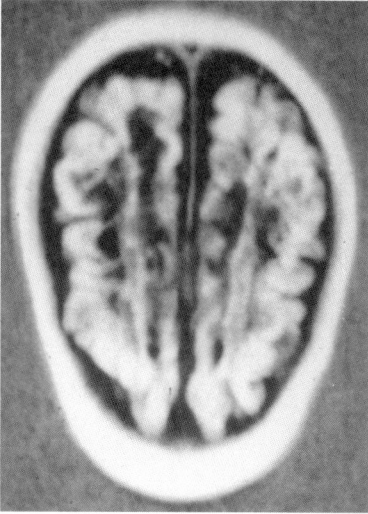

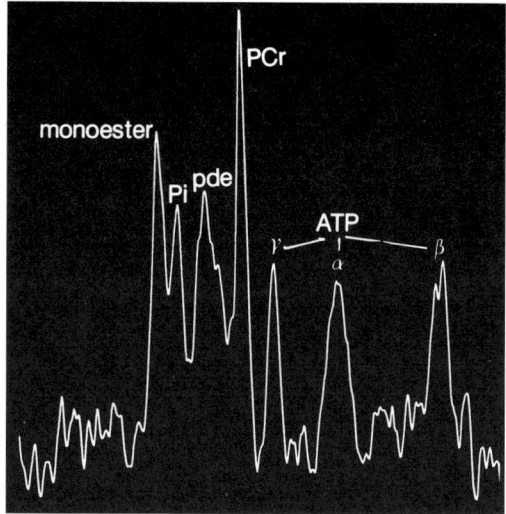

Fig. 12.16. The paradox of 'normal' MRS in an abnormal brain. This figure, from a 3-year-old child, shows the late effects of perinatal asphyxia on MRI, but an unremarkable ^{31}P spectrum, obtained from a volume of interest which included most of the right hemisphere.

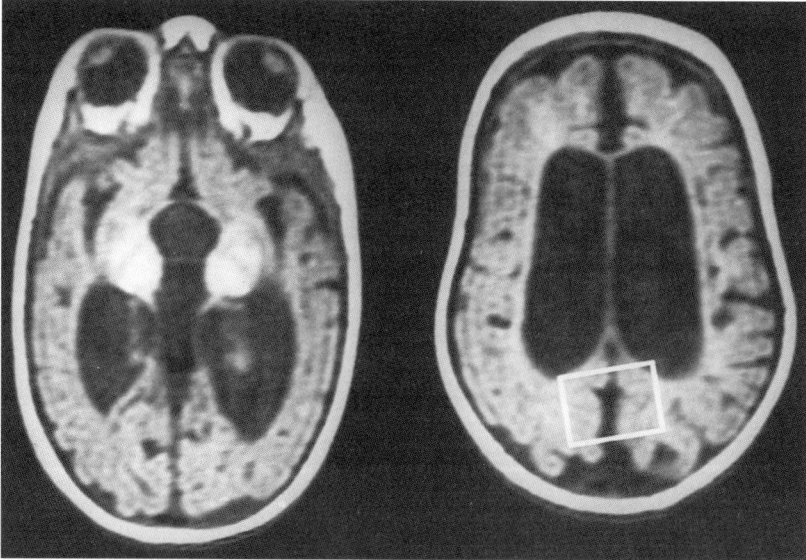

Fig. 12.18. Development of ventricular dilatation and cortical atrophy. Same infant as in Fig. 12.17, at 12 weeks post-partum. MRI now shows the loss of cortical thickness, associated with hypoxic encephalopathy, so that density of surviving 'neurons' in the voxel is somewhat increased. This is one possible explanation for increased NA/Cr in Fig. 12.17D.

300

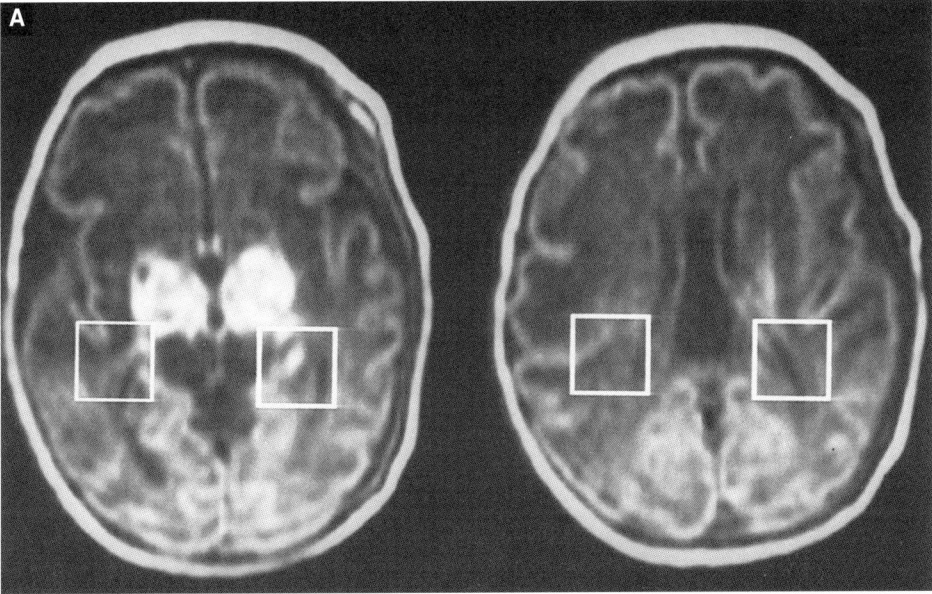

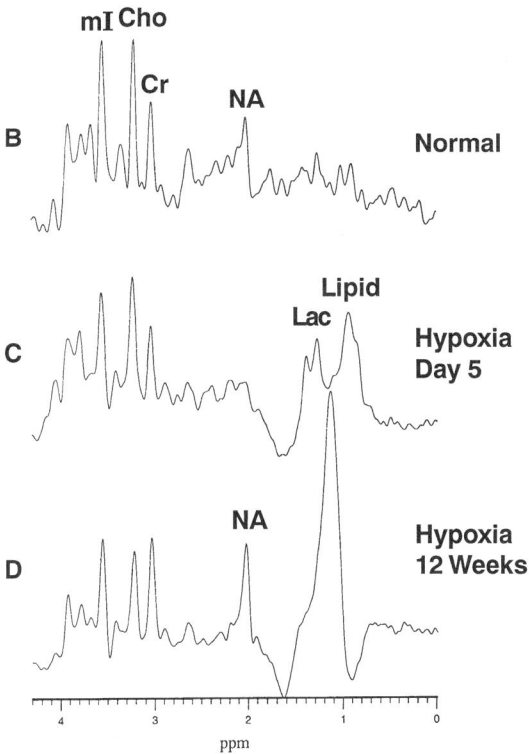

Fig. 12.17. Hypoxic encephalopathy in the immature brain. MRI and MRS of an infant of 31–34 weeks GA at caesarean section performed as emergency after death of the mother. The duration of hypoxia is uncertain. MRI *(A)* appears to reflect hypoxic encephalopathy but is equivocal at this immaturity. MRS on day 5 *(C)* is unequivocally that of hypoxic encephalopathy (low NA/Cr; excess lactate and lipid), when contrasted with that of normal preterm infant *(B)* (GA ~35 weeks at time of MRS). MRS at 12 weeks *(D)* was obtained rom a different brain region to that from the earlier examination (occipital cortex). The paradoxical 'recovery' of NA makes the spectral appearance almost normal, but the explanation for this may be that offered by Figure 12.3. mI/Cr is higher than appropriate for postnatal age 12 weeks, but may be correct for gestational age. The lipid signal is possibly an artifact.

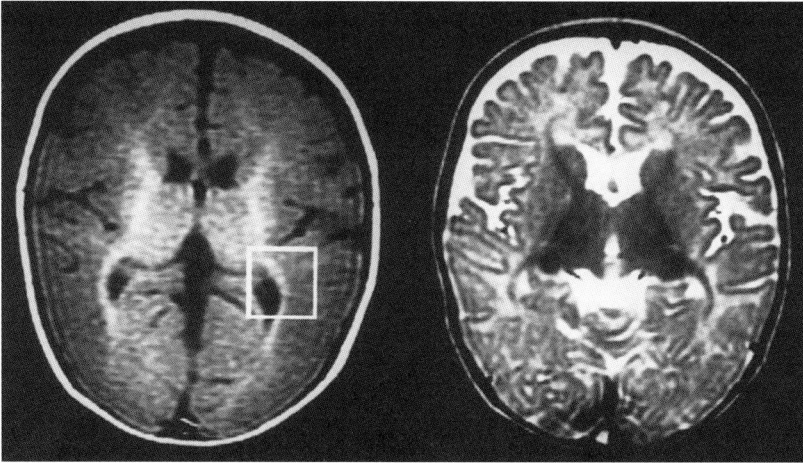

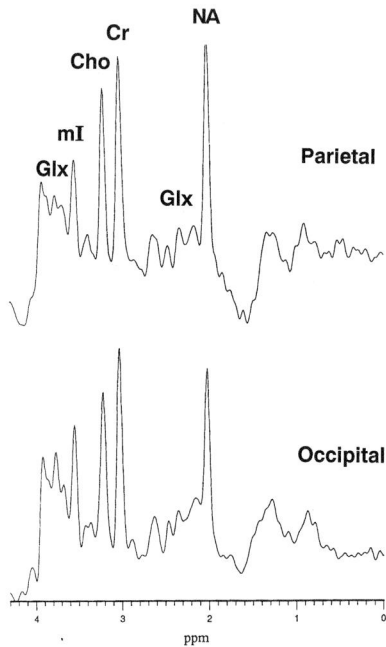

Fig. 12.19. Effect of cardiac arrest on cerebral metabolites in 3-month-old child. Arrest followed asphyxia due to inhalation. Resuscitation followed by bronchoscopy was successful and neurological status was described as normal. MRI performed on day 4 showed no acute changes but some frontal atrophy ?due to an earlier insult. MRS, in contrast, was definitely abnormal, with more marked changes in the occipital (parasagittal) location. In addition to a reduction in NA/Cr, an increase in both α and β–γ regions of the Glx is noted. The Cho/Cr ratio is approximately normal for age (see Fig. 12.6). Absolute quantitation shows low [NA] and [Cr] concentrations. The effect is so marked in the occipital cortex, where NA is 67 per cent of normal, and Cr 86 per cent of normal, that prognosis for full neurologic recovery was guarded. At 1 year there is significant neurologic abnormality.

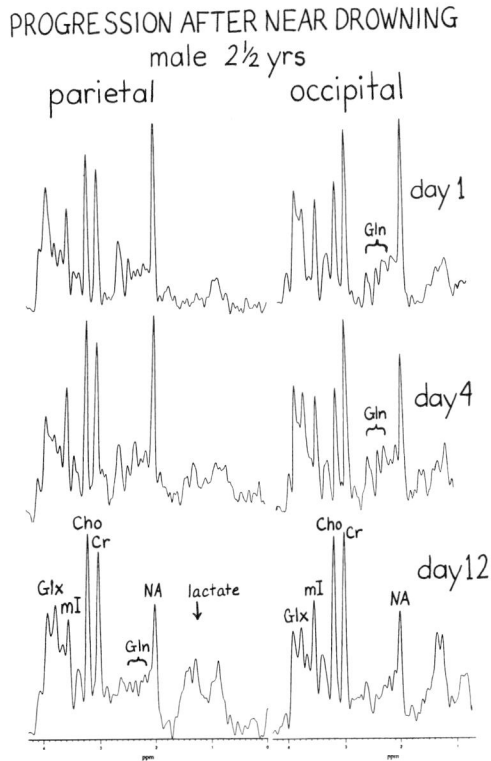

Fig. 12.20. Parasagittal sensitivity to hypoxia. Sequential changes in ¹H MRS from two locations of the brain after submersion injury. Note the progressive loss of NA, which is considerably more pronounced in the occipital (parasagittal) spectra. Spectra obtained from the parietal white matter, on the other hand, can show remarkable preservation of NA at day 4. Excess glutamine (Gln) is most marked in gray matter, days 1 and 4. Lactate appears most marked in gray matter, day 12, in this example. (For a full description of these events see Kreis *et al.* 1992*a*, Ross *et al.* 1992.)

Cerebral hypoxia in older infants and children

Unlike the case with MRI, where very different patterns of response are expected in the brains of newborn infants from those seen in children and adults, in ¹H MRS our experience suggests that an essentially similar spectrum characterizes hypoxia in older children. Figure 12.19 shows loss of NA and Cr in response to asphyxia and arrest in a 3-month-old induced by inhalation of an apple-core. There were minimal neurologic signs, and MRI was essentially normal (showing only some frontal lobe atrophy from an earlier event). MRS in the parietal lobe is distinguished by a small reduction in NA/Cr and modest elevation in Glx, with much more marked abnormalities in the occipital cortex.

Progression of hypoxic events in older children has now been well demonstrated in 16 patients resuscitated after near-drowning. Figure 12.20 shows the sequence of changes in parietal and occipital cortex in a child after near-drowning. Accumulation of glutamine

SUMMARY

MRI	MRS	
–	– ⎫	¹H MRS: Rule out
–	+ ⎭	***
+	+	Infarct; Hemorrhage; Hypoxia
+	–	¹H MRS: Focal; Late

Role of MRI
1) Very early-
   diffusion EPI
2) Late and very
   late neurological
   sequelae

Role of MRS
1) High clinical
   suspicion,
   but -ve image
2) Prognosis
3) Intervention

Fig. 12.21. Hypoxic encephalopathy: role of MRI and ¹H MRS in early diagnosis. (EPI = echo-planar imaging.) Examples are shown to emphasize that ¹H MRS readily confirms the diagnoses when MRI is positive. This is not an important role for ¹H MRS. Similarly, the diagnosis of late damage, which is easily confirmed with MRI, is of largely academic interest for ¹H MRS. The major diagnostic roles are therefore seen as (a) the patient at risk, but clinically negative, (b) the patient with high clinical suspicion, but normal ultrasound and CT, and (c) the patient with equivocal or negative findings on MRI. As summarized here, ¹H MRS is the most sensitive technique currently available for the definition and quantitation of cerebral hypoxic damage.

and glutamate is obviously present on day 1 and day 4, but lactate appears somewhat later. Loss of NA is apparent on day 1, but becomes obvious first in the occipital cotex on day 4, and only later in the parietal cortex. In more severe cases, the accumulation of intracerebral lactate is obvious (Kreis *et al.* 1992*a*), as in neonatal hypoxia. At present, it is not clear whether hypoxia in these older children results in either of the other two biochemical changes, the loss of mI and the accumulation of lipid, so prominent in infants.

Conclusions

Clinical ¹H MRS can now be performed with safety in circumstances as varied as perinatal asphyxia and near-drowning. The information obtained from well-localized, quantitative spectroscopy is best understood on the basis of a simplified model of the biochemical and histopathologic consequences of hypoxia, with some further elucidation based on knowledge of the MRI or CT patterns. The possible place of ¹H MRS in clinical management of the hypoxic child is suggested in Figure 12.21.

From the pattern of biochemical changes, their anatomic distribution and their evolution over time, we are gaining some new insights into cerebral hypoxia. In clinical management, it is possible that MRS will find a place in: earlier diagnosis; quantitation and prognosis; therapeutic monitoring; and the development of new therapies.

MRS offers several new avenues for therapeutic advance. The interventions should be designed to correct each of the readily measured abnormalities in the spectrum: (a) elevated glutamate plus glutamine; (b) elevated lactate; (c) loss of PCr; (d) loss of NAA; (e) excess lipid, as well as those changes already documented with ^{31}P MRS, principally acidosis and increased inorganic phosphate. Several older therapies might profitably be re-evaluated using the objective, time-related changes now so easily followed by sequential ^{1}H MRS, to provide more subtle analyses of outcome.

We strongly advocate the use of image guided localized ^{1}H MRS in infants with a high index of suspicion for hypoxic encephalopathy, even if findings with other conventional techniques, including ultrasound, CT, MRI or EEG, are negative.

ACKNOWLEDGMENTS

The members of the Altadena Guild of HMH strenuously supported this program to improve pediatric care in Southern California. We are grateful for financial support from the L.K. Whittier Foundation of California, and for a Boswell Fellowship to R.K. We thank Drs Ricardo Liberman, Ernesto Gangitano, John Vogt and Edgardo Arcinue for permission to examine patients under their care, as well as Drs Carolyn Stevenson and Elizabeth Kovacs and the staffs of the Neonatal and Pediatric Intensive Care Unit at Huntington Memorial Hospital, and the Respiratory Therapy team (Director, Dr Craig Lysy). John Smith of Guardian Ambulance generously donated transportation for many seriously ill infants. We acknowledge the support of Dr Allan Mathias, Executive Director of HMH. Finally, we thank Ms Jennifer Bellinger for preparing the manuscript and illustrations, and Ms Truda Shonk, BS, for assistance with illustrations.

REFERENCES

Behar, K.L. (1991) 'Separation of macromolecules from metabolites in the ^{1}H NMR spectrum of brain.' *In: Proceedings of the10th Annual Meeting of the Society of Magnetic Resonance in Medicine, San Francisco. Vol. 1.* p. 189

Boesch, C., Gruetter, R., Martin, E., Duc, G., Wuthrich, K. (1989) 'Variations in the *in vivo* P-31 MR spectra of the developing human brain during postnatal life.' *Radiology,* **172,** 197–199.

Bottomley, P.A. (1991) 'The trouble with spectroscopy papers.' *Radiology,* **181,** 344–350.

—— (1992) 'Proton MR spectroscopy for diagnosing hepatic encephalopathy?' *Radiology,* **182,** 6–7. *(Editorial.)*

Cady, E.B., de Costello, A.M., Dawson, M.J., Delpy, D.T., Hope, P.L., Reynolds, E.O.R., Tofts, P.S., Wilkie, D.R. (1983) 'Non-invasive investigation of cerebral metabolism in newborn infants by phosphorus nuclear magnetic resonance spectroscopy.' *Lancet,* **1,** 1059–1062.

Ernst, T., Ross, B.D., Flores, R. (1992) 'Cerebral MRS in infant with suspected Reye's syndrome.' *Lancet,* **340,** 486. *(Letter.)*

—— Kreis, R., Ross, B.D. (1993) 'Absolute quantitation of water and metabolites in the human brain. Part I: Compartments and water.' *Journal of Magnetic Resonance Imaging,* **102,** 1–8.

Gadian, D.G. (1982) *Nuclear Magnetic Resonance and its Applications to Living Systems.* New York: Oxford University Press.

Hope, P.L., de Costello, A.M., Cady, E.B., Delpy, D.T., Tofts, P.S., Chu, A., Hamilton, P.A., Reynolds, E.O.R., Wilkie, D.R. (1984) 'Cerebral energy metabolism studied with phosphorus NMR spectroscopy in normal and birth-asphyxiated infants.' *Lancet,* **2,** 366–370.

Kreis, R., Ross, B.D. (1992) 'Cerebral metabolic disturbances in patients with subacute and chronic diabetes mellitus: detection with proton MR spectroscopy.' *Radiology,* **184,** 123–130.

—— Ernst, T., Arcinue, E., Liberman, R., Ross, B.D. (1991*a*) '*Myo*-inositol in short TE ^{1}H MRS: a new indicator of neonatal brain development and pathology.' *In: Proceedings of the 10th Annual Meeting of the Society of Magnetic Resonance in Medicine, San Francisco.* p. 1007.

—— Farrow, N.A., Ross, B.D. (1991*b*) 'Localized ^{1}H NMR spectroscopy in patients with chronic hepatic encephalopathy. Analysis of changes in cerebral glutamine, choline and inositols.' *NMR in Biomedicine,* **4,** 109–116.

—— Ernst, T., Arcinue, E., Flores, R. Ros, B>D. (1992a) 'Proton MRS in children resuscitated after near-drowning: a possible prognostic indicator?' *In: Proceedings of the 11th Annual Meeting of the Society of Magnetic Resonance in Medicine, Berlin.* p. 237.

—— Ross, B.D., Farrow, N.A., Ackerman, Z. (1992b) 'Metabolic disorders of the brain in chronic hepatic encephalopathy detected with H-1 MR spectroscopy.' *Radiology,* **182**, 19–27.

—— Ernst, T., Ross, B.D. (1993a) 'Absolute quantitation of water and metabolites in the human brain. Part II: Metabolite concentrations.' *Journal of Magnetic Resonance,* **102**, 9–19.

—— —— —— (1993b) 'Development of the human brain: *in vivo* quantification of metabolite and water content with proton magnetic resonance spectroscopy.' *Magnetic Resonance in Medicine,* **30**, 1–14.

Peden, C.J., Cowan, F.M., Bryant, D.J., Sargentoni, J., Cox, I.J., Menon, D.K., Gadian, D.G., Bell, J.D., Dubowitz, L.M. (1990) 'Proton MR spectroscopy of the brain in infants.' *Journal of Computer Assisted Tomography,* **14**, 886–894.

Ross, B.D. (1991) 'Biochemical considerations in ¹H spectroscopy. Glutamate and glutamine; *myo*-inositol and related metabolites.' *NMR in Biomedicine,* **4**, 59–63.

—— Kreis, R., Ernst, T. (1992) 'Clinical tools for the 90's: magnetic resonance spectroscopy and metabolite imaging.' *European Journal of Radiology,* **14**, 128–140.

van der Knaap, M.S., van der Grond, J., van Rijen, P.C., Faber, J.A.J., Valk, J., Willemse, K. (1990) 'Age-dependent changes in localized proton and phosphorus MR spectroscopy of the brain.' *Radiology,* **176**, 509–515.

—— Luyten, P.R., den Hollander, J.A., Nauta, J.J.P., Valk, J. (1992) '¹H and ³¹P magnetic resonance spectroscopy of the brain in degenerative cerebral disorders.' *Annals of Neurology,* **31**, 202–211.

Volpe, J.J. (1987) *Neurology of the Newborn.* Philadelphia: W.B. Saunders.

Zimmerman, R.A., Wang, Z. (1992) 'Proton spectroscopy of the pediatric brain.' *Rivista di Neuroradiologica,* **5**, 5. *(Abstract.)*

13
LOCALIZED MR SPECTROSCOPY OF NEURODEGENERATIVE DISEASE AND TUMORS

A. Aria Tzika

Magnetic resonance spectroscopy (MRS), may offer a non-invasive *in vivo* approach to biochemical analysis in humans (Weiner 1988, Radda *et al.* 1989). Furthermore, MRS can supply quantitative as well as qualitative information regarding cellular metabolites, since metabolite signal intensities are linearly related to steady-state metabolite concentration (Chance and Whearly 1985). The lack in biochemical diagnostic specificity of magnetic resonance imaging (MRI) provides justification for the need of such an approach in the clinical environment (Bottomley 1989). Besides, if MRS can detect changes at the cellular biochemical level, which precede the morphological changes detected by MRI and other radiological imaging, further insight into both follow-up assessment and prognosis might be furnished. Radioisotope imaging, in particular positron emission tomography (PET), represents the only alternate approach to the non-invasive *in vivo* metabolite imaging. However, such imaging requires model-dependent data transformations since the different metabolites cannot be directly marked.

MRS has been a challenge to both manufacturers and scientists in its clinical applicability (Bottomley 1989). Until recently, MRS had not been performed in the clinical environment because of the great demands on instrumentation and methodology, and the lack of a clearly defined role. Although the introduction of ^{31}P MRS in biomedicine was encouraging, its limited sensitivity, which translates into large voxels of interest requirements, has discouraged clinical research trials and thus its effective clinical application. Unlike phosphorous-31, proton has a high inherent sensitivity (15-fold improvement in signal-to-noise ratio over phosphorous at the same magnetic field strength). Thus a small voxel of interest provides adequate signal-to-noise in relatively short acquisition periods (a few minutes), offering the opportunity to address tissue heterogeneity within healthy or diseased tissue. Also, due to the enhanced sensitivity of protons, even low-concentration metabolites can be detected.

The diagnostic potential of brain localized proton MRS has been recently evaluated in children; this evaluation, however, has been based solely on long echo time (TE) proton spectra (van der Knaap *et al.* 1990, Bruhn *et al.* 1992). In our recent evaluations we have used both long- and short-TE spectra, to increase the sensitivity to a greater number of metabolites than are routinely detected with long TEs (Tzika *et al.* 1993*a,b,c*). Our goals were first to acquire good quality water-suppressed proton MR spectra from small single voxels in the brains of children, and second to evaluate the combination of MRI and single-voxel localized proton MRS in the clinical setting.

In this chapter, clinical experience with single-voxel localized proton MRS is discussed within the context of the currently available literature. This is prefaced by a brief discussion of methodological aspects pertaining to localized proton MRS. Background knowledge on basic MRS is assumed. This topic is adequately covered in Chapter 12.

Localized proton MRS
Methodology

Implementation of localized proton MRS requires suppression of water and/or lipids so that signals from other mobile metabolites, of a lower tissue concentration range, can be detected. Several methods have been introduced to overcome this dynamic-range problem; these have been reviewed elsewhere (Leibfritz 1992). In addition, *in vivo* proton MRS is inherently limited by factors which decrease spectral and hence metabolite resolution. These factors include the complexity of the spectra and the considerable overlap of the metabolite signals. Spectral resolution (detectable difference between two adjacent signals) depends on: the nucleus of interest; the organ of interest; the field strength; the pulse sequence used; and finally the quality of the field homogeneity. Of these factors the ones that can be controlled in proton MRS are field strength and homogeneity, and the use of signal-to-noise optimized pulse sequences. Increase in the field strength results in increased resolution, but generates additional considerations (besides obvious financial constraints) rendering high-field MRS in the clinical environment disadvantageous. Optimum field homogeneity ('shimming') is still an operator dependent variable, even for state-of-the-art systems such as the ones equipped with superconducting magnets and actively shielded gradients. However, automated routines for shimming have been introduced and are undergoing clinical evaluation, preliminary results of which are promising at the present time (Tzika *et al.* 1994, Webb *et al.* 1994).

A variety of different localization methods have been described and attempted *in vivo* (Aue 1986, Akoka 1992). Of these, single-voxel methods provide easy and accurate control of localization as well as shorter acquisition times. In our experience, a 5 minute acquisition time per spectrum for each voxel renders good quality spectra. In addition, single-voxel methods are less susceptible to motion occurring between acquisitions than multiscan add-and-subtract techniques such as the image-selected *in vivo* spectroscopy (ISIS) technique (Ordidge *et al.* 1986). Certain advantages of single-voxel methods over multivoxel ones emerge from their comparison (Granot 1986). For instance, localized shimming which can be performed with the single-voxel methods is a major advantage, especially for heterogeneous regions of interest with magnetic field inhomogeneities. A disadvantage of multivoxel techniques is the high number of acquisition averages required; on the other hand, the high proton sensitivity offers the capability for acquisition of an adequate quality spectrum with only a few averages. In addition, single-voxel methods are more useful for the *in vivo* determination of relaxation times. This determination requires repetitive acquisitions with different parameters and is needed for the accurate absolute quantitation of metabolites. Nevertheless, multivoxel methods, and especially spectroscopic imaging (Brown *et al.* 1982) or chemical shift imaging (CSI), may be the methods of choice in clinical spectroscopy, principally because they provide multiple spectra from multiple voxels in the same acquisition period. Also, reduction of multivoxel data acquisition time can be achieved when one-dimension chemical shift imaging (1D-CSI) is combined with slice selection.

Data analysis

In vivo MRS data analysis is needed for proper data interpretation and might involve: spectral peak assignments to specific metabolites; qualitative evaluation based on previous experience; and quantitative metabolite evaluation.

Appropriate *in vivo* MRS spectral assignments may be achieved via correlation with *in vitro* data from tissue extracts, surgical specimens and model solutions of metabolites. *In vitro* data should preferably be acquired at a higher field strength so that strong metabolite overlaps can be avoided. Inasmuch as correlation of *in vivo* with *in vitro* MRS data may be helpful in spectral interpretation, it could also be somewhat irrelevant to the actual *in vivo* situation due to the lapse in time between tissue collection and MRS data acquisition (Gill *et al.* 1989, 1990; Michaelis *et al.* 1991). Thus the events occurring before and during *in vitro* MRS should be considered carefully when such correlation is attempted.

Raw data manipulations, except Fourier transformation and phasing of the spectra, such as filtering resolution enhancement and baseline corrections, can affect the appearance of the spectra. In pathologic cases, observed spectral alterations may reflect changes in metabolite concentration and metabolite visibility or mobility, as well as changes in metabolite MR relaxation times. These alterations can result from single or multiple metabolite changes, since more than one metabolite are contained in the broad peaks. Such circumstances, along with the requirement of references (either internal or external), make quantitation difficult. Considering the above, even qualitative evaluation of the proton spectra should be performed with caution.

Accurate quantitative evaluation of metabolites contained in the *in vivo* proton MR spectrum acquired on clinical systems at 1.5 T is hampered by the spectrum's complexity and its limited resolution due to considerable metabolite overlap and strong coupling. Also, the relationship between *in vivo* MR visibility of a metabolite and its actual concentration, which depends on its mobility and/or compartmentalization, needs to be determined. Unfortunately, in the presence of strong coupling of individual metabolite resonances, the resonance areas are not linearly related to the metabolite concentration. Thus absolute quantitation is a remarkably difficult task; nevertheless, it is feasible, especially when performed taking into account all possible relevant factors (Hennig *et al.* 1992, Kreis *et al.* 1992, Christiansen *et al.* 1993, Michaelis *et al.* 1993). Meanwhile, selected metabolite ratios can be used and reflect relative changes of metabolites. In such analysis, ratios of the integrated area of the peaks of interest (not of the peak heights) may be used and represent relative measures of metabolite concentrations (Provencher 1993).

Clinical MRI-guided single-voxel proton MRS of neurologic disorders in children

Methodology

Two different single-voxel localization methods, namely point resolved spectroscopy (PRESS) (Bottomley 1987) and stimulated echo acquisition mode (STEAM) (Frahm *et al.*

1989) have been compared concerning specifications for *in vivo* localized proton MRS (Moonen *et al.* 1989). For long TEs, PRESS offers a factor of 2× increase in signal-to-noise, is less sensitive to motion and diffusion, and is not susceptible to multiple-quantum effects. STEAM is advantageous when shorter TEs are required and can be used to detect coupled metabolites with short T_2 relaxation times. However, half of the potential signal is lost with STEAM as compared to PRESS, due to the use of stimulated echoes instead of spin echoes (Hahn 1950).

Recently improved versions of PRESS and STEAM have been implemented on General Electric 1.5 T Signa systems. These versions make use of optimal frequency selective excitation pulses (Pauly *et al.* 1991). Three-dimensional spatial localization is achieved using three of these pulses in the presence of mutually orthogonal field gradients in a single acquisition. To detect the greatest number of metabolic resonances including short T_2 and/or strongly coupled metabolites (Frahm *et al.* 1989, Kreis *et al.* 1992, Rothman *et al.* 1992), short-TE acquisitions must be performed. Since a short TE is not easily achieved with PRESS, the method of choice is STEAM (Moonen *et al.* 1989). However, to detect and identify lactate, long-TE acquisitions are required (Bruhn *et al.* 1989*b*) to reduce possible interference with lipid resonances. The lactate spectrum is composed of a doublet due to its methyl protons at 1.33 ppm and a quartet due to its methylene protons at 4.3 ppm (in proximity to the water to be observed *in vivo*). At TE of 135 ms, the 1.33 ppm lactate resonance is inverted. Its amplitude, however, is reduced by 40 per cent using PRESS due to incompletely phased magnetization. At a TE of 270 ms, the same resonance is completely refocused and coupling effects do not occur (Ernst and Hennig 1991). Also, the amplitude of the 1.33 ppm lactate doublet is approximately doubled when PRESS is used instead of STEAM (Ernst and Hennig 1991). Thus for long- TE acquisitions, PRESS with TE of 135 ms may be used to identify lactate, and PRESS with TE of 270 ms enhances sensitivity for lactate detection.

Spectra in normal children
Using the STEAM and PRESS sequences described above, proton spectra of normal healthy children in our studies revealed large resonances from *N*-acetylaspartate (NAA, 2.0 ppm), total creatine (Cr) and phosphocreatine (PCr) (3.0 and 3.9 ppm), and choline-containing compounds (Cho, 3.2 ppm) (Fig. 13.1). In short-TE STEAM spectra, additional resonances were observed (Fig. 13.1*b*). Such resonances are due to short T_2 and/or strongly coupled protons in compounds such as: glutamate, glutamine, GABA (Glx, 2.0– 2.55 ppm); inositols (Inls, 3.55–3.68 ppm); and glutamate, glutamine, glucose (Glx, 3.68–3.85 ppm). Resonances observed at 0.8 ppm and 1.3 ppm (due to methyl and methylene protons respectively) may represent mobile moieties of both proteins and short-chain fatty acids in the cell cytoplasm (Behar *et al.* 1983, Behar and Ogino 1991, Kauppinen and Palvimo 1992, Kauppinen *et al.* 1992).

In our setting, control children were divided into separate groups according to age. These age groups were then used in the interpretation of the spectra from similar-aged children with brain abnormalities. This is critical, because proton brain MR spectra also reflect the metabolic changes occurring during the course of early brain development

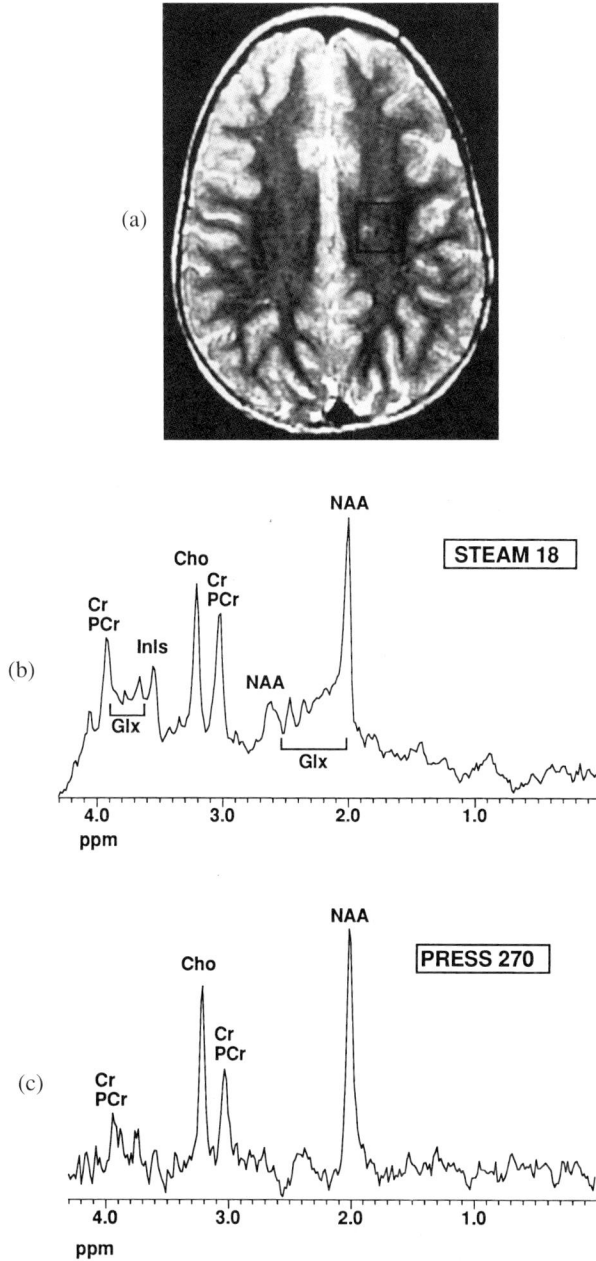

Fig. 13.1. MRI guided single-voxel localized proton MRS of a 2.5-year-old male; 4.9 cm^3 voxel of interest *(square)*. *(a)* T$_2$-weighted MR image (TR/TE = 2,000/100 ms). *(b)* Short-TE proton MR spectrum using STEAM (TR/TE = 2,000/18 ms). *(c)* Long-TE proton MR spectrum using PRESS (TR/TE = 2,000/270 ms): *N*-acetylaspartate (NAA); total creatine (Cr: creatine; PCr: phosphocreatine); choline-containing compounds (Cho); inositols (Inls); glutamate, glutamine, other amino acids (Glx).

311

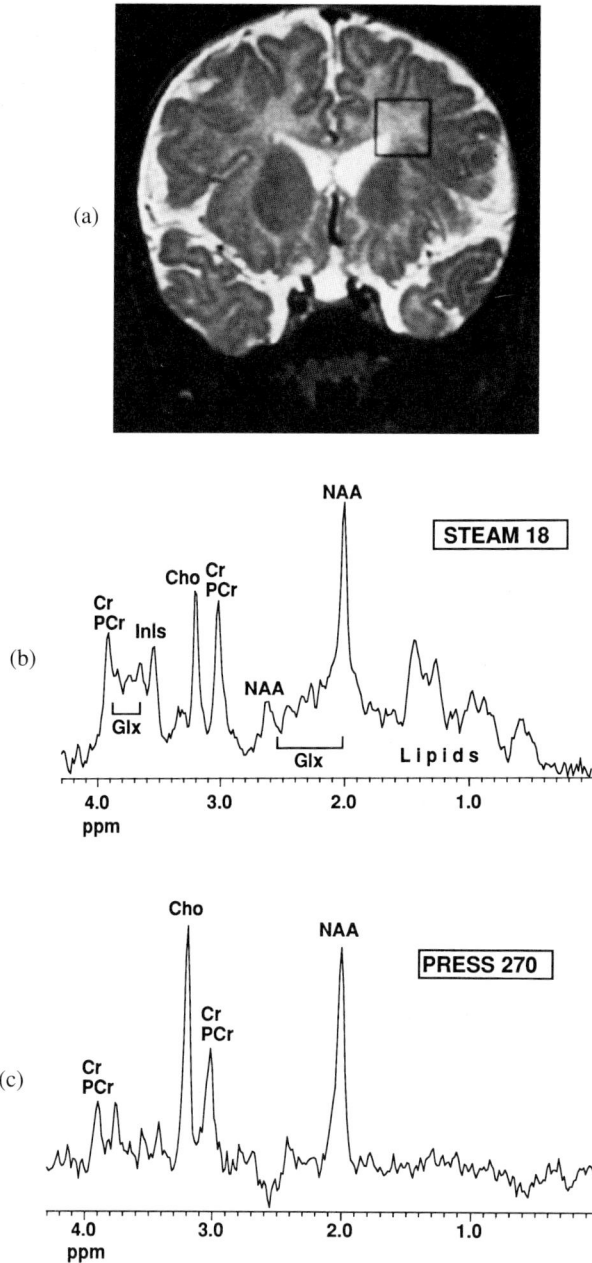

Fig. 13.2. MRI guided single-voxel localized proton MRS of a 6-month-old male; 3.4 cm^3 voxel of interest *(square). (a)* T$_2$-weighted MR image (TR/TE = 2,000/100 ms). *(b)* Short-TE proton MR spectrum using STEAM (TR/TE = 2,000/18 ms). *(c)* Long-TE proton MR spectrum using PRESS (TR/TE = 2,000/270 ms). Note the lower NAA relative to choline-containing compounds (Cho), associated with an immature brain. (Adapted from Tzika *et al.* 1993*c*.)

312

(Bates *et al.* 1989, Burri *et al.* 1990, Peden *et al.* 1990, van der Knaap *et al.* 1990). The difference in the relative prominence of the metabolite peaks during early brain development is demonstrated by comparison of the spectra from a 6-month-old normal infant (Fig. 13.2) to those from the 2.5-year-old normal child shown in Figure 13.1. The most noticeable change is an increase in the relative level of NAA as the brain develops (Michaelis *et al.* 1991). NAA becomes the most pronounced peak in the proton spectra of the brain by approximately 6 months of age. The increase in NAA is nearly complete by 2–5 years of age, and the NAA signal is twice that of Cho by 10–13 years. Also, the Cho peak increases relative to the total creatine peak during brain development.

Spectra in children with intracranial masses
MRS FINDINGS
All low-grade astrocytomas and ependymomas exhibited abnormal proton MR spectra. Low NAA and high choline levels were observed in all cases. Lactate and mobile lipids were detected in certain cases. The Glx peaks were elevated in the short-TE STEAM of all but one case; in a few cases, a single 3.55 ppm peak was identified. Figure 13.3 shows proton MRS findings in a patient with a pilocytic astrocytoma. Mobile lipid peaks seemed to be greater in patients with ependymomas than in patients with astrocytomas. A sample case of ependymoma is illustrated in Figure 13.4. Depressed relative creatine levels and enhanced Glx levels were found in this and other similar cases.

In primitive neuroectodermal tumors (PNETs), elevated mobile lipid peaks were identified. Lactate was found in one PNET, in which Cr and PCr were also greatly reduced (Fig. 13.5).

The spectra from a 23-month-old female with a histologically proven dermoid showed no metabolite peaks other than mobile lipid peaks and possibly lactate in both short-TE STEAM and long-TE PRESS. In two cerebrospinal fluid (CSF) collections or arachnoid cysts, a similar absence of metabolites was observed.

DISCUSSION
Proton MR spectra from pediatric tumors exhibit metabolite profiles that are different from those of normal brain (Sutton *et al.* 1992, Tzika *et al.* 1993*c*). Changes in metabolite levels include: reduction in NAA and total creatine, due to neuronal loss and energetic exhaustion; increase in choline-containing compounds due to altered membrane metabolism; increase in lactate due to metabolic acidosis; and increase in resonances centered at 0.9 and 1.2 ppm which include lipid methyl and methylene groups of mobile lipids and cytosolic proteins. Low NAA has been demonstrated in tissue specimens of astrocytomas by analytical methods (Nadler and Cooper 1972), *in vitro* high resolution MRS (Gill *et al.* 1989) and *in vivo* proton MRS in adults (Bruhn *et al.* 1989*a*, Gill *et al.* 1990, Frahm *et al.* 1991*a*). Furthermore, NAA has been proposed as an endogenous marker for mature neurons since it appears to be lacking from mature glial cells (Nadler and Cooper 1972, Koller *et al.* 1984, Urenjak *et al.* 1992). Thus, proton MR spectra may indicate a neuronal or glial cellular

(Continued on p. 317)

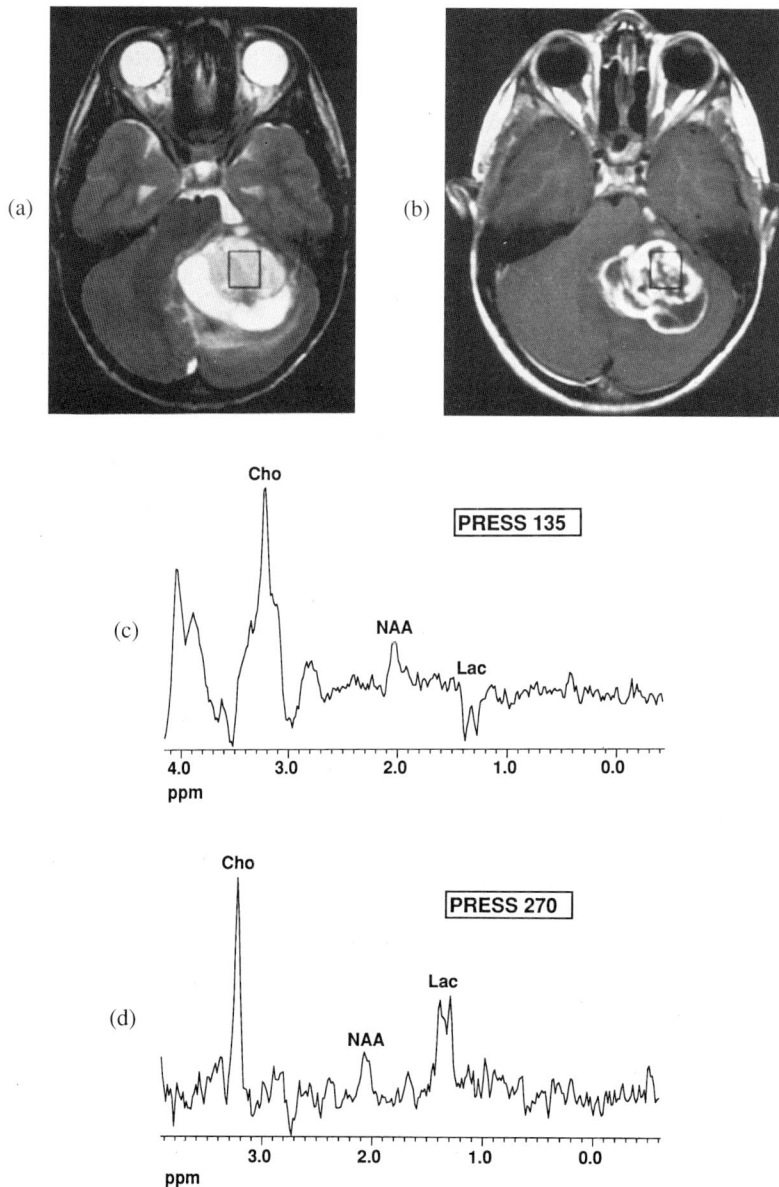

Fig. 13.3. MRI guided single-voxel localized proton MRS of an 8-year-old male with a cerebellar pilocytic astrocytoma; $3.2\,cm^3$ voxel of interest *(square)*. *(a)* T_2-weighted (TR/TE$_{eff}$ = 2,800/120ms) fast spin-echo MR image shows a mass away from the left cerebellar hemisphere with a posterior cystic component brighter in signal than the rest of the tumor. *(b)* T_1-weighted MR image (TR/TE = 500/12ms) following gadolinium-DTPA injection. Note the heterogenous enhancement of the tumor after gadolinium injection. The voxel of interest is placed in the solid portion of the tumor. *(c)* Long-TE PRESS (TR/TE = 2,000/135ms). Lactate is identified as the inverted 1.33ppm resonance, using 135ms echo time. *(d)* Long-TE proton MR spectrum using PRESS (TR/TE = 2,000/270ms). Note decreased NAA and accumulated lactate. (Adapted from Tzika *et al.* 1993c.)

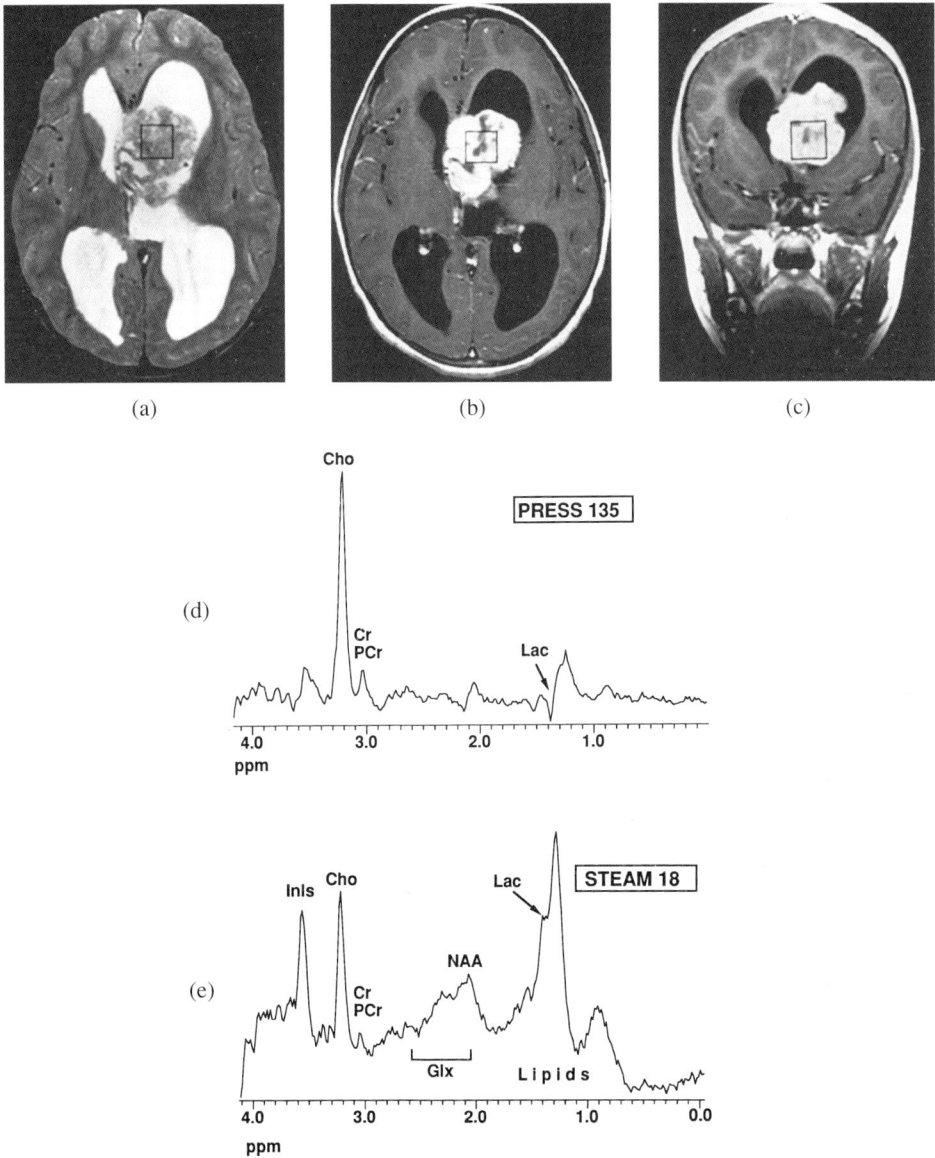

Fig. 13.4. MRI guided single-voxel localized proton MRS of a 5-year-old male with an ependymoma; 5.8 cm³ voxel of interest *(square)*. *(a)* T₂-weighted MR image (TR/TE = 2,500/100 ms). Note presence of an inhomogeneous centrally located mass. *(b)* Axial, and *(c)* coronal T₁-weighted MR images (TR/TE 500/12 ms) following gadolinium injection. The centrally located mass enhances with gadolinium; the voxel of interest is localized within the tumor mass. *(d)* Long-TE proton MR spectrum using PRESS (TR/TE = 2,000/135 ms). Note absence of NAA (2.0 ppm), the reduced total creatine (Cr, PCr), a large choline (Cho) resonance and an inverted lactate resonance. *(e)* Short-TE proton MR spectrum using STEAM (TR/TE = 2,000/18 ms). In addition to the metabolites observed with PRESS *(d)*, mobile lipids, amino acids (Glx), and a 3.55 ppm resonance presumed to be inositol (Inls) are observed. (Adapted from Tzika *et al.* 1993*c*.)

315

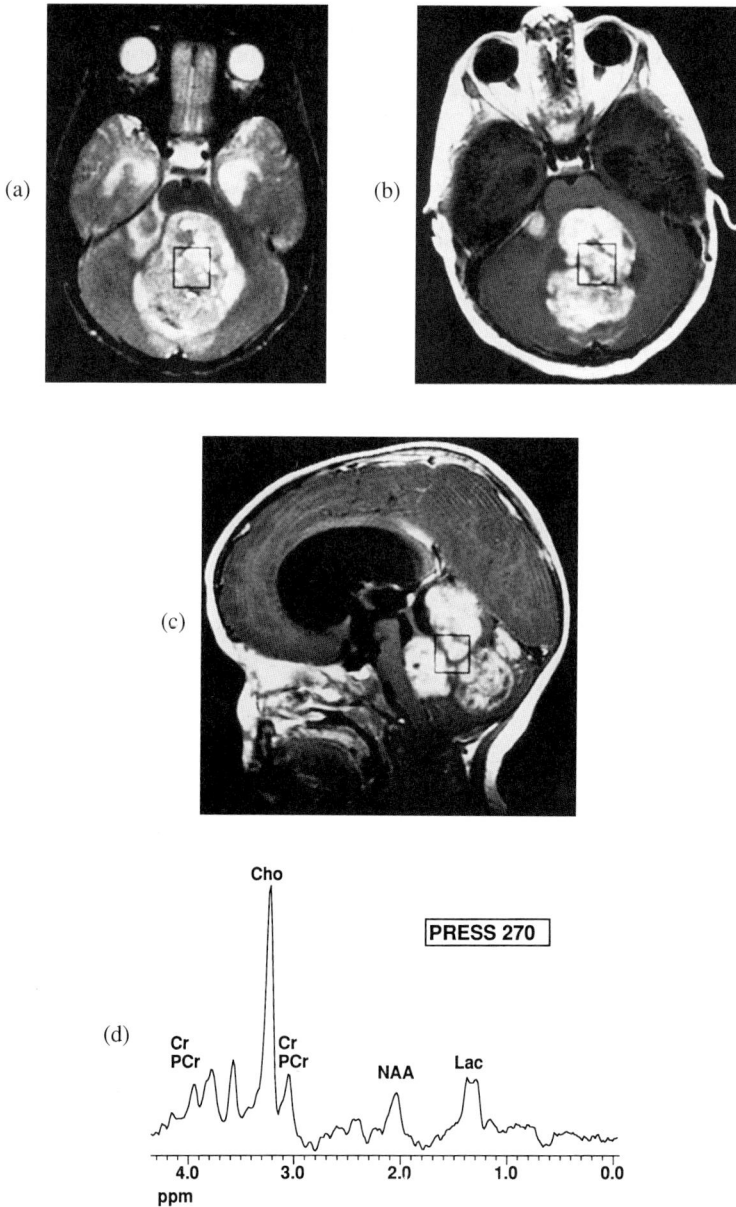

Fig. 13.5. MRI guided single-voxel localized proton MRS of a 17-month-old female with a primitive neuroectodermal tumor (PNET); 5.8 cm³ voxel of interest *(squares)*. *(a)* T_2-weighted MR image (TR/TE = 2,500/100 ms). Note large midline inhomogeneous posterior fossa mass. *(b,c)* T_1-weighted MR images (TR/TE = 500/12 ms) following gadolinium injection. Note enhancement of the posterior fossa mass; the voxel of interest is localized entirely within the mass. *(d)* Long-TE proton MR spectrum using PRESS (TR/TE = 2,000/270 ms). Note detection of lactate (1.33 ppm), low NAA, decreased total creatine (Cr, PCr) and large choline (Cho) peak. (Adapted from Tzika *et al.* 1993*c*.)

316

consistency of a tumor, especially because proton MR spectra from surgical specimens of cerebral astrocytomas resemble the spectra of primary astrocyte cultures (Gill *et al.* 1990). Nevertheless, it has also been suggested that the NAA peak includes contributions from *N*-acetyl-containing compounds other than NAA (Frahm *et al.* 1991*b*). In addition, interpretation of tumor data from immature mammals requires caution since proton spectra of the immature brain change during brain development (Bates *et al.* 1989, Burri *et al.* 1990, Peden *et al.* 1990, van der Knaap *et al.* 1990). Thus for spectral interpretations in the pediatric setting age-matched controls are needed. Reduced levels of total creatine (Cr and PCr) have been observed by ourselves (Fig. 13.3) and others (Lowry *et al.* 1977; Gill *et al.* 1989, 1990). If the total creatine peak includes primarily PCr, reduction of this peak probably represents PCr decrease (Hennig *et al.* 1992). This may be in accordance with an energetic exhaustion of the tumor tissue or a shift in its metabolism. However, it may also reflect a reduction in cellularity indicating cell death. The lactate peak characteristically observed in tumors *in vivo* (Fig. 13.3) is probably associated with tissue necrosis and has also been shown to be elevated in the *ex vivo* extract spectra of surgical tumor specimens (Gill *et al.* 1990). *In vivo* assessment of lactate cannot be replicated by MRS of tumour extracts because of its non-specific accumulation between the surgical specimen removal and freezing. Although high lactate levels have been attributed to malignant and more aggressive tumors (Radda *et al.* 1984, Arnold *et al.* 1990, Gill *et al.* 1990), whether tumor therapy assessment will be assisted by the lactate peak detected *in vivo* is debated. It has been suggested that lactate levels are less specific indicators of malignancy than the broad signals observed in the 0–2 ppm area of the proton spectra (Fulham *et al.* 1992, Kugel *et al.* 1992, Ott *et al.* 1993). In order to detect these signals, shorter TE spectra are needed. The increase in the number of MR-visible metabolites, as seen with short-TE proton MR spectra, may further assist in tumor characterization or determination of their degreee of malignancy. Elevated mobile lipids (Lazeyras *et al.* 1992, Ott *et al.* 1993, Posse *et al.* 1993) and a single resonance at 3.55 ppm presumed to be *myo*-inositol (Frahm *et al.* 1991*a*) are thought to be correlated to tumour grade (see Fig. 13.4).

Cysts exhibit spectra devoid of all the metabolites found in normal or tumorous brain regions, except for low levels of lactate (Bruhn *et al.* 1989*a*, Alger *et al.* 1990, Tzika *et al.* 1993*c*). These show no metabolite resonances due to the sub-millimolar concentrations of the metabolites in CSF (Petroff *et al.* 1986). Also, intracranial dermoids can be differentiated from other tumors by the absence of any metabolite peaks.

Spectra in children with neurodegenerative disorders
MRS FINDINGS
• *Hereditary.* Males with X-linked adrenoleukodystrophy (X-ALD) and neurologic symptoms presented with abnormal proton MR spectra. MR images and proton MR spectra from an X-ALD patient are shown in Figure 13.6. Abnormal bright signal was found in the posterior parietal and occipital white matter on T_2-weighted MR images. Proton MR spectra, acquired from a voxel of interest within the area of the brightest signal in MR images, exhibited greatly reduced NAA, increased inositols and elevated lipid peaks. A lactate peak was also detected by long-TE PRESS spectra, in which lipids

317

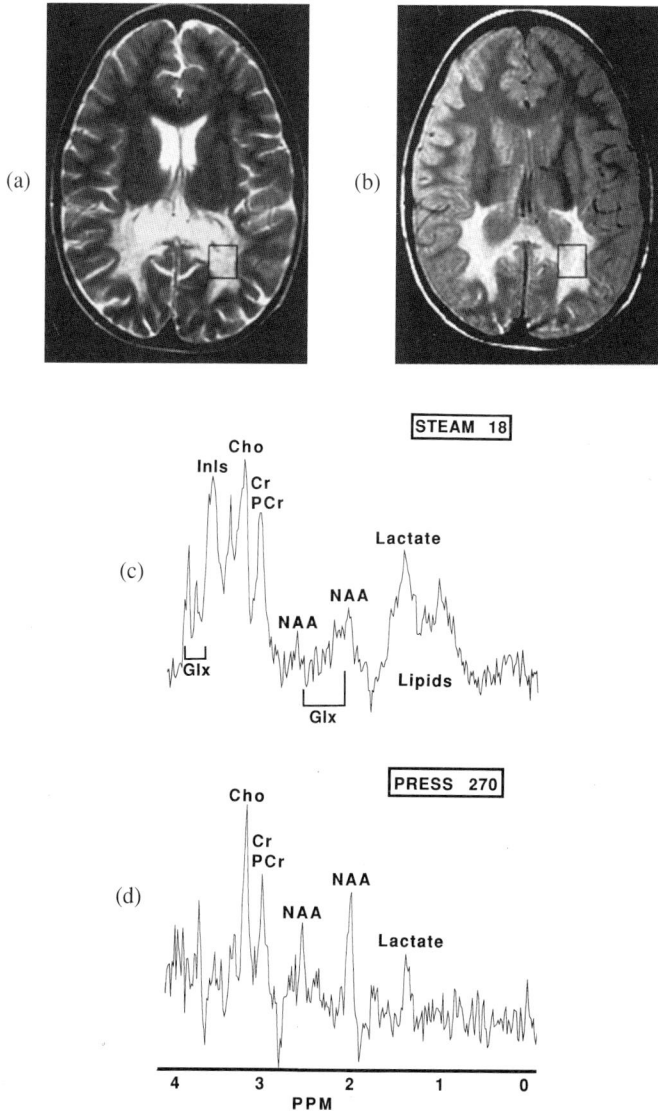

Fig. 13.6. MRI guided single-voxel localized proton MRS of an 8-year-old male with X-linked adreno-leukodystrophy (X-ALD); 3.4 cm^3 voxel of interest *(squares)*. *(a)* T$_2$-weighted (TR/TE = 2500/120 ms) fast spin-echo MR image shows bilateral occipital white matter lesions typical of X-ALD. *(b)* Proton density (TR/TE = 2000/19 ms) fast spin-echo MR image. Better separation of ventricles and white matter permits selection of voxel of interest within the hyperintense abnormal occipital white matter. *(c)* Short-TE proton MR spectrum of an occipital voxel of interest, selected from image *(b)*, using STEAM (TR/TE = 2000/18 ms). Substantial reduction of NAA relative to cholines (Cho) and maintained creatines (Cr, PCr) may indicate neurodegeneration and gliosis. Enhanced inositols (Inls) and lipids may be associated with encephalopathy and demyelination respectively. *(d)* Long-TE proton MR spectrum using PRESS (TR/TE = 2000/270 ms). Relative presence of NAA to cholines (Cho) is observed in addition to a peak at 1.33 ppm presumed to be lactic acid. (Adapted from Tzika *et al.* 1993*a*.)

318

are minimally present. Patients with X-ALD but without neurological deterioration showed normal MR images and near-normal proton spectra. However, quantitative analysis of their spectra revealed an increase in choline-containing compounds (Tzika *et al.* 1993*b*). Newborns with Zellweger syndrome showed low NAA in the anterior cerebral white matter and excessive elevation of mobile lipids and Glx metabolites. Patients with lysosomal storage disease presented NAA reduction to a varying degree and elevated Glx/Inl metabolites in the proton MR spectra of the cerebral white matter. In patients with Leigh's disease, T_1- and T_2-weighted MR images showed abnormal hypo- and hyperintensities in the deep basal ganglia respectively. Proton MR spectra localized within the region of abnormal MR signal exhibited highly increased levels of lactate. Representative images and spectra from a neonate with Leigh's disease are shown in Figure 13.7. Children with neurofibromatosis had lower NAA and higher Glx/Inl than controls of the same age. One child presented normal MRI and proton MR spectra of the white matter, and another had abnormal signal in the globus pallidus in addition to multiple patchy areas of increased signal in the medulla, pons and middle cerebellar peduncles on T_2-weighted MR images. Proton MR spectra localized to signal abnormalities in the deep gray matter showed lower NAA and increased Glx.

• *Acquired.* One 19-year-old hemophiliac male with acquired immune deficiency syndrome (AIDS) showed MRS findings of low NAA and elevated Glx despite a normal MRI examination. Qualitative inspection of the spectra of other patients diagnosed with congenital AIDS showed no abnormality on MRI or MRS. Figure 13.8 displays the MR images and spectra from a patient with subacute stroke. The post-contrast T_1-weighted image depicts enhancement in the region of blood–brain barrier breakdown (Fig. 13.8*a*). The T_2-weighted image (Fig. 13.8*b*) shows edema and abnormal bright signal in the adjacent occipital white matter region. Proton MR spectra acquired from within this region of leukomalacia showed a highly abnormal metabolite profile. Lactic acid, although co-detected with the lipids of the short-TE STEAM spectrum (Fig. 13.8*c*), is better seen in the long-TE PRESS spectrum (Fig. 13.8*d*). In other cases of suspected stroke, NAA to choline was reduced, and in one case, Glx was clearly elevated in the region of infarction. Images and proton MR spectra from an infant with a right cerebellar infarct and progressive encephalomalacia are shown in Figure 13.9. Proton MR spectra of the infarcted tissue in the right hemisphere showed decreased NAA to choline, increased Glx metabolites and increased lipid peaks. Spectra from a contralateral region in the left hemisphere exhibited normal metabolite profiles.

• *Idiopathic.* Patients with idiopathic white matter disease invariably showed bright lesions in the T_2-weighted and proton density MR images. These lesions were probably related either to an hereditary metabolic disease of unknown origin, or to an acquired cause not identified by the clinical history of the patients. An exemplary case is shown in Figure 13.10.

DISCUSSION

The neurodegeneration which occurs in certain fatal disorders of childhood can be either

(Continued on p. 323)

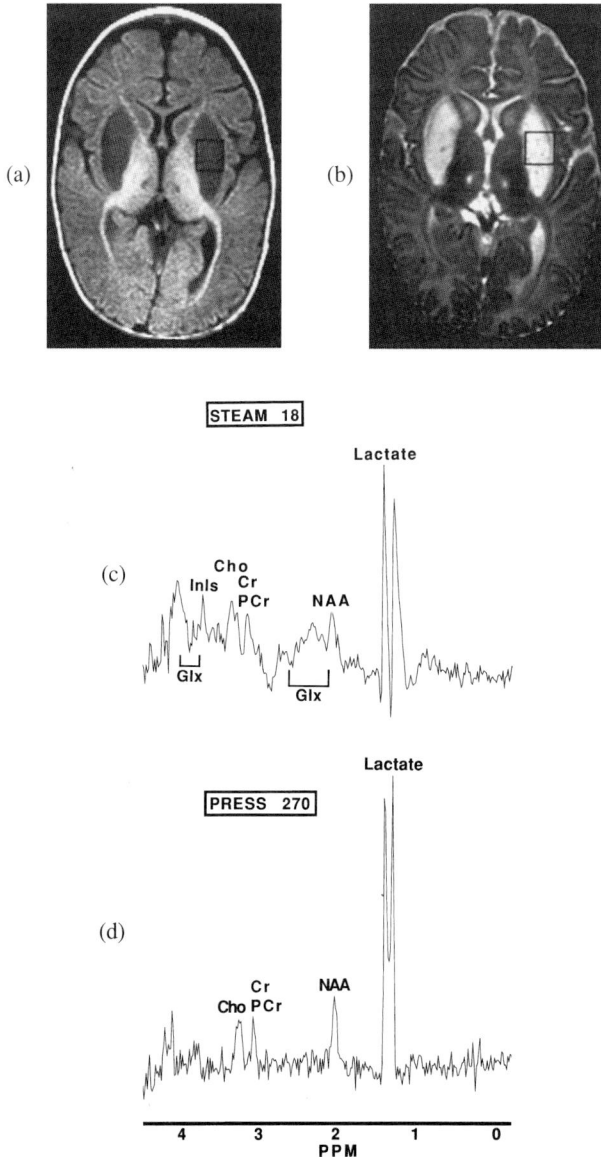

Fig. 13.7. MRI guided single-voxel localized proton MRS of a 4-month-old male with Leigh's disease; 3.4 cm³ voxel of interest *(squares)*. *(a)* Inversion recovery T₁-weighted image (TR/TI/TE = 2000/800/12 ms) shows hypointense lentiform nuclei bilaterally. *(b)* T₂-weighted image (TR/TE = 2500/100 ms) with characteristic pattern of bilateral bright lentiform nuclei. The myelination pattern and the reversed gray–white matter contrast is compatible with an age of 7 weeks. *(c,d)* Localized proton MR spectra from the voxel indicated in images *(a)* and *(b)*. *(c)* Short-TE proton MR spectrum using STEAM (TR/TE = 2000/18 ms). Increased lactic acid is detected. Other metabolites are not clearly resolved due to signal-to-noise considerations. *(d)* Long-TE proton MR spectrum using PRESS (TR/TE = 2000/270 ms). Note an extremely large amplitude of lactate signal as compared to the other resonances. (Adapted from Tzika *et al.* 1993*a*.)

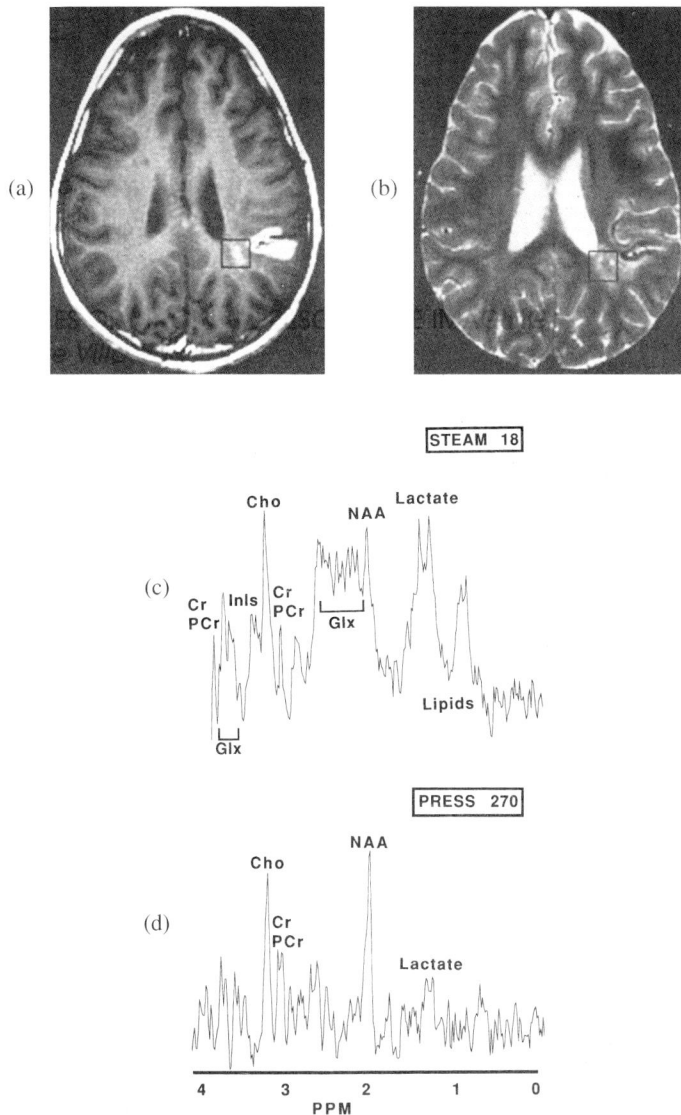

Fig. 13.8. MRI guided single-voxel localized proton MRS of a 9-year-old male with subacute stroke; 2.2 cm³ voxel of interest *(squares)*. *(a)* T₁-weighted image (TR/TE = 500/12 ms) following intravenous Gd-DTPA injection. Note enhancement of a compromised blood–brain barrier. *(b)* T₂-weighted image (TR/TE = 2500/100 ms) shows hyperintensity in periventricular white matter adjacent to area of stroke. *(c,d)* Localized proton MR spectra from the voxels indicated in images *(a)* and *(b)*. *(c)* Short-TE proton MR spectrum using STEAM (TR/TE = 2000/18 ms). Reduced NAA to cholines indicates neuronal degeneration. Increased peaks in the Glx/Inl areas of the spectrum indicates encephalopathy. Enhanced lipid presence indicates demyelination; lactate is detected additionally. *(d)* Long-TE proton MR spectrum using PRESS (TR/TE = 2000/270 ms). Minor accumulation of lactic acid was observed, presumably due to local perfusion deficit detected by dynamic contrast-enhanced perfusion MR imaging. (Adapted from Tzika *et al.* 1993*a*.)

321

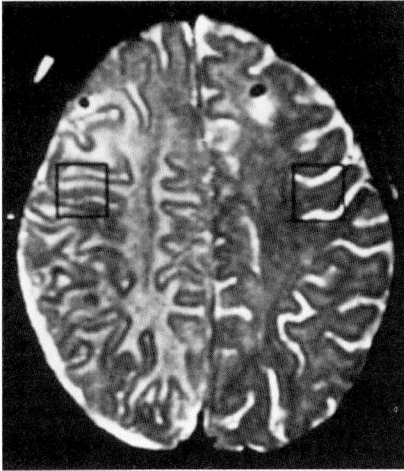

(a)

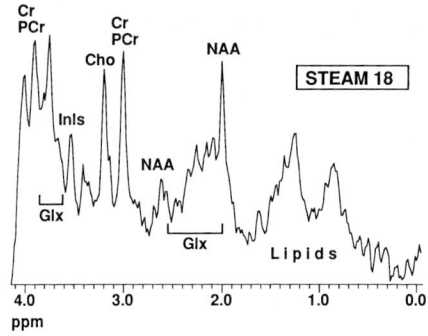

(b)

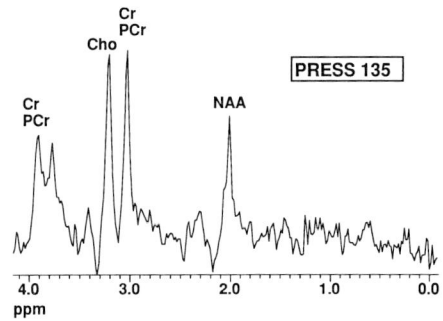

(c)

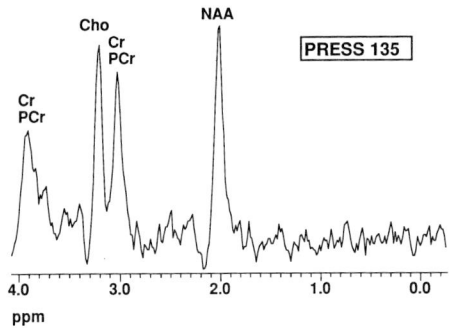

(d)

Fig. 13.9. MRI guided single-voxel localized proton MRS of an 8-month-old male with closed head injury; 3.4 cm³ voxel of interest *(squares)*. *(a)* T$_2$-weighted MR image (TR/TE = 2,500/100 ms). Note asymmetry in MR signal characteristics on the right as compared to the left. *(b)* Short-TE proton MR spectrum of the right cortex using STEAM (TR/TE = 2,000/18 ms). Note decreased NAA, elevated metabolites in the region of the spectra labeled Glx (glutamate/glutamine) and increased mobile lipids. *(c)* Long-TE proton MR spectrum from the right cortical voxel using PRESS (TR/TE = 2,000/135 ms). Low NAA is evident; lactate is not detected. *(d)* Long-TE proton MR spectrum from the left cortical voxel using PRESS (TR/TE = 2,000/135 ms). Normal NAA to choline ratio was found in the contralateral hemisphere as compared to the injured cortex. (Adapted from Tzika *et al.* 1993*c*.)

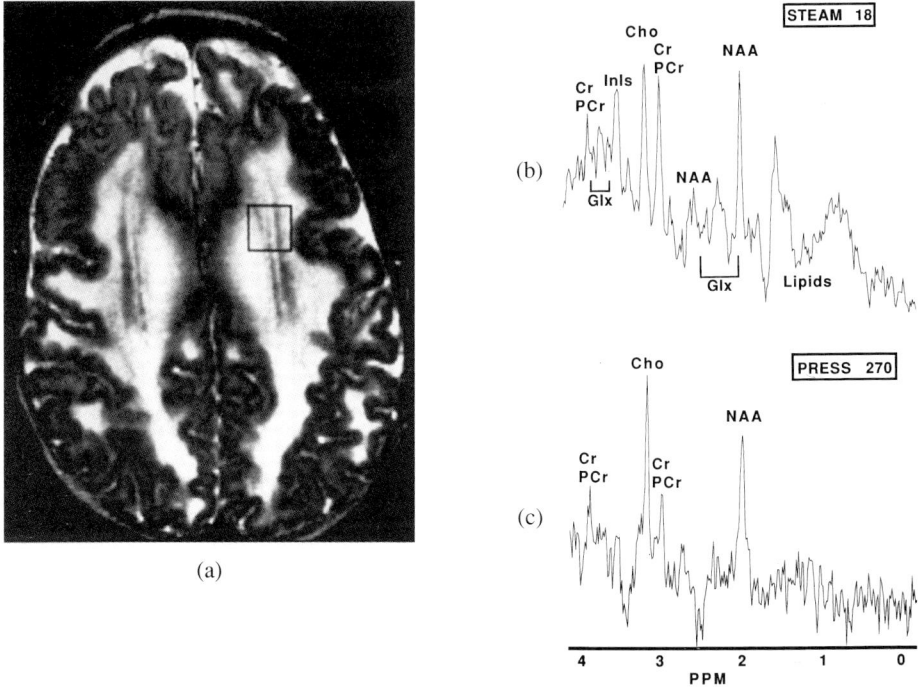

Fig. 13.10. MRI guided single-voxel localized proton MRS of a 12-month-old male with an idiopathic white matter disease; 3.4 cm³ voxel of interest *(squares)*. *(a)* T₂-weighted image (TR/TE = 2500/100 ms) of a 12-month-old male with a possible unknown metabolic disease affecting cerebral white matter. Note abnormal white matter signal. *(b,c)* Localized proton MR spectra from the voxel indicated in image *(a)*. *(b)* Short-TE proton MR spectrum using STEAM (TR/TE = 2000/18 ms). Enhanced lipid presence indicates demyelination. *(c)* Long-TE proton MR spectrum using PRESS (TR/TE = 2000/270 ms). Note that the relative peak heights of NAA to cholines (Cho) is reduced at this age. (Adapted from Tzika *et al.* 1993*a*.)

hereditary or acquired (Valk and van der Knaap 1989, Becker and Yates 1990). Hereditary disorders involve defects in one or more types of cell organelles, such as peroxisomes, lysosomes or mitochondria; these defects may be structural, functional (enzymatic) or both. Organelle defects lead to abnormal cell function and organ malfunction. Acquired hypoxic–ischemic, toxic–metabolic, inflammatory and traumatic disorders can also cause CNS neurodegeneration (Valk and van der Knaap 1989). Recent studies indicate that both hereditary and acquired neurodegenerative disorders include anatomical and neurochemical alterations secondary to excitatory neurotransmitter neurotoxicity (Choi 1988, Freese *et al.* 1990, McDonald and Johnston 1990, Dure *et al.* 1991).

Neuropathologic examination may show either gray or white matter involvement and occasionally no noticeable abnormality (Becker and Yates 1990). Clinical findings often lack specificity, and laboratory tests are of limited value. Imaging modalities demonstrate the impact of abnormal cellular function on organ morphology. Both CT and MRI demonstrate degenerative changes in the CNS (Mirowitz *et al.* 1991). Although MRI is very sensitive, its specificity is limited and is dependent on optimization achieved by improving MR image quality and interpretation (van der Knaap *et al.* 1991). To enhance the specificity of MRI in the assessment of neurodegenerative disease, proton MRS can non-invasively detect metabolite levels, and thus may allow earlier detection of neuro-degeneration.

• *Hereditary*. Peroxisomal disorders are associated with inherited metabolic defects caused by the absence of or erratic deficiencies in one or more of the peroxisomal en-zymes (Moser 1991). The most common disorder involving a single peroxisomal enzyme deficiency is X-ALD (Moser *et al.* 1984). The deficiency prevents breakdown of very long chain fatty acids, which are incorporated in myelin rendering it unstable (Brown *et al.* 1983). Myelinated regions of white matter are therefore replaced by a mesh of glial fibers. Frequently, necrosis with cavitation and/or calcification is concurrently observed. The changes in myelin correlate well with the MR spectroscopy findings. Proton MR spectra from voxels of interest placed within hyperintense areas of the white matter in T_2-weighted images reveal a dramatic decrease in the NAA resonance and sparing of the total creatine resonance. In addition, changes are observed in the profile of the Glx regions primarily in the STEAM spectra. Furthermore, metabolite abnormalities can be observed in regions of normal signal intensity in MR images and more importantly in asymptomatic individuals (Tzika *et al.* 1993b).

Localized proton MRS findings in hereditary metabolic brain disorders correlate with pathophysiology of the lesions and with MR imaging. Decreased NAA resonances may indicate neurodegeneration which parallels disappearance of neurons, if indeed NAA, as implicated, is a neuronal marker (Nadler and Cooper 1972). Neurodegeneration can also result from increasing accumulations in neurons, which eventually degenerate and ultimately lead to brain atrophy. However, metabolic disorders may change the NAA peak independent of neuronal degeneration. This may result in spectral changes prior to neuronal death and may be of predictive value. Sparing of the total creatine resonance in the absence of NAA may signify that cells other than neurons (*i.e.* glia) are present. This is further supported by the gliosis observed in histological specimens. Choline resonances are more prominent than normal and may be due to increased breakdown products of cell membranes, especially myelin sheaths (*i.e.* phosphatidylcholine, glycerophosphocholine, phosphocholine). In another type of metabolic brain disorder, Leigh's disease, MRI demonstrated bilateral lesions in basal ganglia, especially the putamen and caudate. MRS findings (in long-TE PRESS) in the same areas revealed the striking presence of lactate. This presence of lactate correlates with an enzymatic disorder in the mitochondrial elec-tron chain, known to exist for this disease. Impaired aerobic metabolism results in an-aerobic conversion to lactate. Although the detection of lactate by proton MRS in Leigh's disease may be considered a non-specific finding, it is suggestive of the spongy degenera-tion associated with the astroglial and microglial reaction known to occur in this disease. Nevertheless, lactate is also detected in other metabolic disorders and even in regions of normal MR signal intensity and may suggest a mitochondrial defect. Its presence in intense lesions, however, may be due to aggregated microglial cells or local hypoperfusion.

• *Acquired.* Neurodegenerative disorders can be due to acquired etiology. Hypoxic–ischemic damage is associated with depletion of energy storing compounds and increase in local tissue acidity. Proton MRS shows a decrease in NAA and an increase in lactic acid suggesting continued anaerobic glycolysis (Behar *et al.* 1983, Cockard *et al.* 1987, Gadian *et al.* 1987). These changes are depicted in the spectra of Figure 13.9 in a subject with closed head injury. In addition, short-TE STEAM spectra show an increase in mobile lipid peaks, as well as in the Glx/Inl peaks. These changes are representative of the changes observed in stroke, although in acute stroke, accumulation of lactate is marked and total creatine is reduced (Bruhn 1989*b*).

Intrauterine or early postnatal exposure to toxins may have permanent effects on brain development. Thus toxic encephalopathies may result, and such encephalopathy has been suggested by animal data (Wasiewski 1992). Our limited experience with spectroscopy in children with intrauterine cocaine exposure has not yielded any prominent alterations in the proton MR spectra.

• *Idiopathic.* Several patients showed intermittent evidence of neurodegeneration on proton MRS. These presented with white matter lesions and unknown specific diagnosis based on clinical and MRI findings.

According to the discussion above, proton MRS findings are not limited to a particular CNS disorder. They rather indicate a certain metabolic disturbance associated with encephalopathy, and they can thus contribute to the MR assessment of neurologic disorders. Their value may lie in following disease progression and assessing therapeutic intervention since both of these processes may affect the metabolism of the involved tissue and organs. In addition, their prognostic value bears further investigation inasmuch as it may be of importance in the early detection of these conditions. Early changes may be reversed by appropriate pharmacological intervention, thus preventing structural and neuropathologic deterioration, detection of which signifies irreversible damage.

Summary

State-of-the-art high-field superconducting magnets with homogeneous magnetic fields of 1.5 T have been offering the capability for both imaging and spectroscopy studies. The successful clinical evaluation of proton MRS has recently been enabled by technical developments in clinical systems. Proton MRS is not only technically feasible but also safe and may prove to be of complementary value to MRI in the assessment of neurodegenerative disease and tumors of children. Since proton MRS detects certain metabolite profiles in brain disorders, its potential as a clinical tool for diagnosis, prognosis, therapeutic monitoring and treatment follow-up of pediatric neurologic abnormalities deserves well-controlled evaluation.

ACKNOWLEDGMENTS

I thank Dr William S. Ball, MD for his collaboration. I am grateful to Dr Donald R. Kirks, MD for his support. I thank the Signa Spectroscopy group of General Electric Medical Systems. Last, I greatly appreciate the assistance of my research technologist Mr Scott R. Dunn.

325

REFERENCES

Akoka, S. (1992) 'Localization.' *In:* de Certaines, J.D., Bovèe, W.M.M.J., Podo, F. (Eds.) *Magnetic Resonance Spectroscopy in Biology and Medicine.* Oxford: Pergamon Press, pp. 97–109.

Alger, J.R., Frank, J.A., Bizzi, A., Fulham, M.J., DeSouza, B.X., Duhaney, M.O., Inscoe, S.W., Black, J.L., van Zijl, P.C.M., *et al.* (1990) 'Metabolism of human gliomas: assessment with H-1 MR spectroscopy and F-18 fluorodeoxyglucose PET.' *Radiology,* **177,** 633–641.

Arnold, D.L., Shoubridge, E.A., Villemure, J.G., Feindel, W. (1990) 'Proton and phosphorus magnetic resonance spectroscopy of human astrocytomas *in vivo.* Preliminary observations on tumor grading.' *NMR in Biomedicine,* **3,** 184–189.

Aue, W.P. (1986) 'Localization methods for *in vivo* nuclear magnetic resonance spectroscopy.' *Reviews in Magnetic Resonance in Medicine,* **1,** 21–72.

Bates, T.E., Williams, S.R., Gadian, D.G., Bell, J.D., Small, R.K., Iles, R.A. (1989) '^{1}H NMR study of cerebral development in the rat.' *NMR in Biomedicine,* **2,** 225–229.

Becker, L.E., Yates, A. (1990) 'Inherited metabolic disease.' *In:* Becker, L.E., Yates, A. (Eds.) *Textbook of Neuropathology.* Baltimore: Williams & Wilkins, pp. 331–427.

Behar, K.L., Ogino, T. (1991) 'Assignment of resonances in the ^{1}H spectrum of rat brain by two-dimensional shift correlated and J-resolved NMR spectroscopy.' *Magnetic Resonance in Medicine,* **17,** 285–303.

—— Den Hollander, J.A., Stromski, M.E., Ogino, T., Shulman, R.G., Petroff, O.A.C., Prichard, J.W. (1983) 'High-resolution ^{1}H nuclear magnetic resonance study of cerebral hypoxia *in vivo.* ' *Proceedings of the National Academy of Sciences of the USA,* **80,** 4945–4948.

Bottomley, P.A. (1987) 'Spatial localization in NMR spectroscopy *in vivo.*' *Annals of the New York Academy of Sciences,* **508,** 333–348.

—— (1989) 'Human *in vivo* NMR spectroscopy in diagnostic medicine: clinical tool or research probe?' *Radiology,* **170,** 1–15.

Brown, F.R., Chen, W.W., Kirschner, D.A., Frayer, K.L., Powers, J.M., Moser, A.B., Moser, H.W. (1983) 'Myelin membrane from adrenoleukodystrophy brain white matter—biochemical properties.' *Journal of Neurochemistry,* **41,** 341–348.

Brown, T.R., Kincaid, B.M., Ugurbil, K. (1982) 'NMR chemical shift imaging in three dimensions.' *Proceedings of the National Academy of Sciences of the USA,* **79,** 3523–3526.

Bruhn, H., Frahm, J., Gyngell, M.L., Merboldt, K.D., Hänicke, W., Sauter, R. (1989*a*) 'Cerebral metabolism in man after acute stroke: new observations using localized proton NMR spectroscopy.' *Magnetic Resonance in Medicine,* **9,** 126–131.

—— —— —— —— —— Hamburger, C. (1989*b*) 'Noninvasive differentiation of tumors with use of localized H-1 MR spectroscopy *in vivo*: initial experience in patients with cerebral tumors.' *Radiology,* **172,** 541–548.

—— Kruse, B., Korenke, G.C., Hanefeld, F., Hänicke, W., Merboldt, K.D., Frahm, J. (1992) 'Proton NMR spectroscopy of cerebral metabolic alterations in infantile peroxisomal disorders.' *Journal of Computer Assisted Tomography,* **16,** 335–344.

Burri, R., Bigler, P., Straehl, P., Posse, S., Colombo, J.P., Herschkowitz, N. (1990) 'Brain development: ^{1}H magnetic resonance spectroscopy of rat brain extracts compared with chromatographic methods.' *Neurochemical Research,* **15,** 1009–1016.

Chance, B., Whearly, R. (1985) 'Magnetic resonance spectroscopy emerges as a quantitative diagnostic tool and an aid to therapeutic procedures.' *International Journal of Technology Assessment in Health Care,* **1,** 607–613.

Choi, D.W. (1988) 'Glutamate neurotoxicity and diseases of the nervous system.' *Neuron,* **1,** 623–634.

Christiansen, P., Henriksen, O., Stubgaard, M., Gideon, P. Larsson, H.B.W. (1993) '*In vivo* quantification of brain metabolites by ^{1}H-MRS using water as an internal standard.' *Magnetic Resonance Imaging,* **11,** 107–118.

Cockard, H.A., Gadian, D.G., Frackowiak, R.S.J., Proctor, E., Allen, K., Williams, S.R., Ross Russell, R.W. (1987) 'Acute cerebral ischaemia: concurrent changes in cerebral blood flow, energy metabolites, pH, and lactate measured with hydrogen clearance and ^{31}P and ^{1}H nuclear magnetic resonance spectroscopy. II. Changes during ischaemia.' *Journal of Cerebral Blood Flow and Metabolism,* **7,** 394–402.

Dure, L.S., Young, A.B., Penney, J.B. (1991) 'Excitatory amino acid binding sites in the caudate nucleus and frontal cortex of Huntington's disease.' *Annals of Neurology,* **30,** 785–793.

Ernst, T., Hennig, J. (1991) 'Coupling effects in volume selective ^{1}H spectroscopy of major brain metabolites.' *Magnetic Resonance in Medicine,* **21,** 82–96.

326

Frahm, J., Bruhn, H., Gyngell, M.L., Merboldt, K.D., Hänicke, W., Sauter, R. (1989) 'Localized high-resolution proton NMR spectroscopy using stimulated echoes: initial applications to human brain *in vivo*.' *Magnetic Resonance in Medicine*, **9**, 79–93.

—— —— Hänicke, W., Merboldt, K-D., Mursch, K., Markakis, E. (1991*a*) 'Localized proton NMR spectroscopy of brain tumors using short-echo time STEAM sequences.' *Journal of Computer Assisted Tomography*, **15**, 915–922.

—— Michaelis, T., Merboldt, K-D., Hänicke, W., Gyngell, M.L., Bruhn, H. (1991*b*) 'On the *N*-acetyl methyl resonance in localized ^{1}H NMR spectra of human brain *in vivo*.' *NMR in Biomedicine*, **4**, 201–204.

Freese, A., DiFiglia, M., Koroshetz, W.J., Beal, M.F., Martin, J.B. (1990) 'Characterization and mechanism of glutamate neurotoxicity in primary striatal cultures.' *Brain Research*, **521**, 254–264.

Fulham, M.J., Bizzi, A., Dietz, M.J., Shih, H.H-L., Raman, R., Sobering, G.S., Frank, J.A., Dwyer, A.J., Alger, J.R., Di Chiro, G. (1992) 'Mapping of brain tumor metabolites with proton MR spectroscopic imaging: clinical relevance.' *Radiology*, **185**, 675–686.

Gadian, D.G., Frackowiak, R.S.J., Crockard, H.A., Proctor, E., Allen, K., Williams, S.R., Ross Russell, R.W. (1987) 'Acute cerebral ischaemia: concurrent changes in cerebral blood flow, energy metabolites, pH, and lactate measured with hydrogen clearance and ^{31}P and ^{1}H nuclear magnetic resonance spectroscopy. I. Methodology.' *Journal of Cerebral Blood Flow and Metabolism*, **7**, 199–206.

Gill, S.S., Small, R.K., Thomas, D.G.T., Patel, P., Porteous, R., van Bruggen, N., Gadian, D.G., Kauppinen, R.A., Williams, S.R. (1989) 'Brain metabolites as ^{1}H NMR markers of neuronal and glial disorders.' *NMR in Biomedicine*, **2**, 196–200.

—— Thomas, D.G.T., van Bruggen, N., Gadian, D.G., Peden, C.J., Bell, J.D., Cox, I.J., Menon, D.K., Iles, R.A., *et al.* (1990) 'Proton MR spectroscopy of intracranial tumours: *in vivo* and *in vitro* studies.' *Journal of Computer Assisted Tomography*, **14**, 497–504.

Granot, J. (1986) 'Selected volume spectroscopy and chemical-shift imaging.' *Journal of Magnetic Resonance*, **66**, 197–200.

Hahn, E.L. (1950) 'Spin echoes.' *Physical Review*, **80**, 580–594.

Hennig, J., Pfister, H., Ernst, T., Ott, D. (1992) 'Direct absolute quantification of metabolites in the human brain with *in vivo* localized proton spectroscopy.' *NMR in Biomedicine*, **5**, 193–199.

Kauppinen, R.A., Palvimo, J. (1992) 'Contribution of cytoplasmic polypeptides to the ^{1}H NMR spectrum of developing rat cerebral cortex.' *Magnetic Resonance in Medicine*, **25**, 398–407.

—— Kokko, H., Williams, S.R. (1992) 'Detection of mobile proteins by proton nuclear magnetic resonance spectroscopy in the guinea pig brain *ex vivo* and their partial purification.' *Journal of Neurochemistry*, **58**, 967–974.

Koller, K.J., Zaczek, R., Coyle, J.T. (1984) '*N*-acetyl-aspartyl-glutamate: regional levels in rat brain and the effects of brain lesions as determined by a new HPLC method.' *Journal of Neurochemistry*, **43**, 1136–1142.

Kreis, R., Ross, B.D., Farrow, N.A., Ackerman, Z. (1992) 'Metabolic disorders of the brain in chronic hepatic encephalopathy detected with H-1 MR spectroscopy.' *Radiology*, **182**, 19–27.

Kugel, H., Heindel, W., Ernestus, R-I., Bunke, J., du Mesnil, R., Friedmann, G. (1992) 'Human brain tumors: spectral patterns detected with localized H-1 MR spectroscopy.' *Radiology*, **183**, 701–709.

Lazeyras, F., Charles, H.C., Schold, C., Fredericks, R., Coleman, R.E. (1992) 'H-1 spectroscopic imaging in gliomas.' *Journal of Magnetic Resonance Imaging*, **2(P)** (Suppl.), 71.

Leibfritz, D. (1992) 'Water suppression.' *In:* de Certaines, J.D., Bovèe, W.M.M.J., Podo, F. (Eds.) *Magnetic Resonance Spectroscopy in Biology and Medicine.* Oxford: Pergamon Press, pp. 149–168.

Lowry, O.H., Berger, S.J., Chi, M.M-Y., Carter, J.G., Blackshaw, A., Outlaw, W. (1977) 'Diversity of metabolic patterns in human brain tumours—I. High energy phosphate compounds and basic composition.' *Journal of Neurochemistry*, **29**, 959–977.

McDonald, J.W., Johnston, M.V. (1990) 'Physiological and pathophysiological roles of excitatory amino acids during central nervous system development.' *Brain Research Reviews*, **15**, 41–70.

Michaelis, T., Merboldt, K-D., Hänicke, W., Gyngell, M.L., Bruhn, H., Frahm, J. (1991) 'On the identification of cerebral metabolites in localized ^{1}H NMR spectra of human brain *in vivo*.' *NMR in Biomedicine*, **4**, 90–98.

—— —— Bruhn, H., Hänicke, W., Frahm, J. (1993) 'Absolute concentrations of metabolites in the adult human brain *in vivo*: quantification of localized proton MR spectra. ' *Radiology*, **187**, 219–227.

Mirowitz, S.A., Sartor, K., Prensky, A.J., Gado, M., Hodges, F.J. (1991) 'Neurodegenerative diseases of childhood: MR and CT evaluation.' *Journal of Computer Assisted Tomography*, **15**, 210–222.

Moonen, C.T.W., von Kienlin, M., van Zijl, P.C.M., Cohen, J., Gillen, J., Daly, P., Wolf, G. (1989) 'Comparison of single-shot localization methods (STEAM and PRESS) for *in vivo* proton NMR spectroscopy.' *NMR in Biomedicine*, **2**, 201–208.

327

Moser, H.W. (1991) 'Peroxisomal disorders.' *Clinical Biochemistry*, **24**, 343–351.

—— Moser, A.E., Singh, I., O'Neill, B.P. (1984) 'Adrenoleukodystrophy: survey of 303 cases: biochemistry, diagnosis, and therapy.' *Annals of Neurology*, **16**, 628–641.

Nadler, J.V., Cooper, J.R. (1972) 'N-acetyl-L-aspartic acid content of human neural tumours and bovine peripheral nervous tissues.' *Journal of Neurochemistry*, **19**, 313–319.

Ordidge, R.J., Connelly, A., Lohman, J.A.B. (1986) 'Image-selected *in vivo* spectroscopy (ISIS). A new technique for spatially selective NMR spectroscopy.' *Journal of Magnetic Resonance*, **66**, 283–294.

Ott, D., Hennig, J., Ernst, T. (1993) 'Human brain tumors: assessment with *in vivo* proton MR spectroscopy.' *Radiology*, **186**, 745–752.

Pauly, J., Le Roux, P., Nishimura, D., Macovski, A. (1991) 'Parameter relations for Shinnar–Le Roux selective excitation pulse design algorithm.' *IEEE Transactions on Medical Imaging*, **10**, 53–65.

Peden, C.J., Cowan, F.M., Bryant, D.J., Sargentoni, J., Cox, I.J., Menon, D.K., Gadian, D.G., Bell, J.D., Dubowitz, L.M. (1990) 'Proton MR spectroscopy of the brain in infants.' *Journal of Computer Assisted Tomography*, **14**, 886–894.

Petroff, O.A.C., Yu, R.K., Ogino, T. (1986) 'High-resolution proton magnetic resonance analysis of human cerebrospinal fluid.' *Journal of Neurochemistry*, **47**, 1270–1276.

Posse, S., Schuknecht, B., Smith, M.E., van Zijl, P.C.M., Herschkowitz, N. Moonen, C.T.W. (1993) 'Short echo time proton MR spectroscopic imaging.' *Journal of Computer Assisted Tomography*, **17**, 1–14.

Provencher, S.W. (1993) 'Estimation of metabolite concentrations from localized *in vivo* NMR spectra.' *Magnetic Resonance in Medicine*, **30**, 672–679.

Radda, G.K., Bore, P.J., Rajagopalan, B. (1984) 'Clinical aspects of ^{31}P NMR spectroscopy.' *British Medical Bulletin*, **40**, 155–159.

—— Rajagopalan, B., Taylor, D.J. (1989) 'Biochemistry *in vivo*: an appraisal of clinical magnetic resonance spectroscopy. ' *Magnetic Resonance Quarterly*, **5**, 122–151.

Rothman, D.L., Hanstock, C.C., Petroff, O.A., Novotny, E.J., Prichard, J.W., Shulman, R.G. (1992) 'Localized ^{1}H NMR spectra of glutamate in the human brain.' *Magnetic Resonance in Medicine*, **25**, 94–106.

Sutton, L.N., Wang, Z., Gusnard, D., Lange, B., Perilongo, G., Bogdan, A.R., Detre, J.A., Rorke, L., Zimmerman, R.A. (1992) 'Proton magnetic resonance spectroscopy of pediatric brain tumors.' *Neurosurgery*, **31**, 195–202.

Tzika, A.A., Ball, W.S., Vigneron, D.B., Dunn, R.S., Kirks, D.R. (1993a) 'Clinical proton MR spectroscopy of neurodegenerative disease in childhood.' *American Journal of Neuroradiology*, **14**, 1267–1281.

—— —— —— —— Nelson, S.J., Kirks, D.R. (1993b) 'Childhood adrenoleukodystrophy: assessment with proton MR spectroscopy.' *Radiology*, **189**, 467–480.

—— Vigneron, D.B., Ball, W.S., Dunn, R.S., Kirks, D.R. (1993c) 'Localized proton MR spectroscopy of the brain in children.' *Journal of Magnetic Resonance Imaging*, **3**, 719–729.

—— Dunn, R.S., Webb, P.G., Kohler, S.J., Raidy, T., Hurd, R.E. (1994) 'Evaluation of the clinical performance of automated proton MR spectroscopy (^{1}H MRS) in pediatrics.' *Academic Radiology*, **2**, 46–50.

Urenjak, J., Williams, S.R., Gadian, D.G., Noble, M. (1992) 'Specific expression of N-acetylaspartate in neurons, oligodendrocyte-type-2 astrocyte progenitors, and immature oligodendrocytes *in vitro*.' *Journal of Neurochemistry*, **59**, 55–61.

Valk, J., van der Knaap, M.S. (1989) 'Classification of myelin disorders.' *In: Magnetic Resonance of Myelin, Myelination and Myelin Disorders*. Berlin: Springer Verlag, pp. 4–8.

van der Knaap, M.S., van der Grond, J., van Rijen, P.C., Faber, J.A.J., Valk, J., Willemse, K. (1990) 'Age-dependent changes in localized proton and phosphorus MR spectroscopy of the brain.' *Radiology*, **176**, 509–515.

—— Valk, J., de Neeling, N., Nauta, J.J.P. (1991) 'Pattern recognition in magnetic resonance imaging of white matter disorders in children and young adults.' *Neuroradiology*, **33**, 478–493.

Wasiewski, W.W. (1992) 'Central nervous system effects of cocaine in children.' *In:* Miller, G., Ramer, J.C. (Eds.) *Static Encephalopathies of Infancy and Childhood*. New York: Raven Press, pp. 325–330.

Webb, P.G., Sailasuta, N., Kohler, S.J., Raidy, T., Moats, R.A., Hurd, R.E. (1994) 'Automated single-voxel proton MRS: technical development and multisite verification.' *Magnetic Resonance in Medicine*, **31**, 365–373.

Weiner, M.W. (1988) 'The promise of magnetic resonance spectroscopy for medical diagnosis.' *Investigative Radiology*, **23**, 253–261.

INDEX

H

hamartomas
  hypothalamic, 183–4, *183*
  vascular, 229–30, *230*
head trauma *see* trauma
hemangioblastoma, 172
  spinal, 258–9, 265
hemangiomas
  orbital, 229, *230*
  vertebral, 240
hematomas
  epidural, 99–101, *100*
  non-accidental, 110–11, 154
  parenchymal, *107*, 108, 154
  stroke syndromes, 154–5
  subdural, 101–4, *101–3*, 154
hemimegalencephaly, 56, *57*
hemorrhage
  intracranial, 154–5
  subarachnoid, 104, *105*
  see also hypoxic–ischaemic disorders
hepatoblastoma, 190
herpes simplex encephalitis, 119, *120*
  congenital, 135, *136*
heterotopias, 56, *57*
Hippel–Lindau disease, 80, 91–2, *92*
histiocytosis, 232, 264
histoplasmosis, 127
HIV, intracranial infections, 138–41
Hodgkin's disease, 262
holoprosencephaly, 58–62, *60–1*
  corpus callosum defect, 65
human immunodeficiency virus (HIV), 138–41
Hunter's disease, 206
Hurler's disease, *200*, 206, 207, *207*
hypothalamic hamartoma, 183–4, *183*
hypoxic–ischaemic disorders
  differential diagnosis, *211*, 212
  MRS findings, 279–306, 325

I

immunosuppressed patients, 138–41
infections
  intracranial, 116–45
  spinal, 267–8, *268–9*
instrumentation, 22–5
iron material in body, 32, 35
ischaemia *see* hypoxic–ischaemic disorders

J

Joubert syndrome, 75

K

Kearns–Sayre syndrome, 208
Klinefelter syndrome, 220
Krabbe's disease, *200*, *201*, 204

L

lacrimal gland tumors, 231
lap belt injuries, 270
Larmor equation/frequency, 3
Leigh's disease, *200*, 208, 324
  MRS findings, 319, *320*, 324
leukemia, 188
  orbital involvement, *230*, 231
  spinal involvement, 261–2
leukodystrophy
  metachromatic, *199*, *201*, 204–5, *206*
  see also adrenoleukodystrophy
leukokoria, 223, 224
leukomalacia, *211*
lipidosis, 204
lipomas, spinal, 247–8, *247–8*
lissencephaly, 52–6, *53–5*
lupus vasculitis, *151*, 152
lymphangioma, 229–30, *230*
lymphoma
  lymphomatoid granulomatosis, 189–90, *189*
  malignant, 188–9
  orbital, 231
  orbital pseudotumor and, 227
  spinal, 262
lysosomal disorders, 203, 204–7
  Krabbe's disease, *200*, *201*, 204
  MRS findings, 319

M

magnet types, 22–4
magnetic field strength, optimal, 5
magnetic material in body, 32
magnetic resonance angiography, 33–4
  aneurysm diagnosis, 156, 158
  in craniocerebral trauma, 111
magnetic resonance spectroscopy (MRS), 34, 283–6, 307–8
  in hypoxic–ischaemic disorders, 279–306
  neurodegenerative disease/tumors, 307–28
malignant lymphoma, 188–9
maple syrup urine disease, 207, 208
Maroteaux–Lamy disease, 206
mascara, 32
medulloblastomas, 164, 166–7, *166*
  cerebral, 184–5
  in neonates, 165
  spinal, 259, 261, *261*
medulloepitheliomas, 226
melanoma, 231, *231*
MELAS syndrome, *200*, 208
meningiomas, 186–8, *187*
  optic nerve, 232
  spinal, 259
meningitis, 122–4
  fungal, 127